Feline Practice: Integrating Medicine and Well-Being (Part I)

Editor

MARGIE SCHERK

VETERINARY CLINICS OF NORTH AMERICA: SMALL ANIMAL PRACTICE

www.vetsmall.theclinics.com

July 2020 • Volume 50 • Number 4

ELSEVIER

1600 John F. Kennedy Boulevard • Suite 1800 • Philadelphia, Pennsylvania, 19103-2899
http://www.vetsmall.theclinics.com

**VETERINARY CLINICS OF NORTH AMERICA: SMALL ANIMAL PRACTICE Volume 50, Number 4
July 2020 ISSN 0195-5616, ISBN-13: 978-0-323-73403-5**

Editor: Colleen Dietzler

Developmental Editor: Nicole Congleton

Veterinary Clinics of North America: Small Animal Practice (ISSN 0195-5616) is published bimonthly by Elsevier Inc., 360 Park Avenue South, New York, NY 10010-1710. Months of issue are January, March, May, July, September, and November. Business and Editorial Offices: 1600 John F. Kennedy Blvd., Ste. 1800, Philadelphia, PA 19103-2899. Customer Service Office: 3251 Riverport Lane, Maryland Heights, MO 63043. Periodicals postage paid at New York, NY and additional mailing offices. Subscription prices are $348.00 per year (domestic individuals), $705.00 per year (domestic institutions), $100.00 per year (domestic students/residents), $451.00 per year (Canadian individuals), $876.00 per year (Canadian institutions), $488.00 per year (international individuals), $876.00 per year (international institutions), $100.00 per year (Canadian students/residents), and $220.00 per year (international students/residents). To receive student/resident rate, orders must be accompanied by name of affiliated institution, date of term, and the *signature* of program/residency coordinator on institution letterhead. Orders will be billed at individual rate until proof of status is received. Foreign air speed delivery is included in all *Clinics* subscription prices. All prices are subject to change without notice. **POSTMASTER:** Send address changes to *Veterinary Clinics of North America: Small Animal Practice*, Elsevier Health Sciences Division, Subscription Customer Service, 3251 Riverport Lane, Maryland Heights, MO 63043. Customer Service (orders, claims, online, change of address): Elsevier Periodicals Customer Service, Elsevier Health Sciences Division Subscription **Customer Service 3251 Riverport Lane Maryland Heights, MO 63043. Tel: 1-800-654-2452 (U.S. and Canada); 314-447-8871 (outside U.S. and Canada). Fax: 314-447-8029. E-mail: journalscustomerservice-usa@elsevier.com (for print support); journalsonlinesupport-usa@elsevier.com (for online support).**

Reprints. For copies of 100 or more of articles in this publication, please contact the Commercial Reprints Department, Elsevier Inc., 360 Park Avenue South, New York, NY 10010-1710. Tel.: 212-633-3874; Fax: 212-633-3820; E-mail: reprints@elsevier.com.

Veterinary Clinics of North America: Small Animal Practice is also published in Japanese by Inter Zoo Publishing Co., Ltd., Aoyama Crystal-Bldg 5F, 3-5-12 Kitaaoyama, Minato-ku, Tokyo 107-0061, Japan.

Veterinary Clinics of North America: Small Animal Practice is covered in *Current Contents/Agriculture, Biology and Environmental Sciences, Science Citation Index, ASCA, MEDLINE/PubMed (Index Medicus), Excerpta Medica,* and *BIOSIS.*

Contributors

EDITOR

MARGIE SCHERK, DVM
Diplomate, American Board of Veterinary Practitioners (Feline Practice), catsINK Feline Consultant, Vancouver, British Columbia, Canada

AUTHORS

MELISSA BAIN, DVM, MS
Professor of Clinical Animal Behavior, Department of Medicine and Epidemiology, UC Davis School of Veterinary Medicine, Davis, California, USA

C.A. TONY BUFFINGTON, DVM, PhD
Clinical Professor, Department of Medicine and Epidemiology, UC Davis School of Veterinary Medicine, Davis, California, USA

KIMBERLY COYNER, DVM
Diplomate, American College of Veterinary Dermatology; Dermatology Clinic for Animals, Olympia, Washington, USA

TERRY MARIE CURTIS, DVM, MS
Diplomate, American College of Veterinary Behaviorists; Clinical Behaviorist, University of Florida College of Veterinary Medicine, Gainesville, Florida, USA

MARK E. EPSTEIN, DVM
Dipl. ABVP (C/F), CVPP, TotalBond Veterinary Hospital, Gastonia, North Carolina, USA

DANIELLE A. GUNN-MOORE, BSc (Hon), BVM&S, PhD, MANZCVS, FHEA, FRSB, FRCVS
Royal (Dick) School of Veterinary Studies and The Roslin Institute, The University of Edinburgh, Roslin, Midlothian, Scotland

SARAH HEATH, BVSc, PgCertVE, CCAB, FHEA, FRCVS
Diplomate, European College of Animal Welfare and Behavioural Medicine (BM); RCVS Veterinary Specialist in Behavioural Medicine, EBVS European Veterinary Specialist in Behavioural Medicine, Visiting Lecturer, Small Animal Behavioural Medicine, University of Liverpool School of Veterinary Science, Liverpool, United Kingdom; Clinical Director and Owner, Behavioural Referrals Veterinary Practice, Upton, Chester, United Kingdom

SALLY LESTER, DVM, MVSc
Diplomate, American College of Veterinary Pathology, Clinical and Anatomic; Pathology Consultant, True North Veterinary Diagnostics, Langley, British Columbia, Canada; Pilchuck Veterinary Hospital, Snohomish, Washington, USA

AMY MIELE, BVM&S, PhD, MRCVS
Royal (Dick) School of Veterinary Studies and The Roslin Institute, The University of Edinburgh, Roslin, Midlothian, Scotland

BEATRIZ P. MONTEIRO, DVM, PhD
Department of Clinical Sciences, Faculty of Veterinary Medicine, Université de Montréal, Saint Hyacinthe, Quebec, Canada

BERNARD E. ROLLIN, PhD
University Distinguished Professor of Philosophy, Animal Sciences, and Biomedical Sciences, University Bioethicist, Colorado State University, Fort Collins, Colorado, USA

MARGIE SCHERK, DVM
Diplomate, American Board of Veterinary Practitioners (Feline Practice), catsINK Feline Consultant, Vancouver, British Columbia, Canada

LORENA SORDO, MSc, MVZ
Royal (Dick) School of Veterinary Studies and The Roslin Institute, The University of Edinburgh, Roslin, Midlothian, Scotland

PAULO V. STEAGALL, MV, MSc, PhD
Diplomate, American College of Veterinary Anesthesia and Analgesia; Department of Clinical Sciences, Faculty of Veterinary Medicine, Université de Montréal, Saint-Hyacinthe, Quebec, Canada

ELIZABETH STELOW, DVM
University of California, Davis, Davis, California, USA

Contents

In the health sciences, stress often is defined in terms of stressors; events that are perceived as threats to one's perception of control. From this perspective, a stressor is anything that activates the central threat response system (CTRS). Recent research shows that the CTRS can be sensitized to environmental events through epigenetic modulation of gene expression. When CTRS activation is chronic, health and welfare may be harmed. Environmental modification can mitigate the harmful effects of chronic CTRS activation by reducing the individual's perception of threat and increasing its perception of control, which improves health and welfare.

Environmental optimisation of the home and the veterinary clinic is important, not only for promoting good emotional and cognitive health for domestic cats but also ensuring good physical health. All three aspects of the feline health triad are interconnected. When the social and physical environment is compromised, emotional challenge can result in behavioural responses that are undesirable and/or detrimental to feline welfare. The physiological responses to compromised emotions and sustained protective emotional motivation can be involved in the triggering, maintenance and increased significance of a range of physical health issues including chronic pain and urinary tract, gastrointestinal and dermatological disease.

When an owner notices a behavior change in their cat that concerns them enough to present the cat to the vet, there are 3 possibilities: the behavior change reflects a change in behavioral health (a change in psychological state), a change in medical health (a change in physical state), or a combination (comorbid medical and behavioral pathologies). Because many behavioral pathologies are diagnoses of exclusion, it is important that the veterinarian rule out all of the likely medical differentials for the changed behavior. This article is a behavior-by-behavior guide to the more common differentials for the most common problem behaviors.

and anxiety as means to promote feline welfare and human-pet bond is discussed.

Veterinary medicine has traditionally functioned as an art and a science, that is, as knowledge of general principles and knowledge of, and relationship with, the individual animal and their caregiver. With the advent of increasing specialization, this intimate knowledge of the individual is being lost. This has great ramifications for diagnosis and treatment. Knowing the particular personality and tendencies of the patient helps differentiate between behavioral issues and fully medical issues. Excessive "scientization" in veterinary medicine needs to be addressed in veterinary medical education.

VETERINARY CLINICS OF NORTH AMERICA: SMALL ANIMAL PRACTICE

SERIES OF RELATED INTEREST

Veterinary Clinics of North America: Exotic Animal Practice
https://www.vetexotic.theclinics.com/

THE CLINICS ARE NOW AVAILABLE ONLINE!
Access your subscription at:
www.theclinics.com

Preface

There's So Much More to Cats...

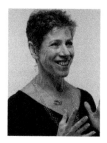

Margie Scherk, DVM
Editor

Our current approach to medicine views the body as a composite of systems. This approach isn't only used in teaching but also, for the most part, in medical specialization. Cats throw a wrench into this approach. They commonly exhibit comorbidities extending beyond 1 organ (eg, triaditis, chronic kidney disease with hyperthyroidism, diabetes with arthritis). In a way, this isn't surprising as the body functions in an integrative manner. Inflammation on 1 body system may be reflected elsewhere as well. But might this "holistic" approach extend further? Cats are restrained and understated: it is easy to miss that they are uncomfortable or unhappy. Caregivers may not notice sickness until their cat is exhibiting clinical signs, such as vomiting, diarrhea, lethargy, rather than more subtle changes. And poor health may, in fact, be a physical manifestation of nonphysical problems, or disease.

The Oxford dictionary defines the adjective holistic as: "Characterized by the treatment of the whole person, taking into account mental and social factors, rather than just the symptoms of a disease."[1] Unfortunately, this term has polarizing connotations within our profession but remains useful with respect to looking at all factors affecting a patient. To a great degree, bodies are designed to heal when basic needs (hydration, nutrition, analgesia, and environmental and social) are met. As practitioners (and researchers), it is important to remember the basic tenet of medicine: "If you can do no good, at least do no harm." It is imperative not to add the challenges of stress/fear, pain/discomfort, unpalatable, unappetizing food, or unnecessary medications to the mix. The idea for this 2-issue issue of *Veterinary Clinics of North America: Small Animal Practice* is to highlight not only exciting medical advances but also clinically relevant understanding of the effects of mental, emotional, and social factors on health, disease, and illness.

The first section of this issue focuses on current understanding of how cats experience and manifest stress through behavior as well as illness and the role of the environment on feline welfare throughout all life stages. An extensive section follows

Vet Clin Small Anim 50 (2020) xi–xii
https://doi.org/10.1016/j.cvsm.2020.04.003
0195-5616/20/© 2020 Published by Elsevier Inc.

addressing differences in pain and meeting analgesic needs, chronic pain, degenerative joint disease, and neuropathic pain. As cats commonly have comorbidities and overlapping clinical presentations, there is an article on complex disease management as well as one on dermatologic lookalikes of the face, nasal planum, and ears.

Sometimes we request diagnostic tests out of a desire to be thorough even though the outcome of that test may not change the outcome for the patient. To this, there is an article on when to use new tests, when to stick with old tests, or whether to run tests at all, which addresses some of these concerns.

Veterinarians (and veterinary nurses) go into animal care because of a love for animals and desire to help them. Part of our ability to be good caregivers is to maintain this passion throughout our careers. The fact that we work for our clients rather than for our patients can lead to medical compromises that cause disappointment, moral distress, or worse. The final article addresses the need to balance the art and the science of veterinary medicine in a moral and ethical way.

I hope you will look forward to the second issue. It includes articles on feline nutrition, updates on infectious diseases, select digestive tract problems and endocrine disorders, use of genetics and stem cell therapies in practice, an update on feline oral health, as well as new neurologic entities in cats that have a stress/environmental component.

I am extremely grateful to every author. Thank you for putting up with my nagging, cajoling, and attempts to fine-tune. Especially as much of this labor of love has been during the COVID-19 pandemic when every one of you has been stressed to the limit, trying to adapt to the rapidly changing requirements, be it in academia or in private practice. I hope that this pair of issues is greater than the sum of its individual parts. Thank you.

Margie Scherk, DVM
catsINK
Vancouver, Canada

E-mail address:
hypurr@aol.com

REFERENCE

1. Hobson A, editor. The Oxford dictionary of difficult words. Oxford: Oxford University Press; 2004.

Stress and Feline Health

C.A. Tony Buffington, DVM, PhD*, Melissa Bain, DVM, MS

KEYWORDS

- Coping • Early life stress • Epigenetic modulation of gene expression
- Perception of control • Perception of threat • Resilience • Threat response system

KEY POINTS

- Stress is often defined in terms of *stressors:* events in the internal and external environment that result in a *stress response.* Stressors increase the ratio of one's perception of threat/perception of control.
- The central stress response system can be sensitized by early adverse experiences, which can leave the individual more susceptible to perceive events in the environment as threats.
- Environmental modifications to reduce perceptions of threat and enhance perceptions of control can promote resilience, which can improve health and welfare.

Everyone knows what stress is, but nobody really knows.

—Hans Selye

INTRODUCTION

Veterinarians strive to improve the health of their patients, and recently there has been a more concentrated effort to understand the relationship among stress, physical health, and emotional health. Recent research has investigated how the effects of stressful environments manifest in cats, expanding from and connecting to research in other species.[1,2]

WHAT IS STRESS?

The term stress can be defined in various ways. From the perspectives of health and disease, stress is often defined in terms of *stressors*, which are events in the internal and external environment that result in a *stress response*. We think of stressors as events that are perceived as threats to one's perception of control. From this perspective, a stressor is anything that activates the central threat response system (CTRS).[3] Stressors can vary along a continuum: positive to negative, duration, acute to chronic,

---

Department of Medicine and Epidemiology, UC Davis School of Veterinary Medicine, Davis, CA 95616, USA
* Corresponding author.
E-mail address: drbuffington@ucdavis.edu

Vet Clin Small Anim 50 (2020) 653–662
https://doi.org/10.1016/j.cvsm.2020.03.001
0195-5616/20/© 2020 Elsevier Inc. All rights reserved.

vetsmall.theclinics.com

and intensity (mild to toxic). For the purposes of this article, we have adapted the "eco-biodevelopmental" framework proposed by the American Academy of Pediatrics, "to stimulate fresh thinking about the promotion of health and prevention of disease across the lifespan,"[4] which provides a helpful way to begin to think about stressors and stress responses. This framework acknowledges that all events that activate the CTRS are not equally threatening, and proposes a conceptual taxonomy comprising 3 distinct types of CTRS responses: mild (positive), moderate (tolerable), and severe (toxic). The taxonomy is based on the differences in their potential to cause enduring physiologic disruptions as a result of the intensity and duration of the response.

Mild stress responses, defined as brief in duration and mild-to-moderate in magnitude, can help develop stress coping skills. Mild stress responses are part of normal development when they occur in the safe, predictable environments of stable and supportive relationships.

Examples of events resulting in positive stress responses in young animals include nonthreatening veterinary visits and exposure to novel environments and foods.

Moderate stress responses result from exposure to experiences that present greater threats, such as lack of stimulation/boredom or household instability, illness or injury, or exposure to a natural disaster. As with mild stress responses, when the event occurs in an otherwise safe environment, recovery to normal is likely. Thus, the essential feature that makes moderate stress response tolerable is the extent to which one's protective surroundings permit retention of sufficient perception of control to permit adaptive coping to occur.

In the most threatening circumstances, severe stress responses can result. Toxic stress responses, strong, frequent, or prolonged, are the most dangerous to long-term health and welfare. Examples of events that can result in severe stress responses include chronic abuse, severe or chronic disease, and adverse early life events like nutritional deprivation,[5] maternal separation, or significant maternal threat during pregnancy (more on this later).[6]

STRESS AND THE LOWER URINARY TRACT

Abnormal signs referable to the lower urinary tract (LUTS) of domestic cats include variable combinations of increased voiding urgency and frequency, decreased volume, blood in the urine, and urination outside the litter box. Although there are many possible causes of these signs, the most common causes include "idiopathic cystitis"; a stone, usually calcium oxalate or magnesium ammonium phosphate; or a urinary tract infection (usually in older cats with upper tract disease). In addition to infection and inflammation, stress responses also can activate the LUT, although some of the fundamental neural mechanisms and pathways linking psychosocial stress to altered behaviors and physiologic disorders are still unclear. Holstege[7] has pointed out that micturition plays a much more important role in the context of the survival of individuals and species in most mammals than it does in humans. For most mammals, urine also signals important messages, such as the demarcation of territory of a specific individual[8] and estrus.[9] These urine functions demonstrate that voiding can occur for reasons other than to empty a full bladder, including the contexts of perception of threat and reproduction. Micturition responses in these situations require, and imply, supraspinal control of micturition.[7]

Part of the interest in feline stress biology arose from studies of cats with severe, recurrent chronic LUTS. LUTS have long been recognized in domestic cats, being described as "very common" in Kirk's 1925 veterinary textbook.[10] Clinicians historically interpreted signs referable to the LUT to suggest an external (eg, infectious agent, urinary stone) or structural disorder of the LUT (eg, stricture or incontinence), although environmental conditions were recognized as a risk factor by Kirk in 1925,[10] and subsequently confirmed to be relevant by other investigators.[11,12]

In 1996, Osborne and colleagues[13] summarized the literature on feline LUTS, identifying some 30 distinct causes of LUTS. That so many potential causes result in similar LUTS demonstrates that the signs in themselves only represent the limited repertoire available to the LUT to respond to any insult. During this time, a syndrome described as "feline interstitial cystitis" (FIC) also was being studied.[14] These studies found that additional problems outside the LUT were commonly present in these cats, and could be mitigated by multimodal environmental modification.[15] Subsequent research has revealed the complex nature of this condition. For example, some cats with severe, chronic LUTS seem to have a functional, rather than a structural, LUT disorder,[1] and that LUTS can occur even in presumably healthy cats exposed to stressful circumstances.[12,16]

These findings suggest that terms such as "feline urologic syndrome,"[17] "feline lower urinary tract disease,"[18] and "feline interstitial cystitis"[14] historically used to describe patients with this syndrome do not describe the extent of the problems occurring in many afflicted cats. Conversely, the narrow focus on the LUT may have precluded thorough evaluation of the entire patient, which might have revealed variable combinations of clinical signs referable to other organ systems such as the gastrointestinal tract, skin, lung, cardiovascular, central nervous, endocrine, and immune systems.[15,19] These comorbidities include some of the most common problems in feline medicine. They also lack a predictable pattern of onset across patients, and often precede the appearance of LUTS. This situation is similar in human beings with "central sensitivity syndromes,"[20] suggesting that individual patterns of comorbidities may represent an amplification of underlying familial sensitivities.[21]

PERCEPTION OF THREAT

The inconsistency of comorbidities observed in cats with chronic LUTS suggests that they may be variable manifestations of a common underlying problem.[22,23] The underlying problem in these patients appears to be a sensitized CTRS,[1] which results in a relative predominance of sympathetic to parasympathetic nervous system responses,[24] increased hypothalamic-pituitary, but not adrenal, activity,[25] as well as variable alterations in immune[26] and endocrine function.[25] Chronic activation of the CTRS seems to result in chronic "wear and tear" on body and brain systems, which can eventually progress to clinical signs referable to those organs most vulnerable in a particular individual.[27]

In addition to alterations in the components of the CTRS distal to the hypothalamus, brain structures that modulate activity of the CTRS also appear to be affected.[28] For example, cognitive factors such as classical and operant conditioning, attention bias, and memory have been shown to play roles in the onset, development, and maintenance of chronic health problems.[28] Moreover, studies have shown that the individual's expectations and ability to cope with potentially traumatic events are more important than the physical events *per se* for determining the immediate and long-term consequences for health.[29]

The sensitization of the CTRS appears to result from genetic disorders, developmental events, environmental threats, or variable combinations of these.[30] A variety of polymorphisms in genes that affect stress responsiveness, including catechol-O-methyltransferase,[31] serotonin transporter,[32] and alpha-2 adrenergic receptor, have been identified in humans.[33,34] In cats, a genetic polymorphism of the alpha-2 adrenergic receptor that appears to enhance stress susceptibility has been reported.[35]

During the past 2 decades, the science of Developmental Origins of Health and Disease[36] has emerged to investigate the role of early life experiences on the sensitivity of the CTRS. Evidence from clinical, epidemiologic, and experimental observations has shown how evolutionarily conserved developmental processes can interact with environmental cues, often transmitted from the mother via the placenta to the offspring, to attempt to match the physiology of the developing organism to its postnatal environment. The sequence of events that has emerged from this research proposes that when a pregnant female is exposed to a sufficiently severe stressor, the neuroendocrine products of the ensuing stress response may cross the placenta and affect the course of fetal development.[37] The biological "purpose" of transmitting such environmental cues to the fetus may be to guide the development of the fetal CTRS and associated behaviors to increase the probability of survival. The fetus may "use" information in its in utero environment to make predictive adaptive response "decisions." If a threatening or nutrient-limiting environment is perceived, the developmental trajectory of the fetus may change in response to the available information to enhance reproductive fitness in the predicted ex utero environment.

Studies of the enduring effects of stressful developmental experiences on health have now been published in a wide variety of mammalian species, from rodents to primates.[6] Problems can arise when the actual ex utero environment does not match the predicted one. Studies in multiple species have found that cardiovascular disease, type 2 diabetes mellitus; metabolic syndrome; and respiratory, gastrointestinal, LUT, dental, and mood disorders all can result from a mismatch between the predicted and actual environment the individual inhabits.[38] Cognitive function, too, is affected by both genetic and developmental influences. Impaired coping to stressful situations, increased fear and anxiety-related behaviors, and dysregulation of the CTRS all have been found in adults exposed to adverse early life experiences.[6]

Recent research also has shown that one mechanism underlying the sensitization of the CTRS involves a process called epigenetic modulation of gene expression.[39] This general biological process results in such commonplace outcomes as sex-specific and organ-specific patterns of gene expression that lead to the final phenotype of the organism by silencing genes not appropriate to the particular tissue environment. The molecular mechanisms of epigenetics are beyond the scope of this review, but detailed explanations are freely available.[40]

The effects of stressors on sensitization of the CTRS seem to depend both on the timing and magnitude of exposure to products of the maternal stress response in relation to the activity of the developmental "programs" that determine the maturation of the various body systems during gestation and early postnatal development. For example, the small adrenal cortices found in some cats with FIC suggest that the event occurred during a time when adrenocortical maturation was occurring.[41] If the developing fetus had been exposed to a stressor before adrenocortical maturation, the effect may not have been observed, whereas if it had occurred later in development, adrenal size and subsequent adrenocortical responses to stress might have been increased. Given the number of orphaned or abandoned kittens obtained from shelters, the risk for sensitization of the CTRS in client-owned cats may be high.

Although sensitization of the CTRS is more likely to occur during growth and maturation of the neural, endocrine, and immune systems, it is not restricted to the developmental period. Moreover, sensitization of the CTRS may be unmasked by another adverse experience later in life, possibly associated with another round of epigenetic modulation of gene expression. Subsequent rounds of alterations in gene expression may be quite stable and resistant to current medical interventions. In addition, sensitization of the CTRS may be part of a more general "survival phenotype" that includes smaller (or larger) size at birth.[42]

PERCEPTION OF CONTROL

Activation of the CTRS appears to depend on the balance between perceptions of threat and perceptions of control. Other recent research has focused on the roles of resilience and choice on stress responsiveness. The American Psychological Association's Web site "The Road to Resilience" (https://www.apa.org/helpcenter/road-resilience) defines resilience as "the process of adapting well in the face of adversity, trauma, tragedy, threats, or significant sources of stress. It means 'bouncing back' from difficult experiences." A recent (September 15, 2019) special issue of *Biological Psychiatry* addressed the topic of the neurobiology of resilience from basic, clinical, and translational perspectives to summarize current knowledge of this important and rapidly expanding topic.[43] For example, Cathomas and colleagues[29] reviewed the physiologic and transcriptional adaptations of specific brain circuits, the role of cellular and humoral factors of the immune system, the gut microbiota, and changes at the interface between the brain and the periphery on the neurobiological mechanisms of stress resilience. They proposed viewing resilience as a process that integrates multiple central and peripheral systems.

Belief in one's ability to exert control over the environment and to produce desired results is essential for well-being, and probably a psychological and biological necessity.

Converging evidence from animal research, clinical studies, and neuroimaging suggests that the need for control is a biological imperative for survival. The ability to choose permits animals to increase their perception of control over their surroundings, which helps reduce activation of the CTRS.[44,45] In fact, 1 of the 5 Freedoms, freedom from fear, recently has been operationalized as the opportunity for choice and control[46]; and Rochlitz[47] has declared that, "Provided extremes are avoided, if the cat has a variety of behavioral choices and is able to exert some control over its physical and social environment, it will develop more flexible and effective strategies for coping with stimuli."

The negative effects of adverse early life events mediated by severe stress responses on the long-term health and welfare of cats demonstrate the importance of identification of risk factors and provision of effective education of clients by clinicians about appropriate environments for indoor or otherwise confined cats throughout their lives.[48] From this perspective, initial vaccination appointments are anything but "routine," and may in fact be the most important appointments of the animal's life. This is because such visits present opportunities to teach husbandry appropriate for the animal based on the environment it is confined to at a time when owners are likely to be most motivated and responsive to recommendations (see also the article by Heath, "Environment and Feline Health: At Home and in the Clinic," elsewhere in this issue). These needs remain but modifications may be required as cats age (see the article by Gunn-Moore, "Feline Aging: Promoting Physiologic and Emotional Well-being," elsewhere in this issue).

Shonkoff[4] described 3 foundational domains to promote long-term health and welfare that can be adapted to preventive veterinary care for confined cats. These include the following:

1. A stable and responsive environment that provides consistent, nurturing, and protective interactions that enhance learning and support development of adaptive capacities (resilience and coping) that promote a well-regulated CTRS

2. A safe and supportive physical, chemical, and built environment that is free from toxins and fear, allows active exploration without significant risk of harm, and offers support for families caring for the cat
3. Satisfactory nutrition for the cat's age, including feeding management practices that maintain an appropriate body condition (beginning with the future mother before conception if possible) while providing safety, choice, and mental stimulation to the extent possible[49] (see also the article by Dantas and Delgado, "Feeding Cats for Optimal Mental and Behavioral Well-Being Part 2," elsewhere in this issue).

Consideration of the role of a sensitized CTRS also has important therapeutic implications. For example, drugs to modulate gene expression are under active investigation in oncology[50] and psychiatry[51] that may become available in veterinary medicine. Given that these drugs also may modulate expression of other genes in potentially unpredictable ways, the availability of a naturally occurring animal model of a disease likely influenced by these mechanisms offers the opportunity to test these compounds before they are introduced to human medicine.[21] Recent research also suggests that drugs, like some of the psychedelics[52] and low doses of ketamine,[53] might prove therapeutic for patients with central sensitivity syndromes.

Environmental modification also can modulate gene expression,[54,55] which may explain the effectiveness of behavior-based approaches for treatment in humans[56] and multimodal environmental modification for therapy of cats with FIC.[12,15] Effective environmental modification has been found to result in significant resolution of signs of comorbid disorders as well as LUTS in treated cats suffering from FIC,[12,15] and to reverse the effects of maternal separation on stress reactivity in rodents.[57]

The roles of environmental modification on feline health and welfare can be visualized in the illustration (**Fig. 1**). Cats' perceptions of threat may be reduced by increasing safety through provision of separate sets of resources, opportunities to

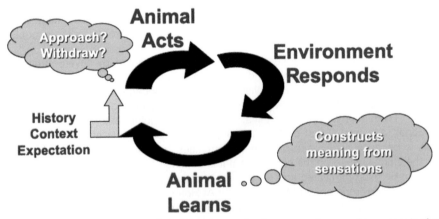

Fig. 1. The "circle of behavior" illustrating how animals sense and respond to events in the environment. Starting at the top, when an animal acts (eg, a cat jumps up onto a counter), the environment may respond (eg, a shout or swat from a person to remove the cat from the counter). The sensations arising in the cats nervous system enter the cat's brain to form a perception of the response, which is then compared with events in the cat's history (genetic, epigenetic, and environmental), the context in which the response was received, and its expectation of future events. These result in subsequent acts, depending on the threat or reward potential of the response. The circle is completed on a time constant of milliseconds throughout the life of the animal.

express species-typical behaviors, and elimination of conflict,[58] and their perception of control can be enhanced by offering resources as choices, and providing only those the cat chooses.[59] Changing the environment changes the context and the cat's expectations, which over time changes its history, permitting it to cope with its environment and benefiting its health and welfare.

SUMMARY

Changing our view of some chronic diseases from that of isolated organ-originating diseases in otherwise healthy individuals to one that considers the role of a sensitized CTRS (and the potential roles of early adverse experiences) has at least 2 important implications. First, it provides a more parsimonious explanation for many findings that previously were quite difficult to account for, including the unfortunate lack of beneficial effect of therapies directed at the peripheral organ of interest by a particular medical subspecialty, the presence of multiple comorbid disorders in many patients with chronic disorders, but not in patients with other individual organ diseases, the unpredictable order of appearance of the comorbidities, and the altered functioning of the CTRS. Second, and more importantly, it opens whole new areas of therapy that may escape consideration from the individual medical specialty perspective. The currently available data only suggest this possibility, however, but they do permit generation of the hypothesis.

DISCLOSURE

The authors have nothing to disclose.

ACKNOWLEDGMENT

The research on cats with FIC was supported by the National Institutes of Health P50 DK64539 Women's Health and Functional Visceral Disorders Center, and DK47538.

REFERENCES

1. Buffington CA. Idiopathic cystitis in domestic cats—beyond the lower urinary tract. J Vet Intern Med 2011;25(4):784–96.
2. Buffington CAT. Pandora syndrome in cats: diagnosis and treatment. Today's Veterinary Practice 2018;8(5):31–41.
3. Elman I, Borsook D. Threat response system: parallel brain processes in pain vis-à-vis fear and anxiety. Front Psychiatry 2018;9:29.
4. Shonkoff JP. Building a new biodevelopmental framework to guide the future of early childhood policy. Child Dev 2010;81(1):357–67.
5. Bouret S, Levin BE, Ozanne SE. Gene-environment interactions controlling energy and glucose homeostasis and the developmental origins of obesity. Physiol Rev 2015;95(1):47–82.
6. Guzman DB, Howell B, Sanchez M. Early life stress and development: preclinical science. In: Bremner JD, editor. Posttraumatic stress disorder: from neurobiology to treatment. Hoboken (NJ): Wiley-Blackwell); 2016. p. 61–80.
7. Holstege G. Micturition and the soul. J Comp Neurol 2005;493(1):15–20.
8. Pryor PA, Hart BL, Bain MJ, et al. Causes of urine marking in cats and effects of environmental management on frequency of marking. J Am Vet Med Assoc 2001; 219(12):1709–13.
9. Hart BL. Facilitation by estrogen of sexual reflexes in female cats. Physiol Behav 1971;7(5):675–8.

10. Kirk H. Retention of urine and urine deposits. In: Kirk H, editor. The diseases of the cat and its general management. London: Bailliere, Tindall and Cox; 1925. p. 261–7.

11. Caston HT. Stress and the feline urological syndrome. Feline Pract 1973;3(6): 14–22.

12. Stella JL, Lord LK, Buffington CA. Sickness behaviors in response to unusual external events in healthy cats and cats with feline interstitial cystitis. J Am Vet Med Assoc 2011;238(1):67–73.

13. Osborne CA, Kruger JM, Lulich JP. Feline lower urinary tract disorders. Definition of terms and concepts. Vet Clin North Am Small Anim Pract 1996;26(2):169–79.

14. Buffington CAT, Chew DJ, Woodworth BE. Feline interstitial cystitis. J Am Vet Med Assoc 1999;215(5):682–7.

15. Buffington CAT, Westropp JL, Chew DJ, et al. Clinical evaluation of multimodal environmental modification in the management of cats with lower urinary tract signs. J Feline Med Surg 2006;8:261–8.

16. Westropp JL, Kass PH, Buffington CA. Evaluation of the effects of stress in cats with idiopathic cystitis. Am J Vet Res 2006;67(4):731–6.

17. Osbaldiston GW, Taussig RA. Clinical report on 46 cases of feline urological syndrome. Vet Med Small Anim Clin 1970;65:461–8.

18. Osborne CA, Johnston GR, Polzin DJ, et al. Redefinition of the feline urologic syndrome: feline lower urinary tract disease with heterogeneous causes. Vet Clin North Am Small Anim Pract 1984;14(3):409–38.

19. Buffington CA, Westropp JL, Chew DJ, et al. Risk factors associated with clinical signs of lower urinary tract disease in indoor-housed cats. J Am Vet Med Assoc 2006;228(5):722–5.

20. Yunus MB. Editorial review: an update on central sensitivity syndromes and the issues of nosology and psychobiology. Curr Rheumatol Rev 2015;11(2):70–85.

21. Buffington CA. Developmental influences on medically unexplained symptoms. Psychother Psychosom 2009;78(3):139–44.

22. Yunus MB. Central sensitivity syndromes: stress system failure may explain the whole picture reply. Semin Arthritis Rheum 2009;39(3):220–1.

23. Neblett R, Cohen H, Choi Y, et al. The Central Sensitization Inventory (CSI): establishing clinically significant values for identifying central sensitivity syndromes in an outpatient chronic pain sample. J Pain 2013;14(5):438–45.

24. Elbers J, Jaradeh S, Yeh AM, et al. Wired for threat: clinical features of nervous system dysregulation in 80 children. Pediatric Neurology 2018;89:39–48.

25. Heim C, Newport DJ, Heit S, et al. Pituitary-adrenal and autonomic responses to stress in women after sexual and physical abuse in childhood. JAMA 2000;284: 592–7.

26. Sturmberg JP, Bennett JM, Martin CM, et al. 'Multimorbidity' as the manifestation of network disturbances. Journal of Evaluation in Clinical Practice 2017;23: 199–208.

27. Danese A, McEwen BS. Adverse childhood experiences, allostasis, allostatic load, and age-related disease. Physiol Behav 2012;106(1):29–39.

28. Ursin H. Brain sensitization to external and internal stimuli. Psychoneuroendocrinology 2014;42:134–45.

29. Cathomas F, Murrough JW, Nestler EJ, et al. Neurobiology of resilience: Interface between mind and body. Biol Psychiatry 2019;86(6):410–20.

30. Buffington CAT. Comorbidity of interstitial cystitis with other unexplained clinical conditions. J Urol 2004;172:1242–8.

31. Stein DJ, Newman TK, Savitz J, et al. Warriors versus worriers. The role of COMT gene variants. CNS Spectr 2006;11(10):745–8.

32. Jacobs N, Kenis G, Peeters F, et al. Stress-related negative affectivity and genetically altered serotonin transporter function - Evidence of synergism in shaping risk of depression. Arch Gen Psychiatry 2006;63(9):989–96.

33. Wüst S, Federenko IS, van Rossum EFC, et al. A psychobiological perspective on genetic determinants of hypothalamus-pituitary-adrenal axis activity. Annals of the New York Academy of Sciences 2004;1032:52–62.

34. Rosmond R, Bouchard C, Bjorntorp P. A C-1291G polymorphism in the alpha(2A)-adrenergic receptor gene (ADRA2A) promoter is associated with cortisol escape from dexamethasone and elevated glucose levels. J Intern Med 2002;251(3):252–7.

35. Lu P, Owens T, Buffington CAT. Association Between Alpha-2a adrenergic Receptor Gene Polymorphisms and Feline Idiopathic Cystitis Paper presented at: NIDDK International Symposium: Frontiers in Painful Bladder Syndrome and Interstitial Cystitis 2006; Bethesda, MD, October 26–27, 2006.

36. Penkler M, Hanson M, Biesma R, et al. DOHaD in science and society: emergent opportunities and novel responsibilities. J Dev Orig Health Dis 2019;10(3): 268–73.

37. Miranda A, Sousa N. Maternal hormonal milieu influence on fetal brain development. Brain Behav 2018;8(2):e00920.

38. Gluckman PD, Buklijas T, Hanson MA. The developmental origins of health and disease (DOHaD) concept: past, present, and future. In: Rosenfeld CS, editor. The epigenome and developmental origins of health and disease. Cambridge, MA: Academic Press; 2016. p. 1–15.

39. Aristizabal MJ, Anreiter I, Halldorsdottir T, et al. Biological embedding of experience: a primer on epigenetics. Proc Natl Acad Sci U S A 2019. https://doi.org/10.1073/pnas.1820838116.

40. Wikipedia. Epigenetics. Available at: http://en.wikipedia.org/wiki/Epigenetics. Accessed December 20, 2019.

41. Westropp JL, Welk KA, Buffington CAT. Small adrenal glands in cats with feline interstitial cystitis. J Urol 2003;170(6 Pt 1):2494–7.

42. Parlee SD, MacDougald OA. Maternal nutrition and risk of obesity in offspring: The Trojan horse of developmental plasticity. Biochim Biophys Acta 2014; 1842(3):495–506.

43. Murrough JW, Russo SJ. The neurobiology of resilience: complexity and hope. Biol Psychiatry 2019;86(6):406–9.

44. Leotti LA, Iyengar SS, Ochsner KN. Born to choose: the origins and value of the need for control. Trends Cogn Sci 2010;14(10):457–63.

45. Falk JH. Born to choose: evolution, self, and well-being. New York: Routledge; 2017.

46. Greggor A, Vicino GA, Swaisgood RR, et al. Animal welfare in conservation breeding: applications and challenges. Front Vet Sci 2018;5:323.

47. Rochlitz I. A review of the housing requirements of domestic cats (Felis silvestris catus) kept in the home. Appl Anim Behav Sci 2005;93:97–109.

48. Ellis SL, Rodan I, Carney HC, et al. AAFP and ISFM feline environmental needs guidelines. J Feline Med Surg 2013;15(3):219–30.

49. Dantas LM, Delgado MM, Johnson I, et al. Food puzzles for cats: feeding for physical and emotional wellbeing. J Feline Med Surg 2016;18(9):723–32.

50. Mummaneni P, Shord SS. Epigenetics and oncology. Pharmacotherapy 2014; 34(5):495–505.

51. Mahgoub M, Monteggia LM. Epigenetics and psychiatry. Neurotherapeutics 2013;10(4):734–41.

52. Murnane K. The renaissance in psychedelic research: what do preclinical models have to offer. Prog Brain Res 2018;242:25.

53. Nowacka A, Borczyk M. Ketamine applications beyond anesthesia–A literature review. Eur J Pharmacol 2019;860(172547). https://doi.org/10.1016/j.ejphar.2019.172547.

54. Sale A, Berardi N, Maffei L. Environment and brain plasticity: towards an endogenous pharmacotherapy. Physiol Rev 2014;94(1):189–234.

55. Sale A. A systematic look at environmental modulation and its impact in brain development. Trends Neurosci 2018;41(1):4–17.

56. Kohrt BA, Jordans MJ, Koirala S, et al. Designing mental health interventions informed by child development and human biology theory: a social ecology intervention for child soldiers in Nepal. Am J Hum Biol 2015;27(1):27–40.

57. Francis DD, Diorio J, Plotsky PM, et al. Environmental enrichment reverses the effects of maternal separation on stress reactivity. J Neurosci 2002;22(18):7840–3.

58. Herron ME, Buffington CAT. Environmental enrichment for indoor cats. Compend Contin Educ Pract Vet 2010;32(12):E1–5.

59. Herron ME, Buffington CA. Environmental enrichment for indoor cats: implementing enrichment. Compend Contin Educ Vet 2012;34(1):E1–5.

Environment and Feline Health: At Home and in the Clinic

Sarah Heath, BVSc, PgCertVE, DipECAWBM, CCAB, FHEA, FRCVS[a,b,*]

KEYWORDS

- Environmental optimization • Emotional health • Cognitive health • Physical health
- Species-specific needs • Health triad • Welfare

KEY POINTS

- The health triad of non-human animals involves the three equally important components of emotional, cognitive, and physical health.
- The veterinary profession is charged with safeguarding the health of non-human species, and traditionally, the emphasis has been on striving to optimize physical health.
- Because of the complex interconnections between all three aspects of the health triad, physical health cannot be optimized unless emotional and cognitive health is also considered.
- The physical and social environment needs to meet the species-specific requirements of the individual in order for physical, emotional, and cognitive health to be optimized.
- Cats need choice and a perception of control over their experiences.

INTRODUCTION

Feline health is often considered in terms of the absence or presence of physical illness or injury, but this limited perspective leads to a lack of consideration of how health is affected by a wide range of factors, including the social and physical environment in which the individual lives. In the 49th edition of the Basic Documents publication from the World Health Organization,[1] health is defined as "[a] state of complete physical, mental and social well-being and not merely the absence of disease or infirmity," and in the Merriam-Webster online dictionary,[2] the term health care is defined in a human context as "efforts made to maintain or restore physical, mental, or emotional well-being especially by trained and licensed professionals."

The author proposes that health care for non-human animals is also a multi-dimensional process and that health of veterinary species should be considered as a triad of equally important aspects that are inextricably linked to one another.[3] This health triad

[a] University of Liverpool School of Veterinary Science, Liverpool, UK; [b] Behavioural Referrals Veterinary Practice, 10 Rushton Drive, Upton CH2 1RE, Chester, UK
* Behavioural Referrals Veterinary Practice, 10 Rushton Drive, Upton CH2 1RE, Chester, UK.
E-mail addresses: office@brvp.co.uk; heath@brvp.co.uk

Vet Clin Small Anim 50 (2020) 663–693
https://doi.org/10.1016/j.cvsm.2020.03.005
0195-5616/20/Crown Copyright © 2020 Published by Elsevier Inc. All rights reserved.
vetsmall.theclinics.com

is composed of physical, emotional, and cognitive health and comprehensive health care involves acknowledging and optimizing all three. The veterinary profession is charged with safeguarding the health of non-human species, and traditionally the emphasis has been on striving to optimize physical health. Because of the complex interconnections between all three aspects of the health triad, this aim cannot be achieved unless emotional and cognitive health is also considered. It has long been acknowledged that providing appropriate human health care involves considering the context in which people live, and there is extensive literature about the so-called place effect on human health.[4,5] This place effect is equally true for non-human animals. The physical and social environment needs to meet the species-specific requirements of the individual in order for physical, emotional, and cognitive health to be optimized. The concept of species-specific environmental needs has been used in both a human and feline medicine context,[5,6] and providing for these needs in our feline patients is something that needs to be considered in the home as well as in the veterinary clinic.

ENVIRONMENTAL OPTIMIZATION

The environment can be defined as "the surroundings or conditions in which a person, animal, or plant lives or operates"[7] and involves both physical and social features. The term "environmental enrichment" has been used to describe processes by which humans have endeavored to improve the environments of non-human species and has led to some considerable improvements in animal welfare. The definition of "to enrich" is to "improve or enhance the quality or value"[7] of something, and there can be no doubt that changes to environments of non-human animals over the last few decades, in both a livestock and a domestic context, have increased the quality and value of those environments. However, there is an implication that enrichment involves providing an environment that goes above and beyond what is necessary and that although an enriched environment is better, a non-enriched environment is still acceptable. The author has therefore suggested that it is more accurate to speak about the need for "environmental optimization" and strive to ensure that environments are optimal for the species. Optimal is defined as "the best or most favorable",[7] and when something is not optimal, it is defined as being suboptimal or "of less than the highest standard or quality".[7] Environmental optimization involves creating environments that meet species-specific needs, and failing to do this results in non-human animals living in contexts that are not acceptable.

CONSIDERING NATURAL BEHAVIOR

In order to create an optimal environment for domestic cats, it is important to consider the natural behavior of the cat. Artificial selection has played an important role in modifying physical features of the domestic cat, such as coat color, coat length, and facial features, but selection for function has not been part of the domestication process as it has for dogs. As a result, modification of behavior has been more limited, and although changes in relation to sociability have undoubtedly occurred, the domestic cat retains many of the behavioral traits of its wild ancestors. It is also important to remember that the domestic dog is a socially obligate mammal, whereas cats are non-obligate in their social behavior. This fundamental biological difference has significant implications for a species that is living in a domestic context primarily in order to fulfill a role of companionship. The provision of a home environment that meets the species-specific needs of both its feline and human inhabitants can therefore be a challenge. The solitary survivor status of the cat leads to an increased tendency to anticipate threat in novel social and physical environments and to a preference for selection of the behavioral responses of avoidance and inhibition in response to pain and fear-anxiety motivation.[8] This can make the optimization of a veterinary environment from a feline perspective difficult to achieve. When environments fall short of the ideal, there is an increased risk that negative (protective) emotions, such as fear-anxiety and frustration, will predominate and that the physiological impact of those emotions may become chronic in nature. The resulting physiological stress has implications in terms of physical health and therefore warrants increased consideration by the veterinary profession.[9,10]

THE CLINIC ENVIRONMENT

When considering the social environmental impact on feline patients in the veterinary clinic, the main consideration is the interaction between the cats and the veterinary practice staff, but potential for visual and scent impact from other cats and other species should also be taken into account.

In the feline environmental needs guidelines,[6] one of the 5 pillars (**Box 1**) states that cats have a need for "positive, consistent and predictable human-cat social interaction." This requirement is a particular challenge in a veterinary context because administration of veterinary treatment often involves the need for intimate handling, together with a degree of restraint. It can also be occurring when the cat is already in an emotionally compromised state, through the presence of ill health and pain as well as the fact that they are in an unfamiliar and challenging physical environment. Veterinary intervention may evoke negative emotional responses in patients, and an understanding of the full range of feline emotional motivations is vital if the veterinary personnel are going to adjust their social interactions with the cats in the most beneficial way.[8]

Over recent years, there has been a great deal of emphasis on the need to reduce negative emotions in the veterinary clinic, and it is essential that such emotions are never induced unnecessarily, for example, through inappropriate handling, such as scruffing, or hostile environments, such as where cats are unnecessarily housed in direct visual contact with canine, or other feline, patients. The aim of increasing positive emotional motivation wherever possible is also desirable, and provision of positive scent signals, through commercial pheromone products, is one example of how this may be achieved. However, the terms negative and positive in the context of emotions do not equate to bad and good, but rather to being protective or engaging,

---

Box 1
Five pillars of a healthy feline environment

1. Provide a safe place

2. Provide multiple and separated key environmental resources: food, water, toileting areas, scratching areas, play areas, and resting or sleeping areas

3. Provide opportunity for play and predatory behavior

4. Provide positive, consistent, and predictable human-cat social interaction

5. Provide an environment that respects the importance of the cat's sense of smell

These have been identified as core requirements for feline welfare.

From Ellis SLH Carney HC, Heath S, et al. AAFP and ISFM Feline Environmental Needs Guidelines. J Feline Med Surg 2013;15(3):221;with permission.

---

respectively. It must be acknowledged that negative emotional motivations are essential for survival, and it is both unrealistic and undesirable to live in a world that is free of fear. An aim to make domestic pet environments devoid of negative emotions also suggests a lack of understanding of the vital role that all emotional motivations play in overall survival.

Suppressing expression of negative emotion when it is justified has potentially serious consequences in terms of the long-term emotional health of the individual but also increases the risk of more undesirable behavioral responses to those emotions becoming apparent. Inducing positive emotional motivation, for example, by exposing patients to a trigger for the desire-seeking system, such as a food, while they are experiencing something that they perceive as being aversive does not necessarily remove any justified negative emotion and can increase overall emotional arousal and emotional conflict, thus making the individual less emotionally stable.

Although positive, engaging, emotions are desirable, and one should work to promote these wherever possible, there are times when negative, protective, emotions are both necessary and appropriate. Learning to recognize, acknowledge, and cater to these emotions is an essential part of providing an appropriate veterinary clinic environment. When cats are in pain or feeling justified fear-anxiety or frustration, the aim is not to replace that emotion with positive emotion, with the goal of triggering them to engage with the veterinary staff, but rather to provide the opportunity for the cat to use its natural behavioral responses to those emotions and disengage. The negative emotion is still present, but the patient has the ability to cope, and as a result, its welfare is optimized. The concept of low-restraint handling[11] is an excellent example of this principle at work. The aim of using a towel to handle a fearful or frustrated feline patient is to provide a context in which the cat can continue to respond emotionally to the challenging situation in which it finds itself, while enabling the veterinary professional to get their job done.[12,13] There are a variety of ways in which the towel can be used. For example, it may be placed over the top of a cat in a carrier in such a way that the cat can continue to hide (using avoidance in response to its emotional motivation of fear-anxiety) while the veterinary surgeon auscultates the chest or examines the relevant parts of the body in turn (**Figs. 1–3**). Alternatively, the towel may be used to loosely hold the cat while a procedure, such as venipuncture, is carried out. The cat is able to move and to hide, thus using its behavioral response of avoidance, and can gather sensory information about the experience via inhibition (**Fig. 4**). None

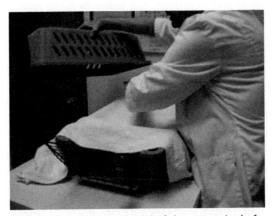

Fig. 1. Sliding a towel between the base and lid of the cat carrier before removing the lid can create a sensation of safety for the cat. (*Courtesy of* I. Rodan, DVM, Madison, WI.)

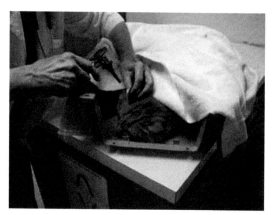

Fig. 2. The towel can be moved to expose only the part of the cat that is being examined, thereby enabling the cat to retain a sensation of being protected. (*Courtesy of* I. Rodan, DVM, Madison, WI.)

of the cats in these figures have altered their emotional response to the veterinary experience; they are still in a state of negative emotion, but they are coping and using species-specific behavioral responses to those emotions in order to do so.

For the intermittent and infrequent feline visitors to a clinic, the emotional impact of social interactions within the veterinary environment is likely to be acute, and long-term effects on the patient's overall health are minimal. However, it is important to remember that negative experiences of handling in a veterinary context can have longer-lasting consequences through the process of learning. It has already been stated that any form of handling that actively induces negative emotions of fear-anxiety, pain, or frustration should be avoided, and examples of unacceptable handling techniques would include scruffing, pinning, and intense or rough restraint.

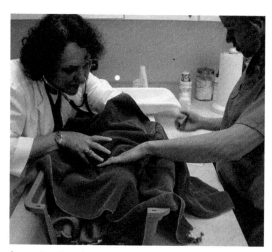

Fig. 3. If the type of examination does not necessitate visual access to the cat, such as auscultation, the towel can be used to completely cover the cat during the procedure. (*Courtesy of* I. Rodan, DVM, Madison, WI.)

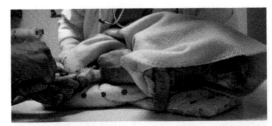

Fig. 4. Loosely cradling in a towel during venepuncture allows the cat to also use an inhibition response to its fear-anxiety and gather information about the situation and avoidance by hiding within the towel. (*Courtesy* of E. Sundhal, DVM, DABVP, Kansas City, MO.)

All of these have the potential to lead to a conditioned emotional response to human handling that can extend beyond the veterinary context and lead to cats being unable to cope with social interaction from people in general. It must also be remembered that just one intensely challenging experience has the potential to lead to formation of emotional associations that persist over time. For this reason, it is not advisable to persist with attempts to handle feline patients, however appropriately, if they are in an exaggerated negative emotional state. When the negative emotional responses are intense and/or unjustified, the use of chemical restraint should be considered. In addition to this short-term solution to the immediate problem, it is also appropriate to offer advice to the caregivers in terms of more in-depth behavioral medicine investigation so that the emotional challenges of the patient can be addressed.

One context in which working to promote positive emotional bias in the veterinary context is appropriate is when emotionally naïve patients are presented. For example, young healthy kittens coming to the practice for the first time for an elective appointment, such as a vaccination, will not have pre-established emotional associations. In these cases, working to increase positive emotional associations with the veterinary practice context and experience is important, and passive delivery of food on the consultation room table can be a useful tool. Allowing the kitten to explore the novel location in its own time will also be beneficial, and selection of appropriate consulting environments is therefore essential. Any feline consulting room should be safe for a cat to be free to wander, and ideally, the cat should be examined in the location where it feels most comfortable. This location may be on the caregiver's knee, in the bottom of the cat carrier, or on the weighing scales (**Fig. 5**). The important thing is the cat has choice and a perception of control over its experience.[13]

Although social challenges from humans in the clinic environment are primarily associated with the delivery of veterinary care, it is also important to ensure that the delivery of recreational social interaction for hospitalized patients is also consistent with feline needs. As non-obligate social creatures, cats can have widely varying requirements for social contact, and it is important to know the needs of the individual patient. For many cats, intense handling is not desirable, and provision of verbal social interaction may be sufficient. However, some highly socialized domestic cats have a high requirement for social interaction with people. Provision of appropriate interactions during extended periods of hospitalization will be important. Decisions as to whether caregivers should be given the opportunity to visit their pet are often subject to multiple factors, which are individual to the practice, but in general terms, it is important to consider the needs of the individual cat and client and try to provide for their social needs as appropriately as possible.

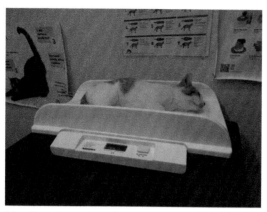

Fig. 5. Where possible allow the cat to select its preferred location in the consulting room. Scales are often chosen as they offer some sense of enclosure and protection and this kitten feels safe enough to rest during the consultation! (*Courtesy of* S. Heath, FRCVS, Chester, UK.)

In the context of the veterinary clinic, social interactions with other non-human animals will generally be something that is kept to a minimum, and the main consideration is how to limit the potential for visual or scent interactions that may induce negative emotions in feline patients. This leads to consideration of the physical clinical environment, and the ways in which the environmental needs pillars of "providing a safe place" and "an environment that respects the importance of the cat's sense of smell" can be met.[6]

The two areas where visual challenge from other animals has the highest potential to impact the feline patient are the waiting room and the hospitalization areas. This challenge is highlighted in the literature produced by the charity iCat-Care as part of their Cat Friendly Clinic initiative whereby they advocate the provision of separate waiting rooms and hospital wards for feline patients.[14] Although this is undoubtedly the ideal situation, it is not practical in every existing veterinary practice, and compromises often need to be made. Provision of visual barriers within the waiting room, the use of blankets or towels over cat carriers, and chairs or stands to allow cat carriers to

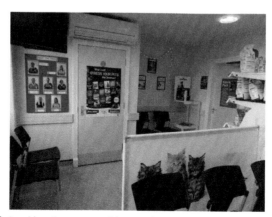

Fig. 6. The use of visual barriers can enable practices to create cat-only areas within a single air space waiting room. (*Courtesy of* S. Heath, FRVCS, Chester, UK.)

be placed in elevated locations, can all help to make cats feel more secure (**Figs. 6** and **7**). It is also important to remember that cats may arrive at veterinary practices in a high state of emotional arousal due to the impact of the cat carrier experience and the car travel. It is therefore very important to work to reduce the negative emotional associations with the carrier and the car and this is emphasised in the Cat Friendly Practice guidelines from iCatCare.

When providing visual safety, it is important to consider the need for cats to retain control, and completely removing visual access can lead to the emotion of frustration, particularly in some hospitalized patients. Rather than placing a towel over the entire of the front of the enclosure, it can be better to place it over half of the front or to place it over an internal shelf so that the cat has the option to look out or to remain hidden (**Fig. 8**A-C). It is important to ensure that cats are not in enclosures that put them in direct visual sight of other cats or other species in the hospitalization area where possible, and the provision of structures inside the enclosures that give the opportunity to hide can also be hugely beneficial. When no suitable "furniture" is made available, it is commonly reported that cats will sit inside the litter tray in an attempt to feel enclosed (**Fig. 9**). Examples of suitable structures to place within the pen include the Hide and Sleep®, produced by the UK charity Cats Protection (**Fig. 10**A, B), or a

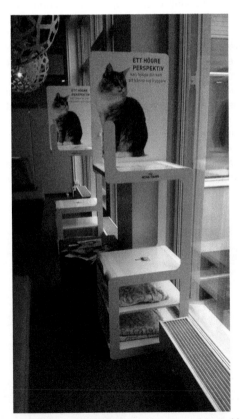

Fig. 7. Providing places for clients to place cat carriers in an elevated location prevents cats from being placed on the floor where they will feel more vulnerable. (*Courtesy of* S. Heath, FRCVS, Chester, UK.)

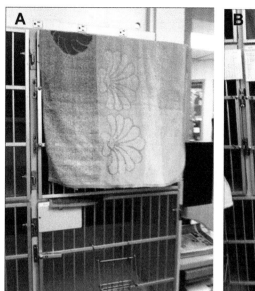
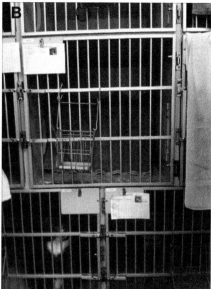
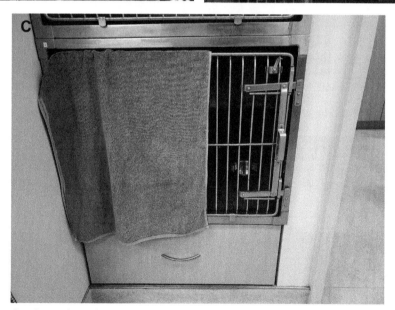

Fig. 8. (*A–C*) Towels can be used to provide a sensation of safety in kennels, but if the towel is over the entire front of the cage, it removes the cat's ability to choose to look out if it is motivated to do so. Putting the towel over half of the cage front or over an internal shelf in the cage can offer the cat choice and thereby reduce the risk of frustration being triggered. (*Courtesy of* [A, B] S. Heath, FRCVS, Chester, UK, [C] M. Scherk, DVM, Dip ABVP (Feline Practice), Vancouver, Canada.)

homemade version (**Fig. 11**), or a simple cardboard box (**Fig. 12**). These structures have the added advantage of providing an elevated surface on which to perch if the cat feels confident enough to do so and a protected location to put the cat's feeding bowl to increase their sense of being safe enough to eat during their hospital stay.

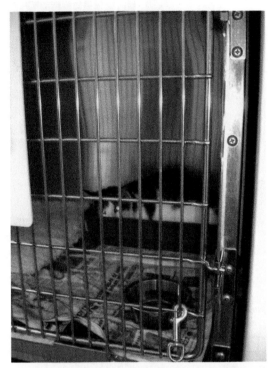

Fig. 9. If no suitable hiding structures are provided in hospitalization cages, cats will frequently sit in the litter tray, which offers some sensation of protection. (*Courtesy of* S. Heath, FRCVS, Chester, UK.)

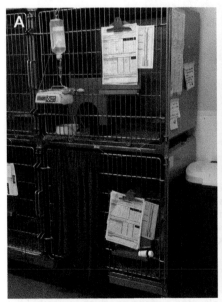
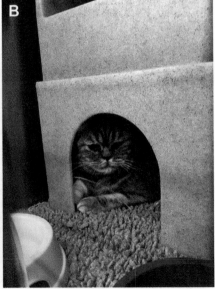

Fig. 10. (*A, B*) The Hide and Sleep® by Cats Protection can be a useful addition to the hospital cage offering somewhere to hide inside or rest on top of. (*Courtesy of* National Cat Centre, Haywards Heath, UK.)

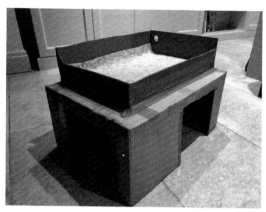

Fig. 11. A talented client was able to make homemade versions of a structure to offer their fearful cat a hide and sleep facility at home. (*Courtesy of* D. Ashton-Martin, Frodsham, UK.)

According to the feline environmental needs guidelines,[6] cats need multiple and separated key environmental resources. One of the biggest challenges in a veterinary hospital environment is lack of space, and purpose-built hospital pens for cats are often so small that appropriate distribution of resources, such as food, water, and latrines, is severely compromised. When patients are in the enclosure for a limited time, for example, for elective procedures or short-term hospitalization for diagnostic work, this is less likely to have a profound impact on them, but when cats are hospitalized for extended periods, moving them to larger enclosures should be considered (**Fig. 13**). Provision of access to adjacent pens and use of enclosures with side "rooms" for litter trays are also possible (**Fig. 14**).

Ensuring a safe scent environment is a challenge within the veterinary context because cats are not only exposed to scent challenges from the proximity of unrelated and incompatible felines but also exposed to scent challenges from other species. In addition, there are a range of potentially hostile scents associated with the veterinary

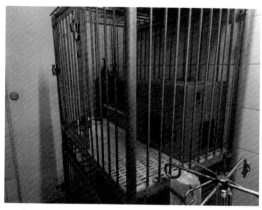

Fig. 12. In situations whereby finances are restricted and existing hospitalization cages are not ideal, the addition of a simple cardboard box can make a big difference to the welfare of patients. (*Courtesy* of S. Heath, FRCVS, Chester, UK.)

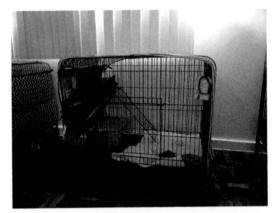

Fig. 13. For longer-stay feline patients, it can be helpful to find ways of providing increased space and an ability to rest in an elevated location. (*Courtesy of* S. Heath, FRCVS, Chester, UK.)

environment, and protecting feline patients from these is also important. Careful selection of cleaning products and considering alternatives to alcohol swabs can be simple but effective ways of optimizing the clinic from a feline perspective. Minimizing exposure to alarm pheromones is also desirable, and it can be beneficial to ask clients to

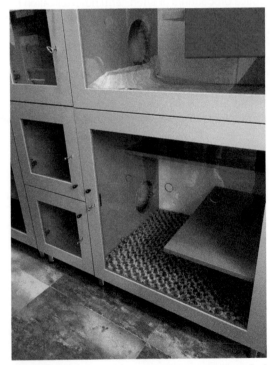

Fig. 14. In this veterinary hospital the cats have access to an upper and a lower side compartment. The litter tray is housed in the lower section and a bed in the upper section. (*Courtesy of* S. Heath, FRCVS, Chester, UK.)

bring a spare towel with them to consultations so that these can be placed onto the consult table to absorb the alarm pheromone secretions from the paw pads. The towel can then be taken away from the clinic by the client at the end of the consult in order to help to minimize the lingering of alarm pheromones in the clinic environment. It is very important that the towel is not placed inside the cat carrier after the consultation and that it is placed in a carrier bag and taken home separately and then washed. Adequate and appropriate cleaning of the tables is also obviously important.

In order to increase the positive olfactory profile of the practice, the provision of synthetic analogues of naturally occurring feline pheromones, such as the F3 portion of the facial pheromone complex and the feline-appeasing pheromone, has been shown to be beneficial. There are several publications regarding the benefits of using the facial pheromone within a veterinary context.[15,16] Use of the feline-appeasing pheromone is also likely to be beneficial, but at the time of publication, there have not been any specific studies using this relatively new product in the clinic setting.

THE HOME ENVIRONMENT

On first consideration, the aim of optimizing the home environment from a feline perspective may seem more easily achievable than in a clinic setting. Certainly, there are some advantages, such as the availability of more physical space and the fact that the cat is in a familiar location. However, meeting the five pillars of environmental needs can still be challenging, and, when they are not met, there is more potential for chronic emotional disturbances and resulting physiological stress because the cat is in the home environment on a consistent basis.

Within the home, the main social environment considerations are the manner of interactions from human caregivers, extended family or friends, and visitors as well as the social encounters with other cats or other non-human species within the household. The same principle of providing "positive, consistent, and predictable human-cat social interaction" applies, but within the home context, these interactions are going to be primarily of the recreational variety rather than for the purposes of administering veterinary care (unless the cat needs home administration of medical treatments). This may lead to assumptions that it will not be problematic, but the difference in social structure between cats and humans can lead to miscommunication that can have negative consequences. Humans (like dogs) are socially obligate and engage in social contact that is low in frequency but high in intensity. In contrast, cats interact with low intensity and high frequency and value social contact that can appear superficial and dismissive from a human perspective. Learning to interact with less intensity can be particularly challenging for people because hugging is an important human signal of affection and one that many caregivers wish to engage in with their cats (**Fig. 15**A-C). Appreciating the value of a brief verbal interaction or casual stroke is an important part of becoming an effective caregiver for cats, and directing that contact to areas of the body that are more acceptable for the cat, such as the temporal region rather than the caudal parts of the body, is also important.[17] Kittens can learn to accept certain aspects of human handling, such as being picked up and gently restrained, but it is essential that such interactions are encountered as early as possible and preferably before 7 weeks of age. Gradual introduction to such handling is also needed, and it is always essential to respect the fact that cats need to feel that they have some element of control (**Fig. 16**).

Social encounters with other non-human species can be a source of emotional challenge for cats, and the potential for the arrival of a dog or other companion animal species into the household to negatively affect the perception of the home as a safe place

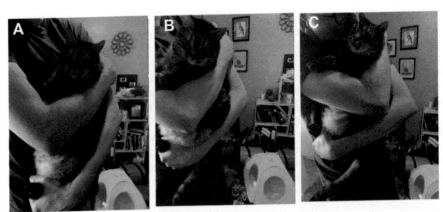

Fig. 15. (*A–C*) Hugging is an important human signal of affection and one that many care-givers wish to engage in with their cats - however intense physical handling and restriction can be challenging for cats as illustrated here, Notice the cat's facial expression and ear po-sition consistent with protective (negative) emotions and attempts to get away. (*Courtesy* of E. Sundhal, DVM, DABVP, Kansas City, MO.)

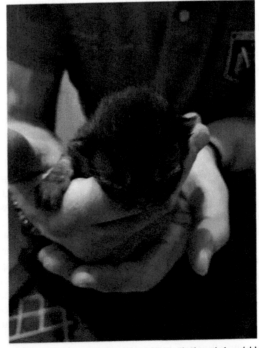

Fig. 16. Gradual introduction to human handling is needed and should be started as early as possible, preferably before 7 weeks of age. (*Courtesy* of A. Franklin, Husdjurshälsan, Göte-borg, Sweden.)

needs to be considered beforehand. The presence of other cats that are not of the same social group can also be a significant source of stress. An understanding of social relationships is crucial when designing the home environment from a feline perspective. Provision of a safe place, of multiple and separate resources, and of opportunities for play and predatory behavior are essential for all cats and are just as relevant for single cats as for those living in multi-cat environments. However, they can all be made more difficult to achieve in a multi-cat environment where there are individuals from different social groups. Providing an environment that respects the cat's sense of smell is also going to be more challenging in this context.

When optimising the home environment it is important to recognise that negative emotions may arise when they are justified. Therefore aiming for an environment that is free of fear is just as unrealistic and inappropriate at home as it is in the veterinary clinic. Instead, the goal is to provide a home that meets all feline environmental needs, encourages a predominance of positive emotional motivations, and ensures that when negative emotions are triggered the cat can respond to them appropriately. Such emotional intelligence enables the cat to maintain optimal emotional health that in turn reduces the risk of chronic physiological stress and resulting concerns in terms of physical health.[18] The three main areas of concern when physiological stress is unresolved are the impact on immune function, mucosal integrity, and perception of pain. Compromised immune function raises concerns in relation to the potential for infectious diseases but also has implications in terms of healing and recovery from illness. Loss of mucosal integrity can impact various systems and lead to a wide variety of reported illnesses, including problems of urinary tract disease, oral health, gastrointestinal compromise, dermatological conditions, and respiratory disease.[19] The emotional impact on the perception of pain may further complicate some of these disease states and makes behavioral consequences more likely. In addition, the potential for emotional compromise and resulting physiological stress to increase the perception of pain from degenerative joint disease and osteoarthritis and other painful conditions in feline patients must not be underestimated.

The use of pheromone products can be part of providing a home environment that respects the feline sense of olfaction. These products have been advocated as part of the approach to improving environmental factors in cases of reported problematic behavior.[20] Use of feline-appeasing pheromone in the environment has been specifically advocated in cases whereby there is tension in multi-cat households[21]; use of the F3 faction of the facial pheromone complex is recommended in cases of urine marking.[22] The range of applications of these products is broad, and the facial pheromone product has also been advocated for the management of unwanted scratching behavior.[23] In the author's experience, the use of feline-appeasing pheromone has been beneficial in single-cat households where compromised feline self-confidence is contributing to anxiety-related behavioral problems.

The provision of a safe place for all cats in a household and of multiple and separate resources will be affected by the social composition of the household as well as the physical space available. Resting places that are elevated, providing some sensation of being enclosed and hidden, not only afford the necessary safe space but also give cats the possibility of using their species-specific preference of avoidance when justified negative emotions occur. Such resting places may be provided by existing furniture, such as wardrobes and shelving (**Fig. 17**), or through the installation of purpose-built structures, such as cat towers (**Fig. 18**). It is important to consider the location of these resting places and ensure that they offer a sensation of safety. Positioning cat towers in windows can make sense in terms of offering something to look out at. However, there is the potential for such positions to feel visually vulnerable from a feline

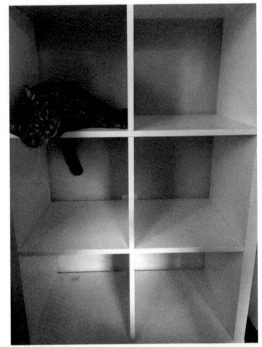

Fig. 17. Resting places that are elevated can give cats the possibility of using their species-specific preference of avoidance when justified negative emotions occur. (*Courtesy* of M. Scherk, DVM, Dip ABVP (Feline Practice), Vancouver, Canada.)

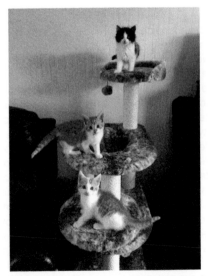

Fig. 18. There are a vast array of cat tree products on the market designed to offer elevated resting and observation locations for cats. (*Courtesy of* S. Heath, FRCVS, Chester, UK.)

perspective, and it can be better to place them in positions that offer the cat the choice to look out or to feel visually protected (**Fig. 19**A-C). Selection of appropriate feline furniture is not as easy as it may seem, and there is a vast range of products on the market. Some of these can unintentionally increase tension in multi-cat households

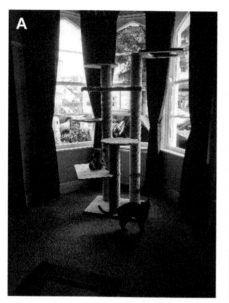
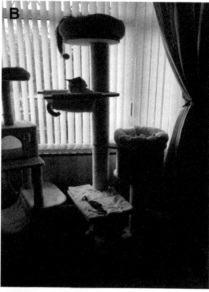
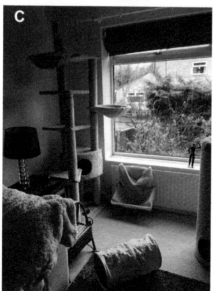

Fig. 19. (*A–C*). Positioning of a cat tower in a bay window can lead to sensation of vulnerability for cats and contribute to negative emotional motivations and chronic physiological stress. The use of blinds or the positioning of the tower slightly to the side of the window can decrease the potential visual impact and offer the cat more choice over whether it looks out at the world (*Courtesy* of S. Heath, FRCVS, Chester, UK.)

and contribute to the negative emotions of fear-anxiety and frustration. For example, when the structure provided offers elevated platforms with only one route up and down, cats can become stuck on those platforms in closer proximity to incompatible cats (**Fig. 20**). In order to avoid this, it is essential to create safe places that offer more than one point of entry and exit and to position shelving and furniture in ways that ensure that spatial blocking does not occur (**Fig. 21**). It is also important to differentiate between platforms that give the cat access to three-dimensional space for the purpose of observation (**Fig. 22**A) and those that provide platforms that give a sensation of enclosure and thereby enable cats to truly rest (**Fig. 22**B, C). Provision of safe places at ground level within the home is also beneficial and can be achieved in various ways. Cat beds are one potential, and some cats will really appreciate them (**Fig. 23**A, B). However, providing opportunities for safety and privacy does not have to cost a lot of money, and cats will often take advantage of unintentional safe places as well (**Fig. 24**A,B). It is also possible to use the cat carrier as a safe haven at home (see **Fig. 24**C); this has the advantage of helping to reduce stress associated with visits to the veterinary clinic because the cat already views the carrier as a safe location. If the cat can go into the carrier voluntarily and feel safe and secure during the car trip, this can significantly reduce the level of negative emotional arousal on arrival at the veterinary practice.

The environmental pillar of multiple and separate resources is particularly important in multi-cat households, but separation of resources is also relevant when cats live alone. There are two aspects to fulfilling this feline need. One aspect is to ensure segregation of the different types of resources, such as water, food, and latrines,

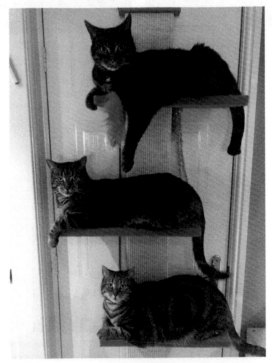

Fig. 20. When elevated locations are only accessible in one direction, cats can find themselves in closer proximity to incompatible house mates, and this can increase chronic social tension within the household. (*Courtesy* of S. Heath, FRCVS, Chester, UK.)

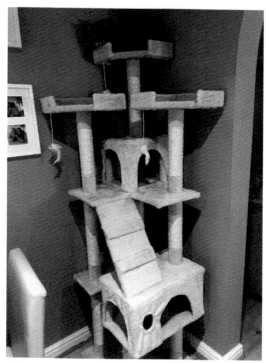

Fig. 21. In multi-cat households it is important to ensure that cat furniture that provides safe places, such as these boxes, offer more than one point of entry and exit. (*Courtesy* of S. Heath, FRCVS, Chester, UK.)

and the other aspect is separation of resources of the same type to ensure suitable provision for individual cats.

In the modern world where living space is often at a premium and time is precious, it can be tempting for caregivers to place all of the essential feline resource types in one location, both in order to save space and in order to make it easier for people to manage them (**Fig. 25**). Doing this can lead to behavioral issues, such as house soiling when the cat self-selects a latrine location that is segregated from the food and water, and can also contribute to physical health concerns, such as by restricting water intake when cats are reluctant to drink from water bowls placed too close to food or food intake when feeding stations are in busy traffic areas. Placing each resource in a distinct physical location, such as another room, is ideal, but when space is restricted, imaginative placement to ensure visual segregation can be a workable compromise, and pieces of furniture can act as visual barriers.

When there are multiple cats living in the same household, the placing of multiple resources of the same type side by side in the same location can make perfect sense from a human perspective (**Fig. 26**). However, the fact that cats are solitary survivors influences their need to have free and immediate access to essential resources at all times. Depending on the size of the feline household, the number of social groups within it, and the physical space available, facilitating this need can be a significant challenge. Inappropriate resource distribution is a significant factor in a range of feline behavioral medicine cases and in physical health cases where chronic physiological stress is playing a role.

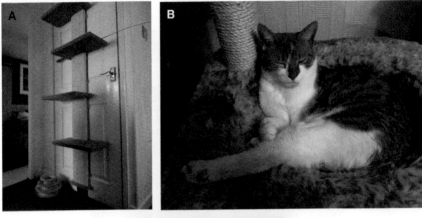

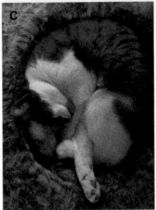

Fig. 22. Some cat tower structures only offer the rigid flat observation platforms (A). Resting platforms should offer some sense of protection and enclosure, creating sufficient securiry for the cat to completely relax (B,C). (*Courtesy of* S. Heath FRCVS, Chester, UK.)

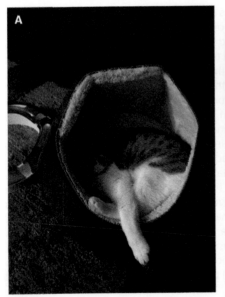

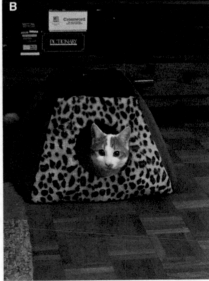

Fig. 23. (*A, B*) Cat beds can create safe resting places. (*Courtesy of* S. Heath FRCVS, Chester, UK.)

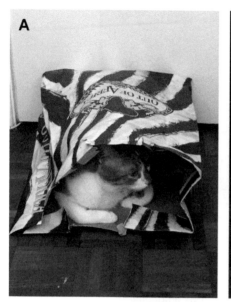
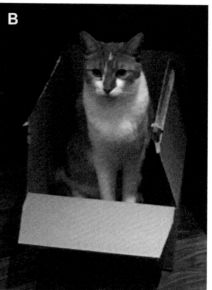
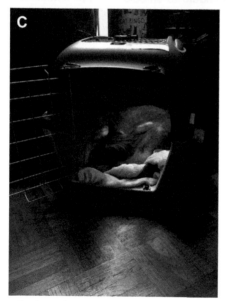

Fig. 24. (A–C) Providing safe places for cats does not need to cost a lot of money. Boxes and bags can be beneficial and cats can be given access to their cat carriers as a resting location, which can also help to reduce stress associated with visits to the veterinary practice. (*Courtesy* of S. Heath, FRCVS, Chester, UK.)

The inability of cats to wait patiently for a resource to become available necessitates provision of sufficient resources such that, should all of the cats in the household need to access a particular type of resource at the same time, they could do so without running the gauntlet of another cat. When this is not possible, the negative impact may be readily apparent, for example, when cats avoid using litter trays that are lined

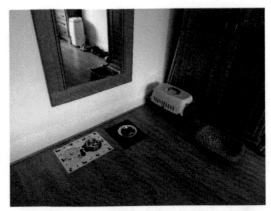

Fig. 25. It is common for caregivers to put all feline resources neatly together in one location. (*Courtesy of* S. Heath, FRCVS, Chester, UK.)

up side by side (see **Fig. 26**) and toilet in other locations in the home. However, when a resource is only available in locations determined by humans, cats can find themselves having to access essential survival resources in a context of social pressure, which can in turn contribute to chronic negative emotional bias and physiological stress. Probably the best example of this is feeding locations. Humans are socially obligate animals for whom nurturing of others is a strongly motivated behavior. This is the very basis of the desire to live with companion animals, and the act of feeding

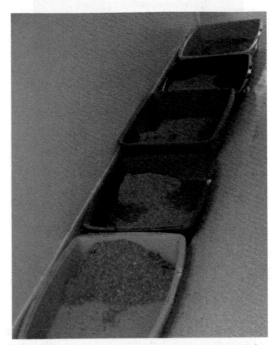

Fig. 26. Placing all litter trays in the same location can increase social pressure in multi-cat households, and cats may self-select an alternative location in which to toilet as a result. This is even more likely if the litter trays do not meet feline requirements in terms of the size of the trays and depth of litter available. (*Courtesy of* I. Rodan, DVM, Madison, WI.)

pets is an important part of the nurturing process. In addition, human animals are so-cial feeders for whom eating with company is a source of pleasure and a symbol of social security,[24,25] and therefore, provision of food bowls in a communal feeding sta-tion makes perfect sense (**Fig. 27**A, B). In contrast, the cat is a non-obligate social mammal and a solitary survivor with individual responsibility for self-nurturing in adult-hood. As a result of this social behavior, cats have a heightened motivation to protect survival resources and to seek access to them in locations that are safe and pro-tected.[26,27] In the context of food, this leads to them being solitary feeders and neces-sitates the provision of individual feeding stations for all cats, regardless of their social compatibility. Safe and protected feeding locations also encourage a grazing pattern of food consumption that is more in keeping with natural feline behavior. (See Mikel Del-gado and Leticia M. S. Dantas's article, "Feeding Cats for Optimal Mental and Behav-ioral Well-Being," in the next issue.) Failure to provide these can lead to cats experiencing emotional conflict when they are simultaneously motivated by desire-seeking to approach the food and by fear-anxiety to avoid an area of potential social tension. When this conflict is occurring once or twice a day, the resulting chronic phys-iological stress can have a significant impact on physical health and be a contributing factor to conditions, such as feline idiopathic cystitis. (See C.A. Tony Buffington and Melissa Bain's article, "Stress and Feline Health," in this issue.) It can also be a contrib-uting factor in cases of obesity,[28,29] because cats eating under social pressure and enhanced sympathetic activity are more likely to lay down adipose storage deposits.[30] The provision of microchip-operated feeding stations can be helpful in multi-cat house-holds (**Fig. 28**), but the location in which this device is placed is still important.

One resource that is often overlooked in feline homes is the ability to access the ter-ritory without conflict. Cats spend a significant proportion of their time exploring their environment, and the ability to move freely around their territory is important to them. Closed doors can lead to feline frustration, and in multi-cat households, blocking of access can be a significant trigger for negative emotional arousal. In some homes, the layout of the house can make blocking more likely, for example, when rooms have only one entrance and exit point or when hallways, staircases, and landings are narrow. Remembering that cats live in a three-dimensional world can be helpful when considering ways to resolve these issues; for example, it may be possible to

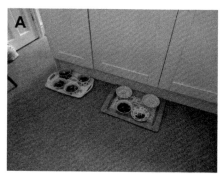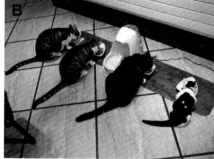

Fig. 27. (*A*) Clients will often feed all cats in the household in a communal feeding location. (*B*). All of these cats are staying at their feed bowls because their desire-seeking motivation to eat is very high. However, their body language shows that they are experiencing fear-anx-iety motivation at the same time. Their ears are scanning for information from the other cats as they remain alert to the possibility of conflict. This will result in them eating in a predom-inantly sympathetic state, which in turn can be a risk factor for developing issues of obesity. (*Courtesy of* [A] S. Heath, FRCVS, Chester, UK. [B] C. Fawcett, Sheffield, UK.)

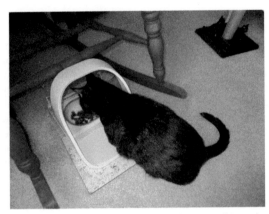

Fig. 28. Providing microchip feeders can be beneficial in a multi-cat households provided they are each positioned in separate safe locations. (*Courtesy of* S. Heath, FRCVS, Chester, UK.)

improve feline access by providing shelving so that cats can move around at different levels or by using hatches, which provide feline access between rooms (**Fig. 29**). When cats live an indoor-outdoor lifestyle, the access point to outdoors is another potential source of tension. Often one cat flap is available, and blocking of entry or exit from the property can be a contributing factor for chronic stress (**Fig. 30**), and provision of a second exit that provides a choice should be considered. It is also important to appreciate the potential for the positioning of entry and exit points to increase a sense of vulnerability for cats as they go outside or re-enter the property. When cat flaps open into visually vulnerable outdoor areas, there is a potential for cats to be intimidated by the presence of other cats or experience anxiety in anticipation of their presence (**Fig. 31**).[31] Likewise, if cat flaps enter into narrow tunnels or passages where non-compatible members of the household can lie in wait, there can be significant issues of emotional conflict (**Figs. 32**A, B and **33**A–C). Desire-seeking motivation, to go outside to explore or come home to a place of safety, can be triggered at the same time as fear-anxiety motivation, related to the anticipation of social confrontation. Repositioning cat flaps or using visual barriers, such as potted plants, to increase a sensation of being protected on leaving the property can be simple but effective

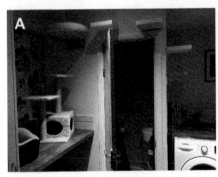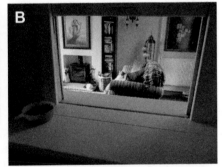

Fig. 29. (*A, B*) Provision of shelving to give access to three-dimensional space or the use of hatches to give additional entry and exit points between rooms can help to reduce bottlenecks in multi-cat households and give cats a sensation of control over their access through their home environment. (*Courtesy of* S. Heath, FRCVS, Chester, UK.)

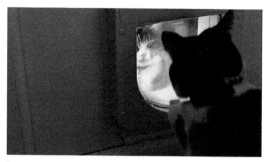

Fig. 30. Blocking of entry or exit from the property can be a problem when there is only one cat flap in a multi-cat household, and this can be a contributing factor for chronic stress. (*Courtesy of* S. Heath, FRCVS, Chester, UK.)

ways of alleviating chronic negative emotional motivation and the resulting physiological stress that can impact physical health.

The final pillar of environmental needs to consider is the provision of opportunities for play and predatory behavior. When kittens first arrive in the household, provision of play usually comes naturally, and most caregivers gain pleasure from the interaction (**Fig. 34**). However, over time, the provision of play by human caregivers decreases. When cats have access to outdoors, they will often satisfy this need by playing with

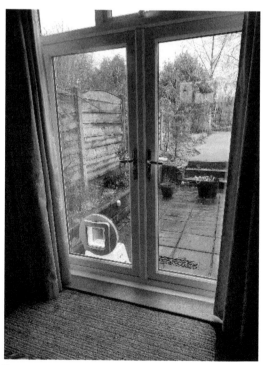

Fig. 31. When cat flaps open into visually unprotected locations, this can contribute to feline anxiety and resulting physiological stress. (*Courtesy of* S. Heath, FRCVS, Chester, UK.)

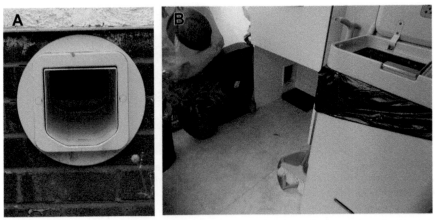

Fig. 32. (*A, B*) If cat flaps are installed in outer walls with connecting tunnels and enter into narrow or restricted locations on the other side, this can contribute to the potential for access blocking and increased social tension. (*Courtesy of* S. Heath, FRCVS, Chester, UK.)

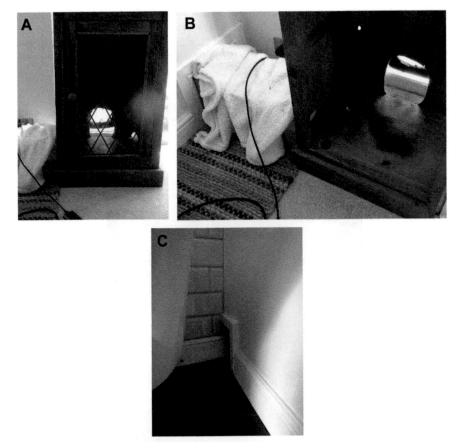

Fig. 33. (*A–C*) This complex access arrangement consisting of a hole allowing cats to enter into a cupboard and then exit through another hole to a tunnel leading through the wall into a very restricted location in a cloakroom contributed to significant social tension in a three cat household. (*Courtesy of* S. Heath, FRCVS, Chester, UK.)

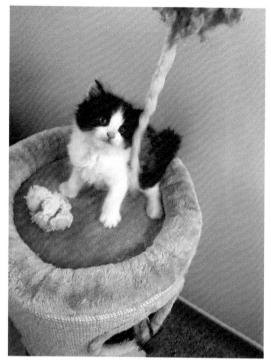

Fig. 34. Kittens readily engage in object play, and caregivers are keen to provide it. (*Courtesy of* S. Heath, FRCVS, Chester, UK.)

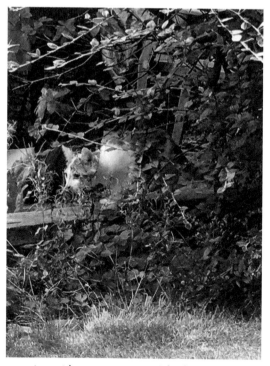

Fig. 35. If given access to outdoors, cats can satisfy their need for predatory and play behavior through playing with leaves or preying on insects, butterflies, or larger prey. (*Courtesy of* S. Heath, FRCVS, Chester, UK.)

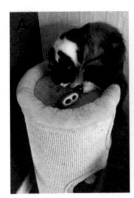 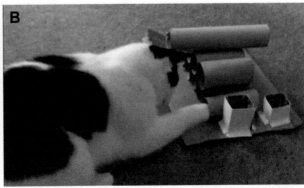

Fig. 36. (*A, B*) Cats can be encouraged to use predatory behaviour when feeding through a range of commercially available feeding products or homemade puzzle feeders. (*Courtesy of* S. Heath, FRCVS, Chester, UK.)

leaves or preying on insects, butterflies, or larger prey, such as birds and small mammals (**Fig. 35**). When self-directed play and predatory behavior in an outdoor context are not available, it is important to remember that access to these activities is a feline need; thus, provision of opportunities is an essential part of the process of environmental optimization.

Predation activity can be catered for by using feeding strategies that encourage cats to search for food and spend more time in the process of food consumption.[27,32] (See Chapter by Dantas: How to Feed in next issue.) There are several commercial products on the market designed to encourage predatory-style feeding, and caregivers can also make feeders from a variety of everyday objects (**Figs. 36**A,B). The other method of providing for this environmental need is through object play. One of the most commonly reported barriers to this provision is caregiver perception that the cat is not interested in play. There are two main reasons for this. First, cats engage in desire-seeking motivated object play in bouts of short duration, and this is contrary to the human perception that worthwhile play is sustained over a period of time. When a cat plays with a toy for one or two minutes, the human interpretation is that they are "not that keen," whereas the cat may have experienced a very worthwhile play experience. Second, the desire-seeking motivation in cats is triggered by sensory change, and they are therefore attracted to toys that offer change in the form of visual or auditory stimulation. Caregivers often report that the cat is very interested in new toys, but that the interest only lasts for a day or two and then the toy is ignored.[33] When this happens, it is important to look at the toy and see if it has the key features necessary to maintain interest. Crinkling, rustling noises, variable texture, reflective surfaces, and unpredictable movement will help to maintain engagement. When these are not present, toys can rapidly appear unchanging and consequently be ignored.

Movement of the toy is a major factor in its ability to engage the cat's interest. Enthusiastic caregivers often move the toy directly toward the cat and wonder why they show no interest or even retreat. It is important to remember that the aim is to trigger predatory-style responses. Mice and birds do not run or fly directly toward the cat, and likewise, the movement of a prey-mimicking toy should either be away from or parallel to the cat.

Another consideration when selecting toys is the ability of the cat to complete the predatory sequence by physically catching the toy.[34] Small toys, offering varying

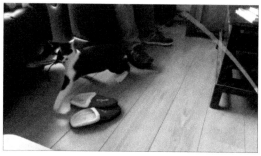

Fig. 37. Lightweight toys enable the cat to easily catch and carry its "prey." (*Courtesy of* S. Heath, FRCVS, Chester, UK.)

textures, are useful, and lightweight toys that the cat can easily catch and carry are also suitable (**Fig. 37**)). Laser pens do not fulfill this requirement and can intensely trigger the desire-seeking system while denying the opportunity to catch the prey, thus resulting in frustration. They are not cat toys, no matter how they are packaged, and they have the potential to create emotional conflict, high emotional arousal, and resulting physiological stress. It is best to advise caregivers to stop using these products, but if they are insistent on doing so, the negative impact can be mitigated to some extent by ensuring that the light lands on a tangible object that the cat can grab at and catch.

The aim of providing suitable toys in short and frequent bouts of play is to trigger beneficial desire-seeking motivation in the moment and also to contribute to the perception of the home as a safe environment. In order for this to occur, it can be important in multi-cat households to provide separate play sessions for individuals so that they can engage in play without anticipating potential social conflict.

SUMMARY

The impact of optimizing the veterinary clinic environment on feline health is primarily a short-term one because veterinary visits are often intermittent and infrequent. Exceptions include when patients have chronic illness, which necessitates repeated visits to the practice as outpatients, and those who need to be hospitalized for the purposes of surgery or inpatient treatment of more complex diseases. The aim is to ensure that the social and physical environment of the clinic fosters enhancement of positive emotion but also provides for appropriate and justified negative emotion to be expressed in ways that are safe for all concerned. Sustained negative emotional motivation can lead to physiological changes that are detrimental to physical health and may delay recovery and healing.

Failure to optimize the home environment has the potential to contribute to chronic emotional compromise and resulting behavioral change as well as physiological stress that can negatively impact the cat's physical health status. Educating caregivers about feline environmental needs and offering practical advice as to how to optimize the home from a feline perspective are therefore part of the professional remit of the veterinary practice. It is not only an important part of preventative health care in its broadest sense but also an essential part of the professional advice that should be given in feline medicine cases where the social and physical environment is impacting the cat's physical as well as emotional and cognitive health.

ACKNOWLEDGEMENTS

The author would like to thank all clients who have given their permission for the use of photographs that she has taken for educational purposes in this paper. In addition, thanks are due to the following institutions for their kind permission to use photographs that the author has taken on their premises.

Figures 5 and 6. J Finney MVB Abbeycroft Veterinary Surgery, Northwich UK.
Figure 7. University Small Animal Hospital at SLU, Uppsala, Sweden.
Figure 10 Davies Referrals Veterinary Practice, Hitchin, UK.
Figure 13. The Pet Project Vet Clinic, Manila, Philippines.
Figure 14. Patiworld Veteriner Klinigi, Ankara, Turkey.

DISCLOSURE

The author has nothing to disclose.

REFERENCES

1. World Health Organization Basic Documents Forty-ninth edition (2020) ISBN-13 978-92-4-000052-0.
2. Merriam-Webster online dictionary. Available at: https://www.merriam-webster.com/dictionary/health%20care. Accessed February 24, 2020.
3. Heath SE (2019) Understanding the Triad of Canine Health and its relevance to training Cognitive, Emotional and Physical Health presented at The National Dog Behaviour Conference, Sheffield, England, May 18, 2019.
4. Diez Roux AV. Investigating neighborhood and area effects on health. Am J Public Health 2001;91:1783–9.
5. Macintyre S, Ellaway A, Cummins S. Place effects on health: how can we conceptualise, operationalise and measure them? Soc Sci Med 2002;44(1):125–39.
6. Ellis SLH, Carney HC, Heath S, et al. AAFP and ISFM feline environmental needs guidelines. J Feline Med Surg 2013;15:219–30.
7. Lexico online dictionary. Available at: https://www.lexico.com/. Accessed February 24, 2020.
8. Heath SE. Understanding feline emotions and their role in problem behaviour. J Feline Med Surg 2018;20:437–44.
9. Hargrave C. Anxiety, fear, frustration and stress in cats and dogs–implications for the welfare of companion animals and practice finances. Companion Anim 2015; 20(3):136–41.
10. Hargrave C. In-practice management of stress in cats and dogs–improving the welfare of companion animals and practice finances. Companion Anim 2015; 20(5):292–9.
11. Yin S. Low stress handling, restraint and behavior modification of dogs & cats cattle. Dog Publishing; 2011.
12. Rodan I and Heath SE (2016) Handling the cat in pain in Feline Behavioural Health and Welfare . Rodan I and Heath SE, editors. p. 287–305
13. Sundahl E, Rodan I, Heath SE (2016) Providing feline friendly consultations in Feline Behavioural Health and Welfare. Rodan I and Heath SE, editors. p. 269–86
14. International cat care Cat Friendly Clinic. Available at: https://catfriendlyclinic.org/. Accessed February 24, 2020.
15. Hewson C. Evidence-based approaches to reducing in-patient stress–part 2: synthetic pheromone preparations. Vet Nurs 2014;29(6):204–6.

16. Pereira JS, Fragoso S, Beck A, et al. Improving the feline veterinary consultation: the usefulness of Feliway spray in reducing cats' stress. J Feline Med Surg 2016; 18(12):959–64.
17. Soennichsen S, Chamove AS. Responses of cats to petting by humans. Anthrozoos 2002;15:258–65.
18. Karagiannis C (2016) Stress as a risk factor for disease in Feline Behavioural Health and Welfare. Rodan I, Heath SE, editors. p. 138–47
19. Buffington CAT. Idiopathic cystitis in domestic cats—beyond the lower urinary tract. J Vet Intern Med 2011;25(4):784–96.
20. Vitale KR. Tools for managing feline problem behaviors: pheromone therapy. J Feline Med Surg 2018;20(11):1024–32.
21. DePorter TL, Bledsoe DL, Alexandra Beck A, Ollivier E. Evaluation of the efficacy of an appeasing pheromone diffuser product vs placebo for management of feline aggression in multi-cat households: a pilot study. J Feline Med Surg 2019; 21(4):293–305.
22. Mills DS, Mills CB. Evaluation of a novel method for delivering a synthetic analogue of feline facial pheromone to control urine spraying by cats. Vet Rec 2001;149:197–9.
23. Beck A, De Jaeger X, Collin J-F, et al. Effect of a synthetic feline pheromone for managing unwanted scratching. Intern J Appl Res Vet Med 2018;16(1):13–27.
24. Fiese B, Schwartz M. Reclaiming the family table: mealtimes and child health and wellbeing social policy report. Soc Res Child Development 2008; 22(4):3–18.
25. Nijs K, de Graaf C, Kok FJ, et al. Effect of family style mealtimes on quality of life, physical performance, and body weight of nursing home residents: cluster randomised controlled trial. Br Med J 2006;332(7551):1180–3.
26. Bradshaw JWS, Casey RA, Brown SL. Feeding behaviour in the behaviour of the domestic cat. 2nd edition. CABI; 2012. p. 113–27.
27. Sadek T, Hamper B, Horwitz D, et al. Feline feeding programs: addressing behavioural needs to improve feline health and wellbeing. J Feline Med Surg 2018;20(11):1049–55.
28. German AJ. The growing problem of obesity in dogs and cats. J Nutr 2006; 136(7):1940S–6S.
29. German A J and Heath S (2016) Feline obesity, a medical disease with behavioural influences in Feline Behavioural Health and Welfare. Rodan I and Heath SE, editors. p. 148–61
30. Tentolouris N, Liatis S, Katsilambros N. Sympathetic system activity in obesity and metabolic syndrome. Ann N Y Acad Sci 2006;1083:129–52.
31. Heath SE, Wilson C. Canine and feline enrichment in the home and kennel: a guide for practitioners. Vet Clin North Am Small Anim Pract 2014;44(3):427–49.
32. Ellis SL. Environmental enrichment: practical strategies for improving feline welfare. Journal of Feline Medicine and Surgery 2009;11(11):901–12.
33. Hall SL, Bradshaw JWS, Robinson IH. Object play in adult domestic cats: the roles of habituation and disinhibition. Appl Anim Behav Sci 2002;79:263–71.
34. Denenberg S. Cat toy play trial: A comparison of different toys. Proceedings of the Annual Scientific Symposium of Animal Behaviour, American Veterinary Society of Animal Behaviour; Denver, CO, July 20–21, 2003.

Behavior as an Illness Indicator

Elizabeth Stelow, DVM

KEYWORDS

- Feline • Behavior • Medical diagnoses • Pain

KEY POINTS

- Behavior change is the primary indicator to owners that their cat may have developed a health problem; the specific behaviors can help the clinician set a rational diagnostic path.
- Many feline behavior changes are caused by underlying medical problems or result from psychological issues that are comorbid with medical problems. Therefore, it is crucial that the veterinarian explore possible medical conditions exhaustively before treating a problem behavior as a "behavior problem."
- To uncover the underlying medical causes for presenting behavior changes, a thorough history is a necessary complement to a thorough physical examination, minimum database, and specialty imaging or laboratory tests.

INTRODUCTION

The behavior of an animal often reflects its physiologic health. A comfortable, well-fed cat presents as relaxed or interested and engages in species-typical maintenance behaviors. The animal that is ill or under physiologic or psychological stress often presents differently.[1,2] And, in fact, nearly every medical problem is first noted by the owner as behavior changes.[3]

So, although owners may be tempted to believe that the cause of their pet's change in behavior is, in fact, behavioral, it is crucial that medical differentials be ruled out.[4] The medical causes of behavior changes may be congenital/developmental, inherited, infectious, inflammatory, immune mediated, metabolic/endocrine, nutritional, degenerative, neoplastic, toxic, and/or traumatic.[3]

Complicating this process of diagnosing and treating our patients is the fact that behavioral and medical diagnoses often coexist.[4]

In order for behavioral changes resulting from medical problems to be addressed, they must first be identified by the owner then diagnosed by the veterinarian.

Some common "behavior" complaints of owners presenting their cats for veterinary care are discussed:

- Toileting outside the litter box
- Urine marking
- Fear/anxiety

University of California, Davis, 1 Shields Avenue, Davis, CA 95616, USA
E-mail address: eastelow@ucdavis.edu

Vet Clin Small Anim 50 (2020) 695–706
https://doi.org/10.1016/j.cvsm.2020.03.003
0195-5616/20/© 2020 Elsevier Inc. All rights reserved.

- Aggression
- Changes in grooming patterns
- Changes in sleeping patterns
- Changes in eating habits
- Changes in cognition
- Changes in vocalization
- Repetitive behaviors

Each of these complaints can have medical and/or behavioral causes that must be explored. For more information on making and treating behavioral diagnoses, please see Behavior Problem or Problem Behavior? in this volume.

Basic Diagnostic Workup of the Problems

For every problem presented in this article, a medical workup consists of the following:

- Acquiring a thorough history, including the onset and progression of the problem and any attempts on the owner's part to correct it
- A comprehensive physical examination
- Blood pressure determination
- Complete blood count, serum biochemistry panel with thyroid analytes, and urinalysis (with culture, when warranted)
- Retroviral serology if the patient's feline immunodefiency virus (FIV) or feline leukemia virus (FeLV) status is unknown

Depending on the specific presenting complaints and examination findings, imaging or additional specialized laboratory tests may be warranted. If a specific diagnosis hinges on specific diagnostic tests, those will be noted in the appropriate sections.

COMMON "PROBLEM" BEHAVIORS AND THEIR MEDICAL DIFFERENTIALS
Toileting Outside the Litter Box: Urine and/or Feces

Toileting outside the litter box refers to the cat urinating or defecating in a place other than the litter box. This is not to be confused with marking (nearly always done with urine),[4] which is discussed in the next section.

Common presentation and history

The owner will often state, as the reason for the appointment, that the cat is "going" outside the box. This can be a new problem, a chronic problem, or a problem of unknown duration in a cat that's new to the household. There's a higher index of suspicion that it is medically related if it is a relatively new problem. There may be a recent history of a urinary tract infection or digestive issue causing pain while using the box, or the owner may note recent increases in vocalization while the cat is in the box, approach/retreat around the box, or possible urination/defecation near the box (just not in it).[5] If both urine and feces are deposited outside the litter box, the index of suspicion for a medical cause is higher.[6]

Medical differential diagnoses
Urination

Degenerative: arthritis, cognitive dysfunction.[4,5,7–11]

Metabolic: polyuria/polydipsia (PU/PD) associated with diabetes mellitus, chronic kidney disease (CKD), hyperthyroidism, diabetes insipidus, and iatrogenic causes of PU/PD.

Neurologic: loss of voluntary control due to central (CNS) or peripheral nervous system lesions.

Inflammatory: lower urinary tract disorders (LUTD) including cystitis, urethritis, urolithiasis, feline idiopathic cystitis and/or Pandora syndrome (see **Box 1** and Stress and Feline Health in this volume).

Defecation

Degenerative: arthritis, pelvic pain.[4,5,7,8,11,12]
Metabolic: hyperthyroidism.
Infectious/inflammatory: colitis, gastrointestinal parasitism.
Other: diarrhea from any cause, constipation from any cause.

Additions to basic diagnostic plan

Changes in urination and defecation warrant a thorough neurologic examination in addition to the basic workup discussed earlier. Surgical exploration may also be warranted, depending on the findings of previous tests.

Urine Marking

Urine marking is the act of leaving small amounts of urine, usually on socially significant vertical surfaces. Although "marking" in cats most typically refers to urine, feces outside the box may be considered marking if it is left in socially significant places.[16] Marking, whether urine or (rarely) feces, should not be confused with toileting, which is discussed earlier. Because urine marking has a more specific purpose than toileting, it is usually more easily diagnosed as having social/behavioral causes. Still, a few medical conditions should be explored.[17]

Common presentation and history

The owners may say that the cat is urinating outside its litter box. On further exploration, the clinician may find that the cat is using the litter box most of the time but is also leaving urine on specific surfaces (mainly vertical) outside the box. There may or may not be a big change in the social or physical structure of the home, including new people or animals, loss of people or animals, moving house or being rehomed, construction, or new furniture.

Medical differential diagnoses

Urine marking can result from the following medical problems[7,18,19]:

Acquired: anal gland impaction, urolithiasis
Metabolic: CKD, hyperadrenocorticism, LUTD, being an intact male. One investigator suggests that up to 30% of cats presented for spraying also have a medical problem[19]
Neurologic: fecal incontinence.
Viral: FIV, FeLV.

Box 1
Feline idiopathic cystitis/Pandora syndrome

Many sickness behaviors can be associated with stress. Manifestations within the home are most often a combination of vomiting food or hair, reduced food intake, and inappropriate elimination.[13] Nearly all of the clinical signs presented in this article have feline idiopathic cystitis/Pandora syndrome as a differential diagnosis. The term "Pandora syndrome" was coined by Dr Tony Buffington to describe an "anxiopathy," a disorder resulting from chronic anxiety (stressors that the cat finds threatening), which can be manifested in any combination of organs.[14,15]

For more information on this important complex in cats, please see Stress and Feline Health.
Data from Refs.[13–15]

Fear/Anxiety

Anxiety (the state of anticipating something scary) and fear (when actually faced with something scary) can cause a variety of behavior changes that may also be seen with certain medical conditions; some of these changes (elimination issues, aggression, changes in grooming, and appetite changes) are addressed separately. Effective treatment depends on a proper diagnosis.

Owners and veterinarians can assess fear and anxiety in cats, in part, by looking at their body postures and facial expressions. A fearful cat may fold its ears back, widen its eyes, lower its head, and tuck its tail. Beyond these body changes, the cat might run away, freeze, attack, or engage in a displacement behavior that seems out of place for the situation (yawning, for instance). There may even be urination and defecation if the fear response is great.[7]

Common presentation and history

The changes caused by anxiety or fear can be quite varied. Owners may report that the cat has started hiding or climbing structures, seemingly to get away; with this, the cat may have started vigilantly scanning the environment. The cat may have become aggressive in certain settings or with certain people/pets. The cat may begin seeking more attention from the owner. There may be greater hesitancy to move around the house or certain rooms or, conversely, there may be pacing. There may be an increased or decreased activity or energy level noted by the owners. The owners may note a crouched body posture and dilated pupils. The cat may have started eating more or less or eating unusual items (pica).[18] Some of the same stressors noted under Urine Marking (discussed earlier) may be noted in the cat's history. Different differentials should be investigated based on specific behaviors in the history.

Medical differential diagnoses

The appearance of "anxiety" in a cat may actually be due to the onset of auditory/visual/mobility changes, hypothalamic-pituitary-adrenal axis disorders, or encephalopathy and other CNS changes due to uremia, liver disease, neoplasia of the frontal lobe/internal capsule/basal nuclei, rabies, toxoplasmosis, or FIP.[5,7,9,11,18,20–22]

More specific signs often associated with anxiety, but that may indicate medical problems, include the following:

- Panting; hyperthyroidism, pain from any cause
- Increased/nighttime vocalization: hyperthyroidism, hypertension, decline in special senses (vision and hearing), pain, and, by exclusion of the others, cognitive dysfunction
- Lip licking: nausea from any number of medical problems, including CKD, gastrointestinal causes, etc.
- Hiding behavior: pain from any cause, arthritis
- Easily startled: cognitive dysfunction
- Reluctance to move throughout the house or certain rooms: arthritis, visual changes (nuclear sclerosis), auditory changes (deafness), cognitive dysfunction
- Increased activity/energy: hyperthyroidism, intracranial neoplasia, hepatic encephalopathy, cognitive dysfunction, rabies
- Decreased activity: general illness, neoplastic processes, hyperthyroidism, hepatic encephalopathy, cognitive dysfunction, arthritis

Additions to basic diagnostic plan

Depending on the specific clinical presentation, the workup should include a thorough neurologic and dermatologic examination, in addition to the workup discussed earlier.

Aggression

Aggression in the cat can be toward other cats, other pets, owners, and/or strangers. It can range from mild (growling) to severe (multiple injuries from bites or scratches). Severity can also be measured by whether the target must be interacting with the cat in some way to trigger the aggression versus the target is simply present when the aggression happens.

Common presentation and history

Because aggression is a nonspecific sign, the history can be varied but often involves the cat attacking another cat or a person in the household. It is important to find out whether the cat must be triggered to elicit the aggression.

Medical differential diagnoses

Degenerative: decline in special senses: vision, hearing.[3,5,9,11,18,20,22]
Developmental: lissencephaly, hydrocephalus.
Anomalous: ischemic encephalopathy.
Metabolic: hepatic or uremic encephalopathy, hyperthyroidism.
Neoplastic: intracranial neoplasia.
Neurologic: psychomotor or partial seizure, peripheral neuropathy.
Nutritional: thiamine, taurine, or tryptophan deficiency.
Infectious: rabies,[1] pseudorabies, toxoplasmosis, *Neospora caninum*, FIV, FIP.
Inflammatory: feline idiopathic cystitis, granulomatous meningioencephalitis arthritis (For more on pain in cats, see **Box 2** and Feline Chronic Pain and Osteoarthritis).
Toxins: lead, zinc, methylphenidate, or heavy metal toxicity.
Traumatic: brain injury, traumatic causes of pain, cerebral infarct.
Vascular: cerebral infarct.

Box 2
Pain as a cause of behavior change

Both acute and chronic pain can have profound effects on an animal's behavior, potentially leading to avoidance and decreased activity, inappetance, irritability, restlessness, and aggression.[3] Therefore, it is very important for the veterinary team to be able to look for pain at each visit by

1. Asking questions of the owner about new—or newly extinct—behaviors related to movement (jumping, climbing, running, walking), feeding/grooming/toileting/social habits, vocalization, and aggression toward family members. These questions should target the timeline and extent to which these behaviors have changed.
2. Observing and examining the cat with an eye toward pain assessment. To assist with its pain assessment, the team should be familiar with the available facial and body pain scales that are in the veterinary literature and from various Internet sites.[3,23]

If pain is identified, the next step is to locate the source and address it with current standard-of-care treatments appropriate for the diagnosis. Pharmaceutical treatment of both acute and chronic pain in the cat continues to be a challenge.

For more on pain in cats, see Feline Chronic Pain and Degenerative Joint Disease.
Data from Landsberg GM, Hunthausen W, Ackerman L. Is it Behavioral or Is it Medical? In: Behavior Problems of the Dog and Cat. 3rd ed. Edinburgh, Scotland: Elsevier Saunders; 2013;75-80 and Brondani JT, Luna SP, Padovani CR. Refinement and initial validation of a multi-dimensional composite scale for use in assessing acute postoperative pain in cats. Am J Vet Res. 2011;72(2):174–183.

Changes in Grooming Patterns (Including Self-Mutilation)

Cats groom for 30% to 50% of their waking time (or 4%–15% of a 24-hour day).[7,24] Grooming removes dirt and parasites, aids in maintaining a comfortable body temperature, and decreases stress.[7] Changes in a cat's grooming habits—either an increase or a decrease—can indicate a problem. Increases in grooming can be localized, generalized, or self-mutilation. Increased localized grooming suggests parasites, pain, and focal dermatopathies. The most common areas of noticeable hair loss are the flank, medial foreleg, tail and dorsal lumbar region, inguinal region, and back legs.[7,24,25] Self-mutilation of the tail can be seen as a side effect of overgrooming in the cat, generally due to anxiety or as a compulsive behavior.[26] Hair can be missing or have a sheared-off appearance. Severe cases of overgrooming can lead to sores in the mouth, which can present as comorbid changes in feeding habits. Reduced grooming leads to an "unkempt" look, with a dirty or greasy hair coat.[7]

Common presentation and history

Owners may or may not notice changes in the amount of time a cat spends grooming or changes in the areas being groomed, but they are likely to notice changes to the hair coat or skin in those areas. They may also note a dirtier, more unkempt coat.[7] In addition, owners may find an increase in hair in the cat's feces or frequency of the cat vomiting hairballs.[27]

Medical differential diagnoses

Several external and internal medical causes are potentially responsible for increased or decreased grooming.

The diagnosis of "psychogenic alopecia" may be made commonly, but it is important to note a few things regarding this condition. The term evolved to describe self-induced alopecia resulting from an underlying behavioral, rather than "organic" cause.[24,25] Generally, overgooming behavior leading to psychogenic alopecia results from the cat attempting to cope with challenging social or environmental stressors.[24] In fact, grooming can often be seen immediately following conflict with another cat. Should these stressors continue, "maladaptive overgrooming" can result.[19]

Dermatologic problems can be complex and multifactorial; so, even when a stress-related cause is suspected in a case of overgrooming, it is important to rule out underlying medical conditions contributing to the problem.[24,25] It should also be noted that more than one differential for overgrooming is a "diagnosis of exclusion," including both psychogenic alopecia and atopic dermatitis.[25] This makes good diagnostics even more crucial.

Decreased grooming

Degenerative: arthritis.[1,22]
Infectious: systemic illness behavior[1]

Increased grooming

Metabolic: hyperthyroidism.[3,7,9,11,25,28–32]
Neurologic: psychomotor seizures, neuropathic pain, feline orofacial pain syndrome.
Infectious: external parasites, skin infections (fungal, bacterial)
Immune mediated: atopic dermatitis, dust mite sensitivity, food allergies and sensitivities, flea bite hypersensitivity, and insect bites.
Inflammatory: urinary tract diseases, trauma, neuropathic.
Trauma.

Additions to basic diagnostic plan

In addition to a basic workup, a thorough dermatologic examination is necessary. Scaling and crusting, especially in areas of hair loss, may direct testing.[29] Examine skin scrapings, tape preps, and plucked hairs under the microscope and submit plucked hair for fungal culture.[25] The hair under the microscope will likely be broken or sheared in cases of overgrooming. External parasiticides should always be administered regardless of whether evidence of fleas is seen. A dietary elimination trial may be indicated.[25]

Changes in Sleeping Patterns (Increases and Decreases, as Well as Quality)

Although considered crepuscular (most active at dusk and dawn),[9] cats are active and "hunt" at all hours.[33,34] But, for owners, who sleep at night, a cat whose primary active time has become nighttime can become a nuisance. There are behavioral reasons a cat may become active at night; some cats wake their owner for interactions, which can be rewarded even with negative interactions. But some savvy owners will note potential medical causes for the overnight sleep disruptions. Conversely however, because of their work habits, owners may not notice when their cats sleep more than usual.

Common presentation and history

Owners are typically intolerant of being awakened from sleep and readily identify when their cat is sleeping less at night.[9] Most commonly, cats will be presented to a veterinary hospital for a sudden increase in waking the owners. The cats may be waking up to scratch themselves, to feed, or to use the litter box at times they historically did not. Owners may also note increased vocalization, which may or may not be easy to interrupt by providing attention.

Medical differential diagnoses

Degenerative: cognitive dysfunction.[3,5,9]
Metabolic: hepatic and uremic encephalopathy, hyperthyroidism.
Neoplastic: thalamic, midbrain tumors.
Infectious: FIV.
Other: medications (prescribed or illicit), pain, or pruritis from any cause.

Changes in Eating Patterns (Including Vomiting, Pica)

There are many reasons that can cause a cat to change its eating habits. Mills notes that cats that are faced with unexpected changes in their management may have decreased appetite and water intake and avoid elimination for 24 hours.[18] Still, because there are many medical causes for these changes, these should be ruled out before owners focus on relieving anxiety.

Common presentation and history

Owners may not notice right away that these behaviors have changed, in part because cats normally consume many small meals throughout the day and night and many owners free-feed kibble.[1,33] If the level of food in the bowl changes unexpectedly or if the cat's weight changes noticeably, the owner will become aware of a problem. This becomes more complicated when the household has 2 or more cats and 2 or more owners: the food may still disappear with one cat not eating it and each owner may assume that the other owner is or is not refilling the bowl. This can result in confusion about exactly how much each cat is eating until a change is weight is noted.[33] At this point, they are more likely to seek medical help. The owners may also report that the cat eats nonfood items, such as fabric, plastic, paper, soil, or ribbon. There seems to be some breed predisposition among Siamese and Burmese to fabric/wool sucking or chewing.[9]

Medical differential diagnoses

Pica Medical and nonmedical causes (**Table 1**) of pica (ingestion of nonnutritional items or those that are not typically thought of as food) include normal exploration or play, living in a deprived environment, natural or pharmacologically induced polyphagia,[9] nutritional deficiency, intestinal parasitism, anemia,[36] chronic small bowel disease, thalamic lesions,[5] or lead intoxication.[7,12,35–41]

Changes in Cognition

Many medical pathologies can result in apparent changes in cognition in the cat. Knowledge of the age at presentation and the history help narrow the differentials. The challenge is that some, as cognitive dysfunction, are diagnoses of exclusion.[42]

Common presentation and history

There is no single presentation or history for cognitive impairment, because the causes and presenting complaints are so varied, and have different ages of onset and progression. The one thing they have in common is the concern on the part of the owner that the cat's brain does not seem to be functioning as expected.

Medical differential diagnoses

Degenerative: decline in special senses: vision, hearing, cognitive dysfunction (see
  Box 3 and Feline Aging: Promoting Physiologic and Emotional Wellbeing in this
  volume.)[5,9,42,43]
Metabolic: hepatic encephalopathy.
Neoplasia of or trauma to the frontal lobe.
Nutritional: taurine or thiamine deficiency.
Infectious: panleukopenia, rabies, toxoplasmosis, bacterial encephalitis, FIP, FeLV,
  FIV, prion-associated diseases.

Additions to basic diagnostic plan

The clinician should focus the thorough history by asking specifically about the "warning signs" of cognitive dysfunction, such as changes in owner interactions, loss of house training, disorientation, and sleep-wake cycle disturbances.

Table 1
Medical differentials for changes in eating habits and digestion

Increased Appetite	Decreased Appetite	Vomiting
1. Exocrine pancreatic insufficiency (EPI)	1. EPI	1. EPI
2. Hyperthyroidism	2. CKD	2. CKD
3. Diabetes mellitus, acromegaly	3. Diabetes mellitus	3. Diabetes mellitus
4. Thalamic lesions	4. Thalamic lesions	4. Pancreatitis
5. Cushing disease	5. Pancreatitis	5. Feline gastrointestinal eosinophilic sclerosing fibroplasia
6. Chronic small bowel disease	6. Feline gastrointestinal eosinophilic sclerosing fibroplasia	
7. Cholangitis	7. Hepatic dysfunction or failure	
	8. Neoplasia	
	9. Viral diseases including FIP, FIV, FeLV, rabies	
	10. Constipation	

Box 3
A note about feline cognitive dysfunction syndrome

Cats can show signs of cognitive change as they age. Although it is convenient to refer to the constellation of signs that include loss of house training, increased vocalization, changes social relationships, increased anxiety, and increased irritability as "cognitive dysfunction," the latter is a diagnosis of exclusion.[42] Diagnostics must rule out other causes such as urinary tract disease for house soiling or hyperthyroidism or hypertension for increased irritability. Other differentials include brain neoplasia, anemia, changes in hearing or vision, and others.[9,43]

Data from Refs.[9,42,43]

Changes in Vocalization

Similar to changes in sleeping patterns, owners are sensitive to increased vocalization in their cats.[9] And, as with sleep changes, there are many medical issues that can cause increased vocalization in cats.

Common presentation and history

There are many possible histories associated with increased vocalization. Of importance are the age of onset, time of day of occurrence, and the timeline of progression. These can help to distinguish among the possible causes.

Medical differential diagnoses

Degenerative: degenerative joint disease, cognitive dysfunction.[7,9,12,44,45]
Metabolic: estrus (including incomplete tissue removal if ovariectomized), uremia, hyperthyroidism, systemic hypertension.
Neoplastic: pain from neoplasia.
Neurologic: hyperesthesia, neuropathic pain.
Infectious: FeLV.
Inflammatory: gastrointestinal pain, urogenital pain, oral/dental pain.
Vascular: hypertension.

Additions to basic diagnostic plan

Depending on findings and specific presenting complaints laboratory work to detect anti-muellerian hormones (AMH) may be warranted.

Repetitive Behaviors

Nearly any behavior may be performed repetitively. Sometimes it is difficult to know the underlying cause. But, with a thorough history, including any relevant triggers, the differentials can be narrowed.[46]

Common presentation and history

Because repetitive behaviors can involve any "normal" behavior, as well as some unusual ones, presentation varies from case to case. Often, cat owners do not perceive these behaviors as troubling until they consume a good deal of the cat's waking time, cause self-harm (as tail chewing),[26] or become annoying to the owner.[46] In cats, the most common repetitive behaviors are associated with grooming,[26,47] pica, and wool sucking.[47]

Medical differential diagnoses

For wool sucking/pica, see "Changes in eating patterns" discussed earlier[3,5]
For grooming, see "Changes in grooming patterns" discussed earlier

For other "ritualistic" behaviors, rule out the following:

Metabolic: hypocalcemia and/or hypomagnesemia.

Neoplastic: lesions in the frontal lobe, internal capsule, or basal nuclei.

Neurologic: partial seizures.

Nutritional: excessively low-protein diet.

Immune-mediated: food hypersensitivity.

Inflammatory: pain from any cause.

Infectious: rabies, tetanus, botulism.

Additions to basic diagnostic plan

Depending on findings of previous tests and specific presenting complaints, advanced imaging or additional specialized laboratory tests may be useful.

The aforementioned are not the only behavior changes that will have clients bringing their cats to the veterinary care team. But they are among the most common.

SUMMARY

Behavior changes (increasing, decreasing, new, or extinct) are indications to owners that something might be wrong with their cat. Sometimes, these changes will have mainly psychological causes. However, in a sizable number of cases, organic health problems will be the underlying cause of (or at least partially responsible for) these changes. The combination of a good history and appropriate diagnostic workup can uncover a wealth of information to guide a diagnosis and effective treatment.

DISCLOSURE

The author has nothing to disclose.

REFERENCES

1. Hart BL. The behavior of sick animals. Vet Clin North Am Small Anim Pract 1991; 21(2):225–37.
2. Gregory NG. Physiology and behaviour of animal suffering. Oxford: Blackwell; 2004. p. 8.
3. Landsberg GM, Hunthausen W, Ackerman L. Is it behavioral or is it medical?. In: Behavior problems of the dog and cat. 3rd edition. Edinburgh (Scotland): Elsevier Saunders; 2013. p. 75–80.
4. Herron ME. Advances in understanding and treatment of feline inappropriate elimination. Top Companion Anim Med 2010;25:195–202.
5. Overall KL. Medical differentials with potential behavioral manifestations. Vet Clin North Am Small Anim Pract 2003;33(2):213–29.
6. Voith VL. Behavioral disorders. In: Davis LE, editor. Handbook of small animal therapeutics. New York: Churchill Livingstone; 1985. p. 519.
7. Seksel K. Behavior problems. In: Little S, editor. The cat: clinical medicine and management. St Louis (MO): Elsevier Saunders; 2012. p. 211–25.
8. Bennett D, Morton C. A study of owner observed behavioural and lifestyle changes in cats with musculoskeletal disease before and after analgesic therapy. J Feline Med Surg 2009;11:997–1004.
9. Horwitz DF, Neilson JC, editors. Canine and feline behavior, Blackwell's five minute veterinary consult. Ames (IA): Blackwell Publishing; 2007.

10. Stella JL, Lord LK, Buffington CAT. Sickness behaviors in response to unusual external events in healthy cats and cats with feline interstitial cystitis. J Am Vet Med Assoc 2011;238:67–73.

11. Reisner I. The pathophysiologic basis of behavior problems. Vet Clin North Am Small Anim Pract 1991;21(2):207–24.

12. Meric SM. Diagnosis and management of feline hyperthyroidism. Compend Contin Educ Pract Vet 1989;11:1053–6.

13. Stella JL, Croney C, Buffington CAT. Effects of stressors on the behavior and physiology of domestic cats. Appl Anim Behav Sci 2013;143:157–63.

14. Buffington CAT. Idiopathic cystitis in domestic cats–beyond the lower urinary tract. J Vet Intern Med 2011;25:784–96.

15. Buffington CAT, Westropp JL, Chew DJ. From FUS to Pandora syndrome; where are we, how did we get here, and where to now? J Feline Med Surg 2014;16:385–94.

16. Overall KL. Diagnosis and treating undesirable feline elimination behavior. Feline Pract 1993;21:11–5.

17. Neilson JC. Feline house soiling: elimination and marking behaviors. Vet Clin North Am Small Anim Pract 2003;33:287–301.

18. Mills D, Karagiannis C, Zulch H. Stress- its effects on health and behavior: a guide for practitioners. Vet Clin North Am Small Anim Pract 2014;44:525–41.

19. Frank D. Recognizing behavioral signs of pain and disease: a guide for practitioners. Vet Clin North Am Small Anim Pract 2014;44:507–24.

20. Clarke SP, Bennett D. Feline osteoarthritis: a prospective study of 28 cases. J Small Anim Pract 2006;47:439–45.

21. Barone G. Neurology. In: Little S, editor. The cat: clinical medicine and management. St Louis (MO): Elsevier Saunders; 2012. p. 734–67.

22. Klinck MP, Frank D, Guillot M, et al. Owner-perceived signs and veterinary diagnosis in 50 cases of feline osteoarthritis. Can Vet J 2012;53:1181–6.

23. Brondani JT, Luna SP, Padovani CR. Refinement and initial validation of a multidimensional composite scale for use in assessing acute postoperative pain in cats. Am J Vet Res 2011;72(2):174–83.

24. Virga V. Behavioral dermatology. Vet Clin North Am Small Anim Pract 2003;33:231–51.

25. Waisglass SE, Landsberg GM, Yager JA, et al. Underlying medical conditions in cats with presumptive psychogenic alopecia. J Am Vet Med Assoc 2006;228:1705–9.

26. Schwartz S. Separation anxiety syndrome in cats: 136 cases (1991–2000). J Am Vet Med Assoc 2002;220:1028–33.

27. Cannon M. Hair balls in cats: a normal nuisance or a sign that something is wrong? J Feline Med Surg 2013;15(1):21–9.

28. Baral RM, Peterson ME. Hyperthyroidism. In: Little S, editor. The cat: clinical medicine and management. St Louis (MO): Elsevier Saunders; 2012. p. 571–84.

29. Moriello KA. Dermatology. In: Little S, editor. The cat: clinical medicine and management. St Louis (MO): Elsevier Saunders; 2012. p. 371–419.

30. Mathews KA. Neuropathic pain in dogs and cats: if only they could tell us if they hurt. Vet Clin North Am Small Anim Pract 2008;38:1365–414.

31. Reiter AM. Dental and oral diseases. In: Little S, editor. The cat: clinical medicine and management. St Louis (MO): Elsevier Saunders; 2012. p. 329–70.

32. Rusbridge C, Heath S, Gunn-Moore DA, et al. Feline orofacial pain syndrome (FOPS): a retrospective study of 113 cases. J Feline Med Surg 2010;12:498–508.

33. Witzel AL, Bartges J, Kirk C, et al. Nutrition for the normal cat. In: Little S, editor. The cat: clinical medicine and management. St Louis (MO): Elsevier Saunders; 2012. p. 243–54.

34. Prospero-Garcia O, Herold N, Phillips TR, et al. Sleep patterns are disturbed in cats infected with feline immunodeficiency virus. Proc Natl Acad Sci U S A 1994;91(26):12947–51.

35. Xenoulis PG, Zoran DL, Fosgate GT, et al. Feline exocrine pancreatic insufficiency: A restrospective study of 150 cases. J Vet Intern Med 2016;30:1790–7.

36. Bartges J, Raditic D, Kirk C, et al. Nutritional management of diseases. In: Little S, editor. The cat: clinical medicine and management. St Louis (MO): Elsevier Saunders; 2012. p. 255–88.

37. Schnauß F, Hanisch F, Burgener IA, et al. Diagnosis of feline pancreatitis with SNAP fPL and Spec fPL. J Feline Med Surg 2019;21:700–7.

38. Quimby JM, Smith ML, Lunn KF. Evaluation of the effects of hospital visit stress on physiologic parameters in the cat. J Feline Med Surg 2003;13:733–7.

39. Weissman A, Penninck D, Webster C, et al. Ultrasonographic and clinopathological features of feline gastrointestinal eosinophilic sclerosing fibroplasia in four cats. J Feline Med Surg 2013;15:148–54.

40. Foley JE, Lapointe JM, Koblik P, et al. Diagnostic features of clinical neurologic feline infectious peritonitis. J Vet Intern Med 1998;12:415–23.

41. Diaz JV, Poma R. Diagnosis and clinical signs of feline infectious peritonitis in the central nervous system. Can Vet J 2009;50:1091–3.

42. Gunn-Moore D, Moffat K, Christie LA, et al. Cognitive dysfunction and the neurobiology of ageing in cats. J Small Anim Pract 2007;48:546–53.

43. Landsberg GM, Nichol J, Araujo JA. Cognitive dysfunction syndrome: a disease of the canine and feline aging brain. Vet Clin North Am Small Anim Pract 2012;42:749–68.

44. Landsberg GM, Denenberg S. Behavioral problems of the senior cat. In: Rodan I, Heath S, editors. Feline behavioral health and welfare. St. Louis (MO): Elsevier; 2016. p. 345–56.

45. Carmichael KP, Bienzle D, McDonnell JJ. Feline leukemia virus-associated myelopathy in cats. Vet Pathol 2002;39:536–45.

46. Tynes VV, Sinn L. Abnormal repetitive behaviors in dogs and cats: a guide for practitioners. Vet Clin North Am Small Anim Pract 2014;44:543–64.

47. Frank D. Repetitive behaviors in cats and dogs: Are they really a sign of obsessive-compulsive disorders (OCD)? Can Vet J 2013;54:129–31.

Behavior Problem or Problem Behavior?

Terry Marie Curtis, DVM, MS*

KEYWORDS

- Feline • Behavior • Problem

KEY POINTS

- What are behavior problems versus problem behaviors? It usually depends on the individual client.
- The goal with objectionable or annoying feline behaviors is to always solve the problem, so creativity is often key.
- It is important to remember that these problem behaviors are normal behaviors for the cat.

INTRODUCTION

For veterinary behaviorists, working with cats with "problem behaviors", it is always the client, the person the cat lives with, that makes the determination of what is a problem. For example, someone can be told that a cat defecating outside the litter box is a problem, but, to the cat's owner, it may not be such a big deal; the owner can pick up the feces with no problem. For another client, a cat scratching the new sofa can mean a death sentence–, but, for another cat owner, the scratching is no big deal. The thing to remember about these problem behaviors, is that they are normal behaviors for cats. Exploring, eliminating, scratching/chewing, jumping/climbing on furniture, destroying things, hunting; these are all things that cats do. Choosing cats to be members of human households does not necessarily make these behaviors lessen or disappear. People are frequently faced with the reality of what their chosen cats do and struggle with what it means to have cats in their homes.

I have lived with cats all my life. Before becoming a veterinary behaviorist, I was a feline-only practitioner. As part of my behavioral training, I did research for my master's degree in feline social behavior. Given all of that, people would think that I know cats. On the contrary: after all this time, I can say with confidence that I do not think that anyone knows cats. However, what I do know is how to solve a problem. And that is what veterinary behavior is: solving a problem (real or imagined) for 1 or more humans living with 1 or more cats.

University of Florida College of Veterinary Medicine, Gainesville, FL, USA
* P.O. Box 100126, Gainesville, FL 32610-0126.
E-mail address: curtist@ufl.edu

Vet Clin Small Anim 50 (2020) 707–718
https://doi.org/10.1016/j.cvsm.2020.03.002
0195-5616/20/© 2020 Elsevier Inc. All rights reserved.

vetsmall.theclinics.com

As stated earlier, all of the behaviors that I have addressed here are normal for cats. In some cases, the behavior is an indicator of a medical problem; for example, house soiling secondary to urinary tract or gastrointestinal tract conditions or nighttime howling secondary to hyperthyroidism. (See Stelow's chapter, "Behavior as an Illness Indicator," in this issue.) However, in most cases, the problem is for the humans they are living with, not the cat.

House Soiling

In one form or another (not using the litter box or urine marking) house soiling is still the number 1 problem I am called on to solve. The key is to realize that the 2 behaviors are different. Not using the litter box to urinate and/or to defecate is typically an issue associated with the litter box itself: the box type (open, covered), the size of the box, the location of the box, and/or what is inside the box (the litter or substrate). With urine marking, it can be more complicated, not only in pinpointing a cause but also in coming up with a treatment that stops the behavior.

When a cat stops (or never starts) using the litter box as its toilet, start there: the litter box. There are number of studies of box type (open versus covered),[1] box size (big),[2] as well as what is inside the box (ie, substrate preferences)[3]. As for location, asking the question: "Where are the accidents?" will provide a great amount of information.

In general, if the "accident" (with cats, there are no real accidents) is next to the litter box, it shows 2 things. First: the cat can get to the box. There is no deterrent. Possible deterrents include other cats, dogs, and children, as well the distance to the box from the cat's core area (ie, where the cat "lives") and location desirability. Second: it shows that the cat does not like the box and/or what is in the box. This bit of information shows that the location of the box is fine. There is no reason to change it and no need to add a litter box elsewhere, the owner can concentrate on the box itself and/or what is inside.

In contrast, if the accident is far away from the box, other things may be at play, such as: The cat cannot get to the box, either because of physical constraints (eg, the cat's core area is on the first floor and the litter box is in the garage or down stairs that the cat can no longer navigate), or social constraints (eg, there is another, hostile, cat lying in between the cat and its toilet; or there is a dog or child doing the same), or the box is located next to an appliance that makes frightening noises. In any case, investigate why the cat cannot, or does not want to, get to the box.

If the cat is eliminating right next to the box, look at the setup. Make sure that:

- The box is big (1.5 times the length of the cat from the head to the tail[4]; **Fig. 1**).
- The box is clean (have the owner scoop the box at least once a day).
- The substrate is one that the cat likes (a soft, sandy, clumping, clay-based litter is what most cats prefer[3]) and is deep (at least 75–100 mm).

If possible, it is important for the owner to observe the cat inside the box. Typically, a cat that straddles the box, standing on the edges, is not happy about what is inside (**Fig. 2**A), whereas a cat that squats in the middle of the box is likely comfortable and happy (**Fig. 2**B).

If the cat is eliminating in a location away from the litter box, set up a new litter box in that location, taking into account all of the box and litter particulars mentioned earlier. At the same time, gather information about this new location. Try to look at things from the cat's perspective. What is it about this place that makes it so desirable? Is it quiet? Is it out of the way of an otherwise chaotic life? Is it right next to where the cat sleeps? Information collected about the inappropriate location can help when setting up an appropriate location.

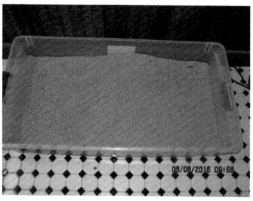

Fig. 1. Large, open plastic storage box.

Keep it simple: big box, clean box, litter that the cat likes, in a location that the cat likes.

Urine marking is typically different. I can say this given that I have shared my life with urine-marking cats for more than 15 years.

There is a lot to read about this topic, but the American Association of Feline Practitioners and International Society of Feline Medicine Guidelines for Diagnosing and Solving House-Soiling Behavior in Cats is an excellent resource[4] that can be accessed free of charge at https://catvets.com/guidelines/practice-guidelines/house-soiling. Discuss with the owner all of the possible contributing factors, such as the social issues that may exist among household cats, or travel/work schedule that could be contributing to separation anxiety. Address the presence of any outside cats using motion detectors, by not feeding strays, by denying them visual access/physical

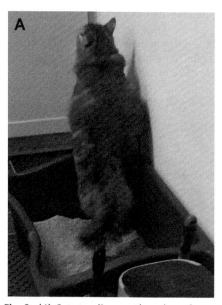
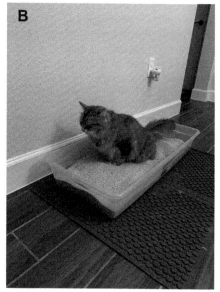

Fig. 2. (*A*) Cat standing on the edge of a normal litter box. (*B*) Same cat as in (*A*) standing inside a large plastic storage box.

access to any cats inside, and so forth. Address environmental enrichment: food, toys, three-dimensional space, individual territories with the proper number of "toilets" and so forth.[5] All of these are important, but they are important in every cat household, not just those with 1 or more urine-marking cats (see also Stress and Feline Health and Environment and Feline Health).

Once the environmental components have been addressed, it often comes down to medicating the cat that is urine marking. There seems to be an association between anxiety and urine marking. Although some cats appear anxious while urine marking (eg, pacing, vocalizing), not all do. Whether or not the cat appears anxious while urine marking - or in general - antianxiety medications typically reduce, if not completely resolve, urine marking.

There are several medication options,[4,6] but my first choice is fluoxetine (generic Prozac). I generally start with 2.5 mg per cat once a day by mouth and work up to 5 mg per cat per day by mouth if necessary. When it comes to medicating cats for urine marking, my advice is always to use the lowest dose that works. For some cats, that is 5 mg every day. For others, it is 2.5 mg every other day (eg, Monday, Wednesday, Friday) and 5 mg on the alternate days (eg, Tuesday, Thursday, Saturday). For others, such as my own 2 males, it is 2.5 mg every 4 to 5 days. I typically start with a daily dose and then work down to a less frequent schedule after a month or so if there is improvement. The dose can always be increased again, if needed.

The most common side effect with fluoxetine is a decrease in appetite, which is usually a dose-dependent effect, so decrease the dose or stop the medication if the cat stops eating. Once the appetite returns, restart the medication at a lower dose, or try a different medication. Medications can always be compounded (liquids, chewable tablets, and so forth) but I prefer tablets. I like to know that the cat is getting the dose I am prescribing. I wrap the pill in half of a Pill Pocket or cover it with some pill paste and administer the medication that way. Some cats will eat the Pill Pocket or pill paste-covered medication which is ideal. Other cats will ingest the pill if it's inside a "glob" of something yummy: cream cheese, salmon-flavored cream cheese, liverwurst, canned cat food, and so forth. The goal is to make the medicating experience as stress free as possible. Although it is attractive to think that transdermal anxiolytic medications can be effective for urine marking, the literature (and personal experience) shows otherwise.[7,8] However, at least 1 study (and, again, personal experience) showed that oral and transdermal buspirone are just as effective in urine-marking cats.[9] In those cases where improvement was seen, the dose of buspirone being absorbed through the skin into the cat's system is therapeutic for those cats.

Cats Have Claws and Teeth for a Reason: Scratching and Chewing

All cats scratch, whether they have claws or not. It is in their nature. Scratching removes the outer layer of the nails. It also hones the nails, keeping them sharp. When cats are unable to scratch, the nails can become thickened and curve inward toward the pads, causing pain, puncture, and infection. Although declawed cats can jump up and climb onto things, sharp claws help with this, allowing the cats to anchor themselves. From watching a cat scratching, it is obvious that the behavior also stretches the entire spine, keeping the cat limber. There are interdigital scent glands, so cats leave behind pheromonal and visual messages where they have scratched (**Fig. 3**).

Because scratching is a normal, and essential, behavior, it is best to address it as such and give the cat an acceptable opportunity to scratch. This approach entails finding the substrate that works best for the cat. Some cats prefer horizontal substrates (eg, mats, expensive rugs, grass; **Fig. 4**), whereas others prefer vertical ones (eg, trees, doorframes, couch corners; see **Fig. 3**). In a recent study,[10] kittens showed

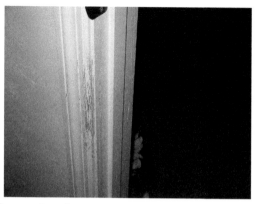

Fig. 3. Scratch marks on a door frame.

a preference for S-shaped corrugated cardboard scratchers. Once the preference has been determined, the goal is to provide the cat with its preferred substrate in places where it will use it. Putting a scratch board in a room that the cat never enters does not help. Typically, cats scratch when they stretch from just waking up. Putting a scratching pad/mat/post near the sleeping area therefore makes sense. It is also important to provide the cat with options where it is currently scratching, so that it chooses the right option. Sprinkling the mat, pad, or post with catnip can make the substrate more attractive, as may the product Feliscratch. If the cat prefers a vertical post, make sure that it is tall and sturdy enough for the cat to fully extend its body and forelimbs without losing its balance.

For some cats, the solution requires more creativity than just purchasing a scratching mat or post from a pet store. For cats who prefer scratching trees, finding a log or tree branch and setting up inside may save bed posts and door frames.

In addition to providing an appropriate scratching substrate, it is also important that the cat's claws be trimmed regularly. Although there are several options when it comes to nail trimming tools, I prefer human nail clippers. I am used to them; they feel good in my hand. This way, I do not have to deal with learning how to use a strange pet nail clipper while I am trying to cut a cat's claws. In addition, cat nails are flat like human nails rather than round in cross section like dog nails - so a human nail clipper works well. I typically have the cat seated in my lap, facing out. This way, all 4 paws are where I need them. It is a quick and easy process, especially if the cat is taught when it is a kitten (**Fig. 5**).

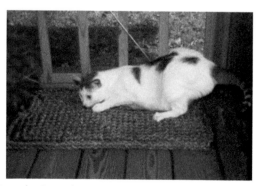

Fig. 4. Cat scratching a horizontal mat.

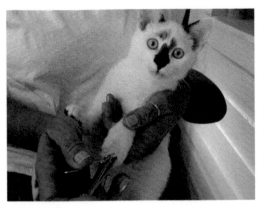

Fig. 5. Trimming a kitten's nails.

For some clients, using nail covers such as Soft Paws is another option (**Fig. 6**). Generally applied by a groomer or veterinarian, the nails are clipped short and the covers are glued on. As the nail grows, the covers generally fall off and are reapplied.

Chewing

Although some cats chew fabrics, sometimes ingesting them, which I define as a behavior problem, more cats eat or chew on house plants, which is normal but can be a problem behavior. If the plants are poisonous/toxic to cats, that poses a danger. However, mostly the chewing is just annoying, preventing the cat's owner from having any plants in the house.

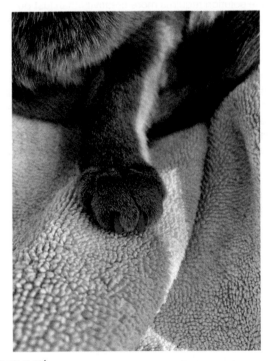

Fig. 6. Nail covers on a cat.

As with most of the problem behaviors discussed here, this one is no different: offer the cat something acceptable to chew on. Cat grass is a delicious option (**Fig. 7**). A combination of wheat, oat, and rye grass, cat grass grows quickly and provides a soft and digestible alternative to house plants. The fresh catnip herb is another option (**Fig. 8**). Some cats will not eat fresh catnip until it is handpicked and rubbed to release the essential oil, and many rub their faces and entire bodies all over the plant before ingesting it.

There is a concern that providing cat grass and/or fresh catnip makes cats vomit. In my experience, this has not been the case.

Climbing and Jumping onto Things

Normally, cats are good climbers, and most can jump very well and high. Cats love to explore. For a cat living outside, they can perform these behaviors on trees, fences, and so forth. Inside, there are counters, refrigerators, book cases, desks, coffee tables, and curtains, all places where they can potentially get into things (**Fig. 9**). All cat owners have had the experience of their cat lying over the computer's keyboard as they attempt to type, or of having their cat "help" them prepare dinner by jumping up on the kitchen counter. Kittens often find that expensive living room curtains are just as much fun to climb as an oak tree. Again, all normal behaviors for cats but annoying for humans.

An ideal goal would be to provide as many and varied perches throughout the house as possible. Perches can be as simple as a cat "condo" (**Fig. 10**) or as complicated as the book The Cats' House shows.[11] Whatever is possible for the individual situation (size of the space, number of cats, patio and/or outdoor access, and so forth), the goal is to provide several levels as well as a variety of surfaces: carpet, wood, tile, sisal rope, and so forth.

Cats can be taught that there are acceptable places to jump up onto and perch, especially if they are properly punished for jumping up onto unacceptable places. Punishment is tricky and, in many cases, very difficult to do. For punishment to work, 3 conditions must be met: (1) it must be immediate, meaning that it happens within a second or so of the behavior; (2) it must be consistent, meaning that it has to happen every time the behavior occurs, otherwise the cat just learns to do the behavior when the owner is not home; and (3) it must be appropriate for the individual, meaning that it stops the behavior without scaring the individual unduly and/or inducing learned helplessness (the cat simply accepts the bad and does not try to

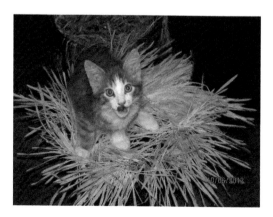

Fig. 7. Cat grass.

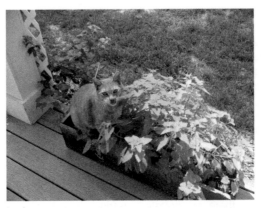

Fig. 8. Fresh catnip herb.

escape). The best form of punishment, one that meets all of those criteria, is remote punishment, which means that the punishment happens whether someone is there to witness the behavior or not. Good options include motion detectors that either emit a stream of air or emit a sound when the cat is nearby. Providing alternative acceptable options nearby helps to solidify the behavior of using the perches that humans want the cat to use, especially if there are rewards such as treats or catnip every time the cat jumps up onto it.

Nighttime Vocalization

Cats are vocal, some more so than others. Oriental breeds, such as Siamese, seem to be particularly "talkative" and many people choose these breeds for that reason: they are "chatty" companions. However, at other times, such as in the middle of the night, a vocal cat is not ideal.

In older cats, nighttime howling may be a result of hyperthyroidism, hypertension, or pain, so be sure to check for these. Another option is cognitive dysfunction (see Stelow's chapter, "Behavior as an Illness Indicator," in this issue).

For other cats, howling at night may also be to solicit food and/or attention. When cats are meal fed, they often only have food in the morning and again when the human returns from work. Although this schedule may work for human caretakers, it is not how cats instinctively behave. Cats are crepuscular, so they are most active (ie, do most of their hunting) at dawn and dusk. When is dawn to a cat? Is it 3:00 AM? Is

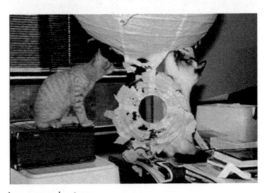

Fig. 9. Cats destroying paper lantern.

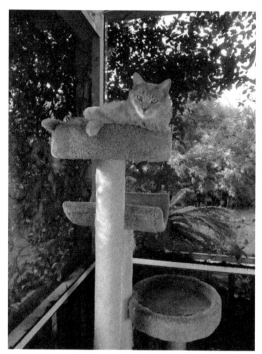

Fig. 10. Cat condo.

it 4:00 AM? It is pretty much when the human is asleep. When the cat howls, if the human wakes up and tends to the cat, the cat learns that this behavior works. Not in a malicious way, but in an operant conditioning way.

When feeding cats, whether they are howling in the early hours for food or not, it is best to stick to their normal behavior. Cats eat about 15 small meals a day, most of them at night. Many cats do very well at maintaining good body weight when fed a good quality diet, free-choice but as frequent small amounts. Others can be given the chance to hunt for their food using a variety of puzzle toys[12] and/or just by putting out several small bowls with tiny amounts of food in each. This way the cat must search for the food, but the food is always available.

For cats that are meowing for attention, if they are successful, they learn through operant conditioning to repeat that behavior. It is what they are being taught. If the cat meows and it gets attention (ie, it is played with, or yelled at: both are equal in a cat's eyes), then it is going to continue to meow.

With attention-seeking behavior there are 2 options. The first is to ignore the behavior. Ignoring is hard because any goal-directed behavior that is ignored/thwarted gets worse before it stops. This behavior pattern is known as the extinction burst and it can be relied on. Therefore, if owners are going to ignore a behavior, they have to see it through. Eventually, the behavior will stop. The cat will learn that there is no good outcome to the mewing. However, if at any time during the ignoring period the cat gets attention, then it reinforces that the extreme and persistent howling is what it needs to do. Bad lesson. The second option involves replacing the undesirable mewing behavior with a more desirable behavior: response substitution. Give the cat attention in a different way, such as with an interactive toy (outside the bedroom), a food puzzle, or by adopting another cat as a playmate. This last recommendation can

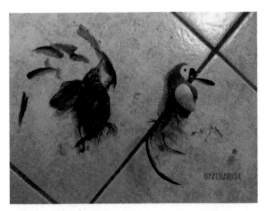

Fig. 11. Teaching cats to hunt birds.

work wonders and should be seriously considered if the human is at all inclined to increase the number of kitties in the household.

Playing with the cat before bedtime can also help, so that the cat learns that there is play and attention but at a time and on a schedule that the human chooses.

Hunting

Cats are hunters. Whether they are inside cats, outside cats, hungry cats, or sated cats, cats hunt. Cats are programmed to follow and go after moving objects: prey. In the wild, cats need multiple small meals (birds, mice, lizards) every day so they hunt many times a day. Again, given their crepuscular nature, cats do most of their hunting at dawn and at dusk. If the cat is hungry, then the prey may become a meal. If not, it may be just be a play thing, with the cat losing interest after the prey stops moving.

As to why the cat brings a dead, half-eaten "present" inside, there are theories. It could be that the cat is storing the bird in a safe place to eat later. It could also be that the cat is soliciting play from its human by bringing in the obviously fun, but dead, mouse. As with so many cat behaviors, there is no definitive answer.

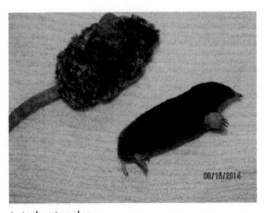

Fig. 12. Teaching cats to hunt moles.

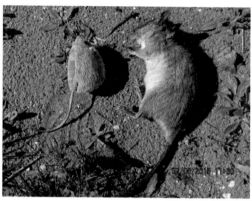

Fig. 13. Teaching cats to hunt mice.

However, what I saw in my own cats is that I Taught Them To Do This. As seen in **Figs. 11–13**, there are toys that I provided my cat alongside the "gifts" my cat gave me.

I'm not offering any solution to the hunting "problem". Other than keeping cats indoors, I do not think that there is one. Cats are mysterious. Personally, I like not knowing the answers to why cats do some of the things they do. It goes back to there being many annoying and/or unacceptable feline behaviors that humans desire to change, and that can be done without fully and completely understanding why the cat does it in the first place. That's problem solving. But there are many behaviors that force us to reflect on the wonderful nature of our kitties and to appreciate the joy that they bring to our lives.

DISCLOSURE

The author has nothing to disclose.

REFERENCES

1. Grigg EK, Pick L, Nibblett B. Litter box preference in domestic cats: covered versus uncovered. J Feline Med Surg 2013;15(4):280–4.
2. Guy NC, Hopson M, Vanderstichel R. Litterbox size preference in domestic cats (Felis catus). J Vet Behav 2014;9(2):78–82.
3. Villeneuve-Beugnet V, Beugnet F. Field assessment of cats' litter box substrate preferences. J Vet Behav 2018;25:65–70.
4. Carney HC, Sadek TP, Curtis TM, et al. AAFP and ISFM guidelines for diagnosing and solving house-soiling behavior in cats. J Feline Med Surg 2014;16(7):579–98.
5. Sadek T, Hamper B, Horwitz D, et al. Feline feeding programs: addressing behavioural needs to improve feline health and wellbeing. J Feline Med Surg 2018;20(11):1049–55.
6. Crowell-Davis SL, Murray TF, de Souza Dantas LM. Veterinary psychopharmacology. 2nd edition. Hoboken(NJ): Wiley-Blackwell; 2019.
7. Mealey KL, Peck KE, Bennett BS, et al. Systemic absorption of amitriptyline and buspirone after oral and transdermal administration to healthy cats. J Vet Intern Med 2004;18(1):43–6.
8. Ciribassi J, Luescher A, Pasloske KS, et al. Comparative bioavailability of fluoxetine after transdermal and oral administration to healthy cats. AM J Vet Res 2003;64(8):994–8.

9. Chávez G, Pardo P, Ubilla MJ, et al. Effects on behavioural variables of oral versus transdermal buspirone administration in cats displaying urine marking. J Appl Anim Res 2016;44(1):454–7.
10. Zhang L, Plummer R, McGlone J. Preference of kittens for scratchers. J Feline Med Surg 2019;21(8):691–9.
11. Walker B. The cats' house. Kansas City (MO): Andrews McMeel Publishing; 2009.
12. Dantas LM, Delgado MM, Johnson I, et al. Food puzzles for cats: feeding for physical and emotional wellbeing. J Feline Med Surg 2016; 18(9):723–32.

Feline Aging
Promoting Physiologic and Emotional Well-Being

Amy Miele, BVM&S, PhD, MRCVS, Lorena Sordo, MSc, MVZ,
Danielle A. Gunn-Moore, BVM&S, PhD, MANZCVS, FHEA, FRSB, FRCVS*

KEYWORDS

• Feline aging • Gerontology • Cognitive dysfunction • Dementia

KEY POINTS

• With more cats living to advanced age, understand changes associated with aging is of growing importance, especially those that result in emotional or physical distress.
• Behavioral changes such as increased vocalization (especially at night) and house soiling are commonly reported in elderly cats and occur for different reasons.
• Diagnosis of illness in elderly cats can be challenging, with many older cats suffering from concurrent medical conditions, often complicated by normal aging changes.
• Elderly cat clinics play a crucial role in educating owners and facilitating early diagnosis and treatment of medical or behavioral problems.
• Adapting the environment of elderly cats to provide all key resources within easy comfortable access can significantly improve their quality of life.

 Video content accompanies this article at http://www.vetsmall.theclinics.com.

INTRODUCTION

Advances in veterinary medicine, nutrition and client education have increased the life expectancy for domestic cats. In the United States, in 2011, approximately 20% of pet cats were 11 years of age or older[1]; and a 2017 study reported a median age of 6.2 years in cats presenting to clinics in the UK, with cats aged more than 8 years representing just more than 40% of feline consultations.[2]

Older cats are classified as mature (7–10 years), seniors (11–14 years), and geriatric or super senior (≥15 years).[3] For the purposes of this article, we refer to all cats 11 years or older as "elderly."

Royal (Dick) School of Veterinary Studies and The Roslin Institute, The University of Edinburgh, Easter Bush Veterinary Campus, Roslin, Midlothian EH25 9RG, Scotland
* Corresponding author.
E-mail address: danielle.gunn-moore@ed.ac.uk

Vet Clin Small Anim 50 (2020) 719–748
https://doi.org/10.1016/j.cvsm.2020.03.004
0195-5616/20/© 2020 Elsevier Inc. All rights reserved.

Box 1
Aging changes in elderly cats—outward changes that owners need to look for plus inward changes that veterinarians need to assess

- The *body condition score* (BCS) and *muscle condition score* (MCS) may decrease—the MCS may indicate the degree of sarcopenia that is common in elderly cats (see **Fig. 1**)
- Aging changes: *eyes* (iris atrophy [**Fig. 13A**], lenticular sclerosis see [**Fig. 13B**],[56] and blindness); *ears* (accumulating wax or deafness); and *coat* (white hairs, browning of a black coat, poor grooming because of underlying OA and/or dental disease).[1]
- *Dental disease*—although not specific to elderly cats, assess gingivitis, periodontal disease, tartar, tooth resorption, etc.
- *Thyroid nodules*—it is essential to palpate for asymmetry or enlargement in elderly cats.
- *Jugular pulse*—this is usually an indicator of incipient or active congestive heart failure (Video 1). The *hepatojugular reflex/reflux* makes it easier to identify this problem. Gently compress the liver to move blood into the thoracic vasculature. If the heart cannot cope, the jugular pulse becomes more obvious and moves up the jugular groove.
- *Auscultation of the apex beat*—this gives heart rate and an indication of the severity of heart murmurs; in elderly cats, the heart falls forward, so auscultate over the sternum to detect murmurs and gallop sounds. Feel for *matched pulses*—because elderly cats often do not like their femoral pulses palpated (owing to OA in the hips and/or stifles) carpal and tarsal pulses are alternate options.
- The *respiratory tract* should be assessed by *looking* (for evidence of inspiratory or expiratory dyspnea, a restrictive, or obstructive pattern), *listening* (to localize any respiratory pathology), *palpation* (the apex beat is usually palpated nearer the sternum in older cats), *compression* (usually reduced in older cats because of costochondral junction mineralization), *percussion* (can be uncomfortable if the cat has bony changes in the thoracic spine), then *auscultation* (listening for all of the potential changes that can occur in cat chests).
- *Abdominal examination*—can be particularly useful in slim, elderly cats.
- *Skeletal examination*—typically reveals OA of many joints; elbow, stifles and hocks often have large bony periarticular exostoses, with elbows held from the body and carpi collapsing inwards (**Fig. 14**). Stifles are also held away from the body, and the hocks and/or tarsi collapse.
- *Nails* may be thickened, brittle, overly long or ingrown (see **Fig. 2**).

Meeting the needs of this aging population can be a challenge for owners and veterinarians alike. This article explores some of the common conditions of elderly cats, with a focus on promoting physiologic and emotional well-being.

THE AGING PROCESS

Aging is a multifaceted process that results in a progressive series of life stages, from conception to senescence. It is influenced by the host's genetics, plus innumerable internal and external factors.[1] It results in the progressive decline in the ability to maintain homeostasis when challenged by physiologic and environmental stressors.[1] Because these factors include previous injuries, disease, nutritional status, and environmental challenges, every cat ages slightly differently.

Although it is important to remember that old age itself is not a disease and clients should promote healthy aging, they also need to recognize often subtle signs of ill-health. Regular health screening can increase the chance of disease being recognized early, so appropriate treatment can be initiated.

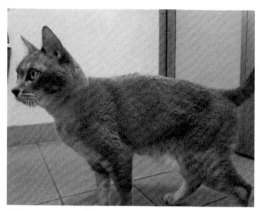

Fig. 1. Elderly cat with sarcopenia of aging.

Common Physiologic and Behavioral Changes in Aging

Although some changes are obvious (**Box 1**) such as a decline in lean muscle mass (sarcopenia; **Fig. 1**), and thickened brittle nails that are prone to overgrowth (**Fig. 2**), others are less apparent, including alterations in digestive physiology, the immune system, kidneys, liver, brain, and skeleton.[1]

Sensitivity to Socioenvironmental Stress

Older cats cope poorly with changes in their daily routine, environment, family, or diet (discussed elsewhere in this article). Their response to stress typically involves hyporexia, hiding, and/or house soiling. It is important to consider the potential for stress when planning changes to a cat's regimen and, when changes are necessary, making them slowly and with much reassurance. All cats, especially elderly cats, should be given a box or bed to hide in—a safe haven[4] (**Fig. 3**). There are many ways to improve the environment for elderly cats, including ensuring that all of their key resources are within easy reach and suitable for an elderly cat to use (**Box 2**).

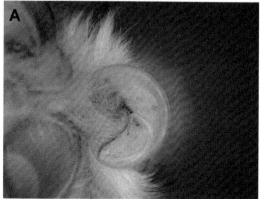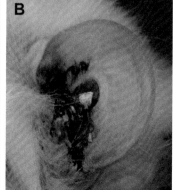

Fig. 2. (*A*) Elderly cats can develop long thick brittle nails (*B*) that become ingrown.

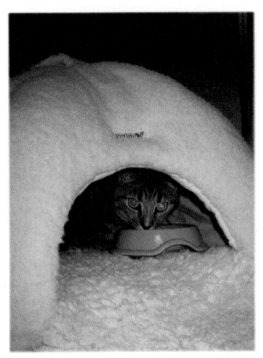

Fig. 3. Elderly cats need somewhere safe to hide in at home—a safe haven.

Changes in Body Weight

A cat should be weighed at each clinic visit (**Fig. 4**); it is essential to calculate the percentage weight change each time (**Box 3**)—it is very easy to miss significant changes in small cats. Significant ($\geq$5%) and/or rapid weight change, especially where muscle mass is lost, can have very serious implications, irrespective of the underlying cause.[5] Cats should be fed to maintain their optimal body weight and muscle mass; long-term studies have shown that both obesity and emaciation increase morbidity and mortality.[6]

Obesity decrease life span, and increases the risk of weight-related diseases, including heart disease, diabetes mellitus (DM), lameness (often owing to osteoarthritis [OA]), liver disease (eg, hepatic lipidosis), and skin problems.[7]

Weight loss is more common in elderly cats than obesity,[8] resulting from physiologic aging changes, pathologic processes, and/or behavioral changes.[9] Most cases are associated with hyporexia, which may result from reduced senses of smell and taste, pain from periodontal disease, and a myriad of illnesses associated with age.[1] However, sarcopenia, the loss of lean muscle mass in the absence of apparent disease,[10] may also occur. Elderly cats digest food inefficiently; they have decreased gastric acid production, pancreatic lipase activity, intestinal motility, and blood flow, as well as changes in bile composition.[11] Digestion and absorption of all dietary components is decreased (particularly fats and proteins), such that individuals may need to increase their intake by up to 25%.[12] Because elderly cats have a limited stomach capacity, they need to eat a highly palatable, highly digestible, energy-dense food, with an increased proportion of protein calories in an attempt to increase (or prevent the loss of), lean muscle mass. Food should be offered frequently, in small amounts

Box 2
Environmental adjustments for elderly cats

Adjustments to the environment and daily routine may promote the psychological well-being of elderly cats. *Key Resources* are food, water, resting places, litter box, scratching substrates, a place to hide and an escape route. All of these should be provided within the cats' *core territory*.

A. Promoting physiologic well-being (provision of key resources)
- There should be at least 1 set of key resources (with the exception of food bowls, which should be per cat) for each social grouping of cats in the household, plus at least 1 extra. A group of cats is one where cats will comfortably groom each other and sleep together (**Fig. 15**).
- Key resources must be easily accessible. If an elderly cat has to walk too far for its food or water or stairs are involved, it may do without, risking weight loss and dehydration. If it has to walk too far for its litter box, it may resort to house soiling.
- Key resources should not be moved from their usual place because this can cause confusion and anxiety in a cat with CDS.
  - Food
    - Elderly cats should be fed separately from conspecifics so they are not stressed by their companions and can eat at their own pace (**Fig. 16**).
    - Food bowls should be away from water bowls and litter boxes.
    - Automatic feeders (to provide additional meals) may help to decrease vocalizations associated with food seeking (**Fig. 17**).
    - Raising food bowls can help to decrease discomfort in cats with OA (**Fig. 18**).
    - Elderly cats have a decrease ability to digest and absorb their food—to reduce the risk of weight loss feed *ad libitum* or increase the frequency of feeding; this can be also be helpful for cats with cognitive decline.
    - Monitor how much food elderly cats eat to make sure that they do not lose weight.
  - Water
    - Elderly cats may prefer a wide bowl if they have poor vision because they can then agitate the water with a paw to help sense the surface—placing a few flakes of fish food on the water can help them to see or sense it if OA prevents them from using their paw in this way.
    - Raising water bowls can help to decrease discomfort in cats suffering from OA.
    - Pet water fountains can help to stimulate elderly cats to drink more (**Fig. 19**) or give fishy water, chicken or meat stock (without onion powder), or commercial soups for cats.
    - Water bowls should be placed away from food bowls and litter boxes.
  - Resting places
    - Ensure resting areas are well-padded and consider providing heated bedding for cats with OA, a thin condition, or a sparse hair coat.
    - Consider ease of access to favored resting areas (or hiding places) and provide steps/ramps where possible, or lower level alternatives.
    - Climbing frames provide welcome high resting places (see **Fig. 20**).
  - Litter boxes or access to outdoor latrine sites
    - Larger litter boxes with a low entrance allow ease of access (**Fig. 21**).
    - Litter boxes need to be easily reached; there should be at least 1 litter box on each floor of the house.
    - Sandy-type litter is usually more comfortable for elderly cats with OA affecting the paws. Litter box liners should not be used because nails may become caught in elderly cats that cannot retract their nails.
    - Elderly cats that go outside to eliminate may find climbing through the cat flap challenging.
    - Elderly cats that go outside may find confronting cats from outside the family group challenging. If cats still want to keep going outside, ensure there is enough "cover" for them to get to the latrine site; place large planters near the cat flap so the cat can go outside under their cover. Alternatively, "cat-proof" the garden with high fencing so that other cats cannot get in (**Fig. 22**). Cats usually have a preferred latrine site—digging in sand will make it easier for an elderly cat to use, especially in winter.

- ○ Scratching places
  - All cats need access to at least 1 scratching post. Whereas younger cats usually prefer vertical posts, elderly cats may prefer horizontal ones (**Fig. 23**).
  - Cats may show preferences for different substrates, for example, carpet, matts.
  - Older cats cannot scratch sufficiently well to remove their overgrown nail sheaths, so they will need to have their nails trimmed to prevent them from getting caught, causing pain in arthritic paws, and confusion in cats with CDS (Section 7).
- ○ Grooming
  - Extra grooming may become increasingly necessary in elderly cats. Although it is well-tolerated by some and can promote the human–animal bond, it is less well-tolerated by others and the preferences of the individual cat should always be respected.
  - Soft grooming brushes are often better tolerated than metal combs, and clipping areas that are getting matted can improve comfort.

B. Increasing environmental security
  - Hiding places
    - ○ Secure indoor hiding places or "safe havens" are very important in elderly cats because the option to escape outdoors may be less accessible or appealing. Hiding places need to be easily accessible for the cat; consider ramps or steps.
    - ○ The cat must have time alone without being disturbed by other animals or owners. Avoid negative associations (eg, medicating), because this will compromise the cat's feeling of security.
  - Changes to core territory
    - ○ Core territory may need to be reduced in cats with reduced mobility, or sensory or cognitive decline, especially with advanced CDS. If this is the case, key resources should be kept within easy reach and in a consistent location.
    - ○ Provide a separate core territory from conspecifics, especially if social dynamics have altered.
    - ○ Install a night light if loss of vision is a concern.
    - ○ A synthetic analogue of feline facial pheromone (eg, Feliway Classic) may help to decrease anxiety.
  - Outdoor access
    - ○ It may be necessary to control access outdoors in cats with decreased mobility, or sensory or cognitive decline.
    - ○ Consider providing a secure outdoor area for cats who are used to having access outdoors.
    - ○ The presence of the owner can help to increase confidence in older cats when outdoors (**Fig. 24**).

C. Optimizing social relationships
  - Human interaction
    - ○ The desire for human interaction varies greatly between cats, but older cats generally seek human contact (see **Fig. 7**).
    - ○ Where human contact is sought, this should be offered in a consistent and predictable way, and never forced. Where a cat is used to being lifted up, this may need to be tailored to cope with progressive OA.
    - ○ Condition owner interaction by using a removable item such as a blanket or towel to help decrease attention-seeking behavior (**Fig. 25**); this can also decrease the risk of overgrown cat nails hurting the owner, making them stop the interaction abruptly, potentially damaging the relationship, and confusing the cat.
  - Interaction with conspecifics and other animals
    - ○ Tolerance of conspecifics and other animals within the household may decrease with age (see **Fig. 7**). Provide separate resources and core territories so that interaction can be avoided when desired. Consider using microchip-controlled cat flaps to allow access to a quiet space (eg, understair cupboard) or adapt an elevated position if the conspecific(s) are not as agile (see **Fig. 16**).
    - ○ Pheromone products (eg, Feliway Friends) may help to decrease tension between conspecifics arising when an elderly cat develops behavioral or physical changes; the provision of space and resources must also be appropriate.

- ○ The loss of a long-time companion may result in grief in some elderly cats, (especially Burmese and Siamese); they will need reassurance and comfort. Introducing a new cat or dog can be very stressful, especially for elderly cats. Do not presume that because a cat is grieving they will welcome a new animal into the household.
- • Routine
  - ○ Routine is particularly important for cats with cognitive decline or chronic medical conditions, which increase susceptibility to environmental stress.
  - ○ Keep feeding times, access to the outdoors (if applicable), and schedule of owner interaction (tailored to cats' individual needs) as consistent as possible.

D. Providing for species-specific and cognitive needs
  - • Outlets for hunting and seeking drive
    - ○ Mental stimulation decreases the rate of decline of cognitive function in aged animals.[57]
    - ○ Provide opportunities for searching, chasing, and pouncing by using a combination of scatter feeding and food puzzles (shop bought or homemade; **Fig. 26**, www. foodpuzzlesforcats.com, Delgado and Dantas, Feeding Cats for Optimal Mental and Behavioral Well-Being, Part 2). Ensure short play sessions involving a range of different toys are incorporated into the daily routine. Ensure all puzzles and play account for mobility issues, especially elbow OA.
    - ○ Toys should be changed regularly to create stimulation and need to be suitable for elderly cats: blind cats will need toys that make a noise (eg, have a bell inside), whereas cats with arthritis will need light-weight, easily lifted toys (**Fig. 27**).
  - • Olfactory enrichment
    - ○ This benefits cats of all ages. It is important to be mindful of the scent profile of the cats' environment. Avoid smoke, scented candles, air fresheners, and chemical cleaning products.
    - ○ Offer access to fresh air, where possible, and consider enclosed outdoor areas ('catios') for indoor cats.
    - ○ Consider providing an herb box containing cat-friendly plants and herbs for elderly cats who have limited exposure to the outdoors.
    - ○ Catnip, silver vine, honeysuckle, and valerian root have all been shown to provoke a positive behavioral response from cats. However, some cats are more sensitive than others to these plants (or their products), so they should be introduced carefully to elderly cats, especially if they have decreased mobility.
    - ○ Cats can quickly habituate to scents within the environment, so intermittent exposure to varied scents is likely to increase engagement

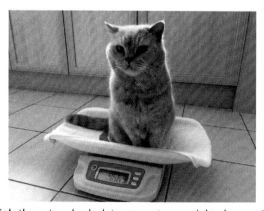

Fig. 4. Always weigh the cat and calculate percentage weight change; if there is a 5% or greater loss, investigation is essential. (*Courtesy of* J. Burn, Congleton, UK.)

> **Box 3**
> **Calculation of the percentage weight loss**
>
> Cat's previous weight (x kg) – cat's current weight (y kg) = z (z/x) × 100 = % weight change
>
> For example, 4.0-3.7 = 0.4/4.0 = 0.1 0.1 × 100 = 10%

with the aim of supporting optimal body weight.[9] Although it is often assumed that elderly cats have a degree of chronic kidney disease (CKD) and may benefit from moderate protein restriction, inappropriate protein decreases risk protein malnutrition, with progressive loss of lean body mass being of particular concern.[9]

Feeding small meals frequently also increases physical activity, which is good for the musculoskeletal system and brain activity.[13]

Diets supplemented with antioxidants and free radical scavengers (eg, glutathione, vitamins A, C, and E, taurine, carotenoids, and selenium), essential fatty acids, and other potentially useful compounds, such as prebiotics, have been shown to benefit elderly cats.[14]

Sensitivity to Thirst

Elderly cats have decreased sensitivity to thirst.[15] This increases their risk of dehydration, especially when combined with the polyuria associated with concurrent CKD, hyperthyroidism, and DM. Dehydration contributes to constipation, which is common in older cats,[16] and exacerbated by concurrent OA if the cat is reluctant to use its litter box or catflap. Where possible, elderly cats should be fed mostly wet food and have easy access to fresh water in a variety of forms (see **Box 2**).

Changes in Immune Function

Immunosenescence with age results in a reduced ability to fight infection and screen for neoplastic cells.[17] For example, in younger cats less than 15% of cystitis is bacterial, compared with approximately 50% in cats 10 years or older.[18] These infections are often associated with CKD, hyperthyroidism, or DM, all of which are common in older cats, and result in less concentrated urine plus local and/or systemic immunosuppression.[19,20]

Changes in Pharmacodynamics

Aging changes affect drug metabolism. Liver disease, low blood albumin concentration, and CKD all occur commonly in elderly cats. When coupled with dehydration, they can result in decreased drug clearance rates and marked increases in drug concentrations.[21] In elderly patients, the dose and dosing intervals of some drugs may need to be altered (**Box 4**).

> **Box 4**
> **Changing drug dosages in cats with kidney or liver disease**
>
> - As a general rule, it is best to *double the dosing interval* or *halve the dosage* in patients with *severe CKD*; and use the least toxic drugs.
>
> - Many factors affect drug clearance by the liver, so it is not possible to apply a simple formula to drug dosing with *severe hepatopathy*. However, there are tables available that have been adapted from human literature.[58]
>
> - A common example is metronidazole, which might be needed, for example, for suppurative cholangitis. It would need to be reduced to 7.5 mg/kg every 12 hours, rather than 10 to 15 mg/kg every 12 hours for cats with normal liver function

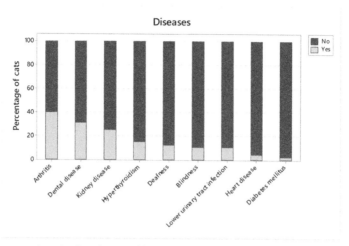

Fig. 5. Common chronic disorders in elderly cats—as per their owners.

Changes in the Musculoskeletal System

Lean muscle loss, joint degeneration, and OA should never be overlooked because their negative effects in elderly cats can be considerable (see **Box 2** in Beatriz Monteiro's article, "Feline Chronic Pain and Osteoarthritism" in this issue).

It is beyond the scope of this article to cover all aging changes; however, 2 detailed reviews of aging in cats have recently been published, describing common physical and functional changes, and describing what is healthy and what is disease.[1,22]

MEETING THE PHYSICAL NEEDS OF AGING CATS

Keeping elderly cats comfortable can require significant environmental modification (see **Box 2**) and management changes, some of which are discussed further in this article.

Nail Care

Elderly cats cannot fully retract their nails, and concurrent OA may decrease their capacity to remove old nail sheaths by scratching. Overgrown nails may pierce the pads (see **Fig. 2**) or get caught in fleecy blankets, causing distress and pain when arthritic

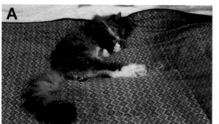
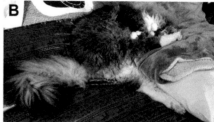

Fig. 6. (*A*) Elderly cat with hip and stifle OA. The fur over his hips has been clipped because he could not groom it anymore. (*B*) Unusual position of his tail and hips because of pain and dysfunction; separated legs to take pressure off hip.

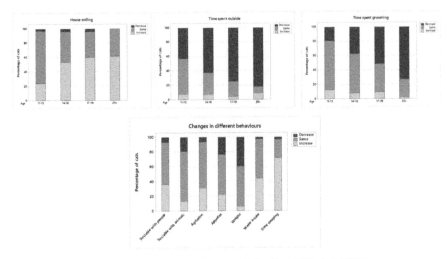

Owner reported changes in behaviour by their cats aged ≥11 y old, n=>800 (Sordo et al 2020a).

Fig. 7. Changes in behavior in elderly cats—as per their owners.

joints are tugged. Owners need to know how to clip their cat's nails (or to have the clinic nurse do so) and monitor for ingrown nails.

Osteoarthritis

Arthritis is common in elderly cats. One study found radiographic evidence of OA in 61% of cats aged 6 years or older; the prevalence increased with age and was associated with decreased mobility and grooming, as well as increased house soiling.[23] A study found owners recognized OA in 40% of cats aged 11 or more years (**Fig. 5**),

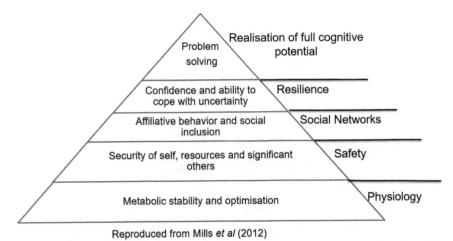

Reproduced from Mills et al (2012)

Fig. 8. Hierarchy of needs for animals adapted from Maslow's hierarchy. (*From* Mills D, Dube MB, Zulch H. How animals respond to change. In: *Stress and Pheromonatherapy in Small Animal Clinical Behaviour.* Chichester, UK: John Wiley and Sons Ltd.; 2013:3-36; with permission.)

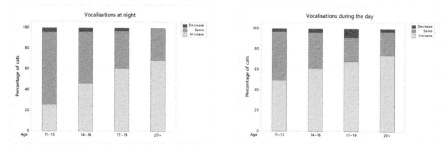

Fig. 9. Changes in vocalization in elderly cats—as per their owners.

Box 5
Common diseases of elderly cats

- Dental disease
  - 68% of cats greater than 3 years, increasing with age[59]
- OA
  - 61% in cats of 6 years of age or older; increasing with age[23]
- CKD
  - Varies from 28% in cats greater than 12 years[20] up to 81% in cats aged 15 to 20 years[60]
  - CKD and OA often occur together[60]
- CDS
  - 36% of 7- to 11-year-old cats, increasing to 88% in cats aged 16 to 19 years[61]
  - 28% of cats aged 11 to 14 years, increasing to more than 50% for cats 15 years of age or older[35]
- Systemic hypertension
  - 13% of apparently healthy cats greater than 9 years of age[52]
  - Less than 25%[50] to 65%[51] with CKD
  - 10% to 90% with hyperthyroidism[48]
- Hyperthyroidism
  - Varies in different countries and increases with age, for example, 12% of cats 8 years of age or older in Southern Germany[62]; 2% cats of all-age cats in Europe and North America[63]
- DM
  - Increasing over the past 10 years or more to 2014: 11.6 cases per 10,000 cat years at risk[64]; approximately 1 in 200 cats, in males, with age, with inactivity, certain lineages of Burmese (Australia, UK), Norwegian Forest cats, Russian Blue, and Abyssinian cats in particular[64,65]
- Gastrointestinal disease
  - Especially low-grade alimentary lymphoma, increased over the past more than 10 years; now the most common gastrointestinal cancer in cats; 60% to 75% of gastrointestinal lymphoma[31]
- Urinary tract infections
  - Common in older cats, especially with CKD, hyperthyroidism, and DM[19]
- Neoplasia—increasingly common in older cats
- Decline of special senses—increasingly common in older cats

Data from Refs.[19,20,23,31,35,48,52,59–61,63–65]

Box 6
Causes of altered behavior and increased vocalization (See also Stelow, Behavior as an Illness Indicator)

A. Medical differentials for common behavioral changes in elderly cats
- Hypertension
- Degenerative disease
- Neoplasia
- Infection
- Metabolic
- Pain or inflammation

B. Social, environmental, and emotional differentials for common behavioral changes in elderly cats
- *Attention-seeking* or resource-seeking behavior
- *Acute frustration* owing to inability to access desired resources
- *Chronic frustration* owing to inability to perform species-specific behaviors
- *Socioenvironmental stress*–change in environment, diet, or owner routine; intercat conflict; traumatic event; owner conflict
- *Generalized anxiety*
- *Separation related problem*
- *Sound sensitivity*
- *Grief* owing to loss of bonded cat, dog or human

---

reporting it as the most common disease in their cats. Environmental modifications help cats cope with OA (see **Box 2**, Monteiro, Feline Chronic Pain and Osteoarthritis).

Management changes include having to groom cats that can no longer groom themselves (especially over the hips, where it is most painful and/or difficult to reach) (see **Box 2**, **Fig. 6**). Grooming decrease with age (**Fig. 7**), whereas house soiling increases,

---

Table 1
Mobility and dementia questionnaire

My Cat	Yes	Maybe	No
Is less willing to jump up or down			
Will only jump up or down from lower heights			
Walks stiffly			
Is less agile			
Is lame or limping			
Has difficulty with the cat flap			
Has difficulty with the stairs			
Cries when lifted			
Has accidents outside the litter tray			
Is grooming less			
Is reluctant to interact			
Plays less			
Sleeps more/is less active			
Cries loudly for no apparent reason			
Appears forgetful			

Adapted from Gunn-Moore DA. Cognitive Dysfunction in Cats: Clinical Assessment and Management. *Top Companion Anim Med* 2011; 26: 17–24; with permission.

Box 7
Behavioral changes in cats with CDS

Cats with CDS display behavioral changes that are summarized by the acronym VISHDAAL:

- Increased *V*ocalizations, especially at night (see Video 2)
- Altered social *I*nteractions and relationships, either with owners or other pets for example, attention seeking, or aggressive behavior toward other animals
- Altered *S*leep/wake patterns
- *H*ouse soiling
- Spatial *D*isorientation or confusion, for example, forgetting the location of the litterbox
- Temporal *D*isorientation, for example, forgetting they have been fed
- Altered *A*ctivity for example, aimless wandering, or decreased activity
- *A*nxiety
- *L*earning and memory for example, forgetting the location of the litterbox, or that they have been fed

---

as reported in the study discussed elsewhere in this article. Although house soiling can be associated with many conditions (such as cognitive dysfunction syndrome [CDS] or behavioral problems) OA plays a pivotal role as affected cats find it painful to climb into the litterbox or out through the cat flap, and to posture to defaecate.

Exercise

Many factors may reduce older cats' willingness or ability to exercise, including muscle weakness associated with sarcopenia or ill health, OA, dehydration, and insecurity. Cats also alter their activity budget (time spent engaging in different behaviors) as they age. Feeding many small, frequent meals with or without feeding puzzles encourages exercise and improves hydration.[24] Lightweight toys help to facilitate play (see **Box 2**).

PROMOTING EMOTIONAL WELL-BEING IN ELDERLY CATS

Veterinary medicine tends to focus on physical well-being; however, the emotional well-being of our patients is just as vital owing to the interplay between emotional distress, behavior problems, and disease (C.A. Tony Buffington and Melissa Bain's article, "Stress and Feline Health," in this issue). A stressor is a physical or socioenvironmental stimulus that triggers an acute or chronic physiologic and/or behavioral stress response within an individual. A state of emotional distress occurs when the

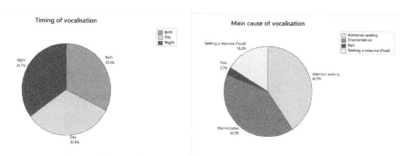

Fig. 10. Increased vocalization in cats with cognitive dysfunction—time of crying and the client speculated reason for the crying.

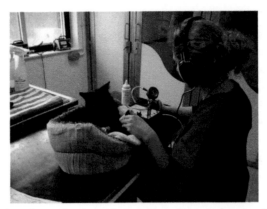

Fig. 11. BP evaluation; the cat is relaxed in its bed, and the student is using headphones so noise does not upset it.

animal is unable to adapt to cope with the cumulative impact of the stressors to which it is exposed. The burden of allostasis (adapting to everyday stressors) is the "allostatic load"; this load increases with advancing age, so elderly animals are less resilient and more susceptible to emotional distress.[25] Many other variables also play an important role in how an animal copes with stress, including genetics and early life experience.

Motivational Theory

Mills and colleagues[26] (2012) modified Maslow's hierarchy of needs (**Fig. 8**) to help explain how animals prioritize their needs to achieve psychological well-being. The motivation to attain physiologic well-being has the highest priority, with security (of self and important resources) and social stability following. Only once these needs have been addressed can the animal devote energy to emotional resilience and the desire to explore and seek information about their environment is reinstated.

Specific needs of individual cats may change over time, being influenced by different factors such as temperament, breed, early life experience, health status, and changes within the home environment, as well as age.[27] **Box 2** explores some of the social and environmental changes that may be required to optimize psychological well-being in the elderly cat, with a focus on creating a secure and accessible core

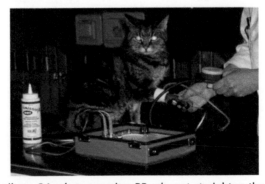

Fig. 12. Consider elbow OA when assessing BP—do not straighten the limb, hold it at a relaxed angle; place the cuff below the elbow in line with the heart.

Box 8
What changes owners should look for as potential signs of ill-health in their mature cat
Food and water consumption

- *Body weight and shape*, for example, loss of weight and/or muscle mass, changing body shape (muscle loss along the back and hips, while the abdomen becomes more obvious)
- *Production of urine*, for example, size of urine ball in litter box (**Fig. 28**) *and feces* (eg, diarrhea or, more commonly in older cats, constipation, and/or house soiling)
- *Behavior*, for example, increased vocalization, confusion, twitching (potential focal seizures), increased hiding, and so on (see **Figs. 7** and **9**)
- *Mobility*, for example, OA affecting the elbows, carpi, hips, stifles, hocks and tarsi, and may even affect the spine, from the neck to the tail
- The *Mobility and Dementia questionnaire* can be very helpful in indication that these problems are present (see **Table 1**).
- *Ask owners to video any behaviors of concern*, for example, locomotion, coughing, altered breathing, regurgitation/vomiting (plus anything the cat brings up), constipation/diarrhea (and what is produced), crying, confusion, and so on, because these can be revealing. Pictures of cats sitting or sleeping in unusual positions can also be helpful (see **Fig. 6**).
- It can be difficult to differentiate behavioral changes caused by behavioral or neurologic diseases from CDS or OA in elderly cats; it is not unusual for an individual cat to have multiple conditions.

Box 9
Minimizing stress associated with visiting the veterinary clinic

- Acclimatize the cat to its carrier from an early age, and with each new carrier. Where possible, leave the carrier out with a soft bed in it, feed the cat treats in it. *It needs to feel a normal and safe place.*
- Clean it out fully after each clinic visit to ensure negative pheromones do not linger
- Place an old favored jumper in the carrier (owners scent is usually calming) and/or spray Feliway Classic into it approximately 15 minutes before placing the cat in it to help calm the cat.[66]
- Acclimatize the cat to car travel so travel does not cause stress.
- If cats become very stressed, either by the cat carrier, the journey, or the clinic visit, give gabapentin[67] or trazadone[68] 50 to 100 mg per cat by mouth or mixed in a little food approximately 90 minutes before travel. These strategies usually result in a much calmer cat, with no negative effects on BP, heart rate, and so on.
- A calmer cat results in a calmer owner, who is more likely to listen to the vet and do as advised, they are also more likely to bring the cat back to the clinic when needed.
- Owners of multiple cats should consider keeping a cat that has just returned from a clinic visit separate (with access to key resources) for a short period of time because the disrupted scent profile of the returning cat can sometimes result in social conflict. Diffuse Feliway Friends and/or use a cloth to gather scent of other cats from the same social group to rub on the returning cat to facilitate reintroduction to the household.

Box 10
Why owners of elderly cats are often reluctant to visit their veterinarian

- The belief that the change is part of normal aging, for example, loss of weight or muscle mass, OA, blindness, deafness, confusion/CDS
- Embarrassment that they cannot cope with their cat's behavioral changes, for example, increased vocalization and/or house soiling
- The misconception that nothing can be done to help their cat
- The stress to owner and cat associated with a trip to the veterinary clinic
- Worries that euthanasia will be suggested

---

territory. These changes may be necessary to support cats suffering from specific health problems or, more generally, to decrease socioenvironmental stress.

WHAT HAPPENS WHEN EMOTIONAL WELL-BEING IS COMPROMISED?

Sustained compromise to the physiologic and/or emotional well-being of an elderly cat increases its allostatic load, further decreasing its ability to cope with socioenvironmental stress, resulting in some degree of emotional distress. This stress can manifest in a range of medical as well as behavioral problems, with a great deal of overlap between the 2 (C.A. Tony Buffington and Melissa Bain's article, "Stress and Feline Health," in this issue). Terry Marie Curtis' article, "Behavior Problem or Problem Behavior?," in this issue. Elizabeth Stelow's article, "Behavior as an Illness Indicator," in this issue. Stress has been shown to accelerate the rate of cognitive decline in humans with early signs of dementia[28] and it seems logical that a similar deterioration may also be seen in cats suffering from CDS.

COMMON BEHAVIORAL PRESENTATIONS OF ELDERLY CATS

Behaviors deemed by the owner to be problematic may be adaptive (eg, urine marking or spraying within the home) or maladaptive (eg, self-mutilation or pica). The true incidence of behavior problems in cats is difficult to quantify, because only those behaviors that represent a problem to the owner (Terry Marie Curtis' article, "Behavior Problem or Problem Behavior?," in this issue.) are presented to professionals.[29]

Owner-reported observations of the behavior of 883 cats aged 11 years and older in the UK included increased vocalization (59%; at night 44%; **Fig. 9**); house soiling

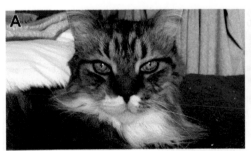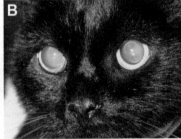

Fig. 13. Ocular changes in cats. (*A*) Iris atrophy. (*B*) Lenticular sclerosis A.

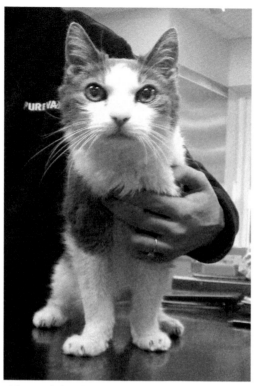

Fig. 14. Elderly cat with OA of the elbows and carpi, resulting in the feet being turned out.

(56%), often despite having a litterbox (in 83% of homes); going outside less (59%); and grooming less (36%). These changes all progressed with age (see **Fig. 7**). Other behaviors present in older cats that did not progress included increased sociability and affection with people (36%), increased agitation (74%), and decreased sociability with cohabiting animals (19%; see **Fig. 7**). They slept more (71%), drank more (44%), and ate less (24%). Of particular note is increased vocalization and sociability and affection with people.

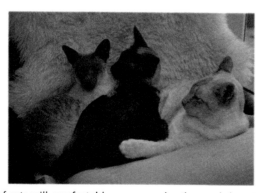

Fig. 15. A group of cats will comfortably groom each other and sleep together.

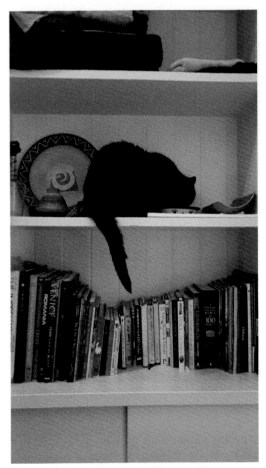

Fig. 16. Elderly cat being fed separately so it is not stressed by its companion—this 18-year-old can still jump to the shelf.

Understanding Behavioral Changes

The reasons for increased affection, sociability, and attention seeking may include an increased dependence on the owner to provide resources, mental stimulation, and social support. Access to resources may be compromised owing to decreased mobility, loss of sensory function, and/or changes to priority of access within a multicat household owing to altered social dynamics. An increased need for social support may also result from changes in relationships with conspecifics or even the loss of a conspecific. Reasons for decreased tolerance to other animals are also likely to be related to concurrent health problems, with pain being a common reason for changes in social interactions[30] within a household.

In the aforementioned study, owners reported that 59% of cats went outdoors less than when they were younger, with cats aged 20 years or older no longer going outside. The reasons for this are likely to be multifactorial, including decreased mobility, pain, decreased sensory function, fear of neighboring cats, and natural changes to activity budgets. Indeed, 71% of aged cats slept more than before, and less than one-third of cats who previously enjoyed hunting still did so.

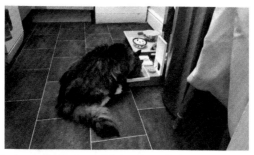

Fig. 17. Elderly with dementia having additional meals from a timed feeder.

COMMON DISEASES OF ELDERLY CATS
Etiologies

Elderly cats may suffer from many diseases (**Box 5**). The most common chronic conditions reported by owners were OA (36%), dental disease (31%), CKD (23%), hyperthyroidism (14%), and deafness (13%) (see **Fig. 5**). Interestingly, some disorders typically considered by veterinarians as common in elderly cats, for example, gastrointestinal disease (inflammatory bowel disease and low-grade alimentary lymphoma)[31] were rarely reported, whereas disorders that veterinarians might not consider, occurred commonly (apparent deafness).

Diagnosis and Management

Diagnosis and management of illness in elderly cats is often complicated. Concurrent diseases can present with similar clinical signs, for example, OA, polyuria (caused by CKD, DM, and/or hyperthyroidism), fecal urgency (caused by chronic gastrointestinal disease), and/or constipation, can all present as house soiling. Concurrent hyperthyroidism and DM can be confusing because their clinical signs are similar, and they complicate each other's diagnosis: unstable DM decreases serum thyroxin concentrations (via euthyroid sick syndrome)[32] and hyperthyroidism decreases serum fructosamine concentrations via increased protein turnover.[33] Treatment of 1 disease may also worsen another; for example, treatment of hyperthyroidism can unmask CKD.[34] A complete investigation is therefore essential if management is to be most effective.

DISEASES THAT CAUSE ALTERED BEHAVIOR AND APPARENT SENILITY

Behavior changes (eg, increased vocalization; Video 2 night crying) and apparent senility are seen frequently in older cats,[35] resulting from many different disorders

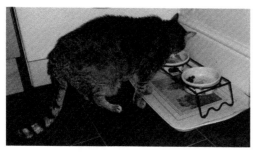

Fig. 18. Elderly cat with severe elbow OA eating from raised food bowls.

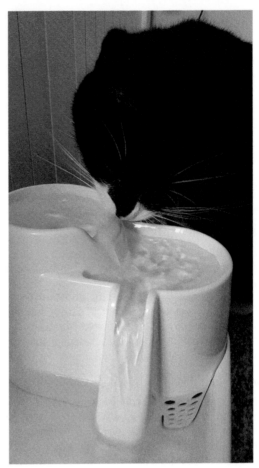

Fig. 19. Elderly cat using a water fountain. (*Courtesy of* S. Miele, Edinburgh, UK.)

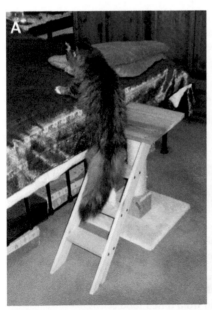

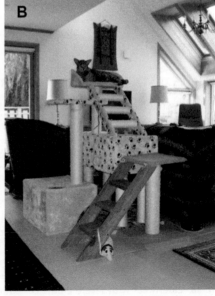

Fig. 20. (*A, B*) Elderly cats with steps to his preferred sleeping place. (*B*) Cats with severe OA may prefer round steps be replaced by flat ones. (*Courtesy of* P. Purves, Walkerburn, UK.)

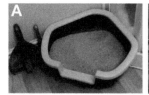 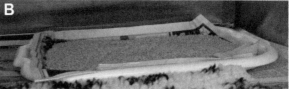

Fig. 21. (*A*) A good litter box for elderly cats, large and high sided, except for the entrance. (*B*) A tray makes a shallow litter box for a cat with severe OA.

(**Box 6**; Elizabeth Stelow's article, "Behavior as an Illness Indicator," in this issue). Of particular importance are CDS, systemic hypertension, and OA (Monteiro, Feline Chronic Pain and Osteoarthritis). Socioenvironmental stress, frustration, or anxiety are other important differentials.

Differentiating between physical and cognitive maladies requires a thorough history to evaluate social and environmental factors, completing a Mobility and Dementia Questionnaire (**Table 1**), and a full investigation looking for underlying illness.

Cognitive Dysfunction Syndrome

CDS and dementia are an age-related deterioration of cognitive abilities, characterized by behavioral changes (**Box 7**) that cannot be attributed to another condition. Antemortem, this is a diagnosis of exclusion, achieved after systemic illness, pain, and other behavioral disorders have been excluded, and environmental issues have

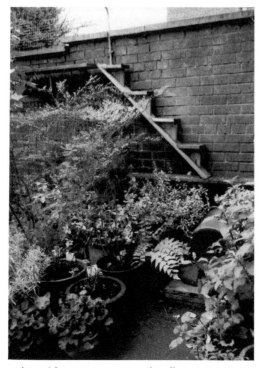

Fig. 22. Cat-proof garden with steps to a covered walkway.

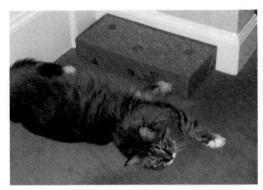

Fig. 23. Elderly cat with a horizontal scratching box playing with the ball inside its base.

been addressed. One study found that 28% of 154 pet cats aged 11 to 14 years develop at least 1 elderly-onset behavior problem, increasing to more than 50% for cats of 15 years of age and older.[35]

Behavioral changes and clinical signs
The behavioral changes comprising CDS are summarized by the acronym VISHDAAL (see **Box 7**). The prevalence of increased vocalization was discussed previously (see **Fig. 9**). Unpublished (Cerna P et al, 2020) data on 37 cats with CDS found that most cried at night (67%); the owners believed the main cause to be disorientation (41%), attention and affection seeking (41%), and looking for food (16%; **Fig. 10**); 67% of the cats had become more affectionate.

Because owners often misinterpret these changes as "normal" aging, especially if they are subtle, veterinarians must ask specific questions (see **Table 1**).

Pathophysiology
Although the pathophysiology remains under investigation, it is believed that oxidative damage, vascular changes (including infarcts and microhemorrhages) and changes in cerebral blood flow (eg, from hypertension, heart disease) play a role in the development and progression of CDS.[36]

Management
There is no licensed treatment for CDS in cats; however, appropriate management can ameliorate clinical signs and improve quality of life. Reassurance and cuddles,

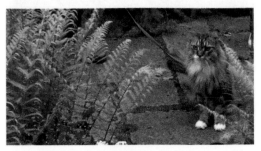

Fig. 24. Elderly cat on a lead with his owner so he feels more confident.

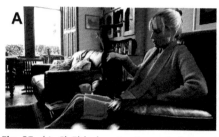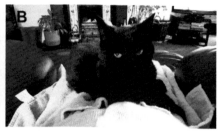

Fig. 25. (*A, B*) Elderly cat using a designated lap cover.

environmental enrichment, dietary supplements, specific diets, and drug treatments may all help; if these fail, owners can use ear plugs.

Dietary supplements Dogs with CDS given *S*-adenosyl-L-methionine (SAMe) showed evidence of improved awareness and activity levels.[37] Both dogs and cats performed better on cognitive tests (reversal learning and object discrimination), with improvement in cats being more evident in the least impaired individuals.[38] SAMe may be beneficial in the early stages of disease.[39]

A study using a supplement containing phosphatidylserine, omega 3 fatty acids, L-carnitine, co-enzyme Q10, selenium, vitamins E and C, plus alpha lipoic acid (Aktivait, VetPlus) resulted in improved social interactions, house soiling, and disorientation in dogs.[40] Because alpha-lipoic acid is toxic in cats, a feline version has been commercially released, but has not been tested for safety or efficacy.

A different supplement, containing phosphatidylserine, pyridoxine, gingko biloba extract, resveratrol and d-alpha-tocopherol (Senilife; CEVA Animal Health, Lenexa, KS) improved memory and reduced signs of CDS in dogs.[41] Although this supplement is labeled for use in cats, no trials have been performed to determine its safety or efficacy in this species.

Specific diets Commercial diets supplemented with essential fatty acids and antioxidants increased activity level,[42] longevity,[6] and improve brain function in cats.[43]

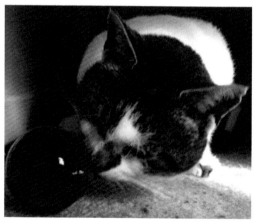

Fig. 26. Puzzles feeders provide mental stimulation and increase exercise. (*Courtesy of* H. Titmarsh, Midlothian, UK.)

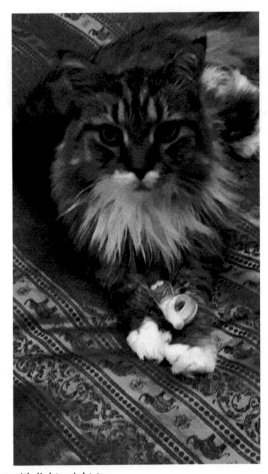

Fig. 27. Elderly cat with lightweight toy.

Environmental enrichment Environmental enrichment provides mental stimulation that can lead to improved cognition (in dogs).[44] To decrease the risk of developing CDS, environmental enrichment should be provided to young cats, especially if they have no outside access (see **Box 2**). In contrast, elderly cats with CDS cannot cope with changes in their environment or routine, causing confusion, increasing stress, and worsening clinical signs.[45] To minimize this negative effect, decrease the size of their environment, ensuring that all key resources are easy to access.

Drug treatments
Although drugs for the treatment of CDS, such as selegiline and propentofylline, have only been studied in dogs,[46] efficacy in cats has been anecdotally reported. Other drugs can be used to decrease specific clinical signs of CDS in cats. Antidepressants and anxiolytics (eg, gabapentin, fluoxetine, trazadone, buspirone), as well as complementary remedies (eg, melatonin, plug-in pheromones, essential oils [although some are toxic to cats]) may help to decrease anxiety and improve sleeping patterns.[47]

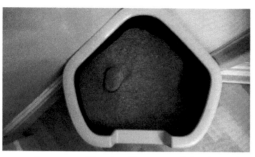

Fig. 28. Urine volume can be assessed by the diameter of the 'litter ball' in clumping litter.

Systemic Hypertension

Clinical signs
Infarcts or aneurisms induced by hypertension (see Rebecca F. Geddes' article, "Hypertension: why it is critical?," in this issue.) can cause cerebrovascular accidents resulting in behavioral changes and neurologic disease in elderly cats.[48] Hypertension can also cause target organ damage to the eyes, heart, and kidneys, resulting in intra-ocular hemorrhage and/or hypertensive retinopathy, congestive heart failure and exacerbation of CKD.[48]

Pathophysiology of hypertension
Hypertension is most commonly secondary to CKD and hyperthyroidism. Prevalence in CKD varies from general practice (<25%)[49] to referral hospital (65%).[50] Prevalence with hyperthyroidism (10%–90%)[48] likely reflects the reactive nature of cats. Situational hypertension (white coat hypertension) can increase blood pressure (BP) by 75 mm Hg,[51] so persistent elevation is needed before diagnosing hypertension. Other diseases or drugs can, less commonly, cause hypertension, including hyperaldosteronism, DM, acromegaly, hyperadrenocorticism, and erythropoietin therapy.[48]

Elderly cats are predisposed to hypertension (because of diseases like CKD and hyperthyroidism); additionally, 13% of apparently healthy cats aged more than 9 years are hypertensive.[52] However, normal BP also increases slightly with age (approximately 1–2 mm Hg per year), making diagnosis confusing.[53]

Unfortunately, hypertension is often only suspected once target organ damage has occurred; that is, cerebral vascular accidents (behavioral changes or seizures), intra-ocular hemorrhage or blindness, CKD, and/or heart failure.

Treatment
Antihypertensive drugs (amlodipine or telmisartan) should be prescribed as per the American College of Veterinary Internal Medicine Guidelines (Figs. **11** and **12**)[48]; a systolic BP of less than 140 mm Hg is considered to carry a minimal risk of target organ damage, 140 to 159 mm Hg [low risk], 160 to 180 mm Hg [moderate risk], and greater than 180 mm Hg [high risk], taking clinic-specific stress factors into consideration before deciding whether or not to treat for hypertension and before substaging patients with CKD.

THE VETERINARY PRACTICE AS A PRIMARY SOURCE OF ADVICE ON AGING
Midlife Clinic Visits

Potential aging changes and geriatric diseases should be discussed with owners of mature cats at routine examinations and vaccination appointments. It is not always easy for owners to recognize the signs of ill health in their cat, so vets must educate them as to what should be monitored (**Box 8**) and explain that changes are not always "normal," and they may result from treatable disease (see **Box 1**). These visits also provide opportunity to discuss minimizing stress associated with clinic visits (**Box 9**), and how best to maintain their aging cats' physical and emotional well-being (see **Box 2**).

Senior Health Care Clinics and Client Education Evenings

Senior health care programs should be offered to all clients with cats greater than 8 years of age. Initially, most cats need only attend 1 to 2 times a year, unless they already have significant disease.[54] Ideally, nurse-led clinics can be alternated with vet-led ones.[55] These provide an opportunity to monitor the cat's weight, percentage weight change, and BP, to collect information on eating and drinking, and for the cat's physical and emotional well-being to be assessed. Owners of elderly cats are often reluctant to enlist the help of veterinarians when they notice a change in their cat's physical or mental health. Veterinarians and nurses need to be aware of these concerns (**Box 10**), and specifically ask about them during elderly cat consultations. Client education evenings are another good way to increase client awareness of low stress handling, common conditions of old age and treatment options.

Ultimately, these interventions increase the likelihood of clients identifying early signs of ill health in their cat (physical or emotional) and they embrace the veterinary clinic as their primary source of information and support, resulting in an increased quality of life for cats and their owners.

Treat the Individual

Although veterinary medicine can offer complex diagnostic and therapeutic options, it is important to remember that elderly cats are often poorly tolerant of physical handling, or the stress of hospitalization. Each cat must be assessed and treated as an individual. Occasionally, investigations or interventions may have to be adapted or even abandoned if they are poorly tolerated for either medical or temperamental reasons. Although old age is not a disease, it is important that we pay particular attention to our older cats, care for them appropriately, and observe them closely so we can keep them well, for as long as possible.

DISCLOSURE

A. Miele, L. Sordo and D.A. Gunn-Moore have no financial relationship with any products named in this article.

SUPPLEMENTARY DATA

Supplementary data related to this article can be found online at https://doi.org/10.1016/j.cvsm.2020.03.004.

REFERENCES

1. Bellows J, Center S, Daristotle L, et al. Evaluating aging in cats: how to determine what is healthy and what is disease. J Feline Med Surg 2016;18:551–70.
2. Sánchez-Vizcaíno F, Noble PJM, Jones PH, et al. Demographics of dogs, cats, and rabbits attending veterinary practices in Great Britain as recorded in their electronic health records. BMC Vet Res 2017;13:218.

3. Vogt AH, Rodan I, Brown M, et al. AAFP-AAHA feline life stage guidelines. J Am Anim Hosp Assoc 2010;46:70–85.

4. Van Der Leij WJR, Selman LDAM, Vernooij JCM, et al. The effect of a hiding box on stress levels and body weight in Dutch shelter cats; A randomized controlled trial. PLoS One 2019;14(10):e0223492.

5. Perez-Camargo G, Patil AR, Cupp CJ. Body composition changes in aging cats. Compend Contin Educ Pract Vet 2004;26:71.

6. Cupp CJ, Kerr WW, Jean-Philippe C, et al. The role of nutritional interventions in the longevity and maintenance of long-term health in aging cats. Int J Appl Res Vet Med 2008;6:69–81.

7. Scarlett JM, Donoghue S, Saidla J, et al. Overweight cats: perspectives and risk factors. Int J Obes 1994;18:S22–8.

8. Harper EJ. Changing perspectives on aging and energy requirements: aging, body weight and body composition in humans, dogs and cats. J Nutr 1998; 128:2627S–31S.

9. Laflamme D, Gunn-Moore D. Nutrition of aging cats. Vet Clin North Am Small Anim Pract 2014;44:761–74.

10. Cruz-Jentoft, Martin FC, Schneider SM, et al. Sarcopenia: European consensus on definition and diagnosis: report of the European Working Group on Sarcopenia in Older People. Age Ageing 2010;39:412–23.

11. Anantharaman-Barr HG, Gicquello P, Rabot R. The effect of age on the digestibility of macronutrients and energy in cats. Proc Br Small Anim Vet Assoc 1991;164.

12. Taylor EJ, Adams C, Neville R. Some nutritional aspects of ageing in dogs and cats. Proc Nutr Soc 1995;54:645–56.

13. Deng P, Iwazaki E, Suchy SA, et al. Effects of feeding frequency and dietary water content on voluntary physical activity in healthy adult cats. J Anim Sci 2014;92: 1271–7.

14. Cupp CJ, Jean-Phillipe C, Kerr WW, et al. Effect of nutritional interventions on longevity of senior cats. Int J Appl Res Vet Med 2006;4:34–50.

15. Carver DS, Waterhouse HN. The variation in the water consumption of cats. Proc Anim Care Panel 1962;12:267–70.

16. German AC, Cunliffe NA, Morgan KL. Faecal consistency and risk factors for diarrhoea and constipation in cats in UK rehoming shelters. J Feline Med Surg 2017; 19:57–65.

17. Day MJ. Ageing, Immunosenescence and Inflammageing in the Dog and Cat. J Comp Pathol 2010;142:S60–9.

18. Lekcharoensuk C, Osborne CA, Lulich JP. Epidemiologic study of risk factors for lower urinary tract diseases in cats. J Am Vet Med Assoc 2001;218:1429–35.

19. Mayer-Roenne B, Goldstein RE, Erb HN. Urinary tract infections in cats with hyperthyroidism, diabetes mellitus and chronic kidney disease. J Feline Med Surg 2007;9:124–32.

20. Bartlett PC, Van Buren JW, Neterer M, et al. Disease surveillance and referral bias in the veterinary medical database. Prev Vet Med 2010;94:264–71.

21. KuKanich B. Geriatric Veterinary Pharmacology. Vet Clin North Am Small Anim Pract 2012;42:631–42.

22. Bellows J, Center S, Daristotle L, et al. Aging in cats: common physical and functional changes. J Feline Med Surg 2016;18:533–50.

23. Slingerland LI, Hazewinkel HAW, Meij BP, et al. Cross-sectional study of the prevalence and clinical features of osteoarthritis in 100 cats. Vet J 2011;187:304–9.

24. Kirschvink N. Effects of feeding frequency on water intake in cats [Abstract]. Lakewood (CO): American College of Veterinary Internal Medicine (ACVIM); 2005.

25. McEwen BS. Sex, stress and the hippocampus: allostasis, allostatic load and the aging process. Neurobiol Aging 2002;23:921–39.

26. Mills D, Dube MB, Zulch H, et al. How animals respond to change. In: Mills DS, Dube MB, Zulch H, editors. Stress and pheromonatherapy in small animal clinical behaviour. Chichester (United Kingdom): Wiley-Blackwell; 2012. p. 15–48.

27. Amat M, Camps T, Manteca X. Stress in owned cats: behavioural changes and welfare implications. J Feline Med Surg 2016;18:577–86.

28. Peavy GM, Jacobson MW, Salmon DP, et al. The influence of chronic stress on dementia-related diagnostic change in older adults. Alzheimer Dis Assoc Disord 2012;26:260–6.

29. Fatjó J, Ruiz-de-la-Torre JL, Manteca X. The epidemiology of behavioural problems in dogs and cats: a survey of veterinary practitioners. Anim Welf 2006;15: 179–85.

30. Monteiro BP, Steagall PV. Chronic pain in cats: recent advances in clinical assessment. J Feline Med Surg 2019;21:601–14.

31. Paulin MV, Couronné L, Beguin J, et al. Feline low-grade alimentary lymphoma: an emerging entity and a potential animal model for human disease. BMC Vet Res 2018;14:306.

32. Lee S, Farwell AP. Euthyroid sick syndrome. Compr Psychol 2016;6:1071–80.

33. Schaefer S, Kooistra HS, Riond B, et al. Evaluation of insulin-like growth factor-1, total thyroxine, feline pancreas-specific lipase and urinary corticoid-to-creatinine ratio in cats with diabetes mellitus in Switzerland and the Netherlands. J Feline Med Surg 2017;19:888–96.

34. Williams TL, Peak KJ, Brodbelt D, et al. Survival and the development of azotemia after treatment of hyperthyroid cats. J Vet Intern Med 2010;24:863–9.

35. Gunn-Moore D, Moffat K, Christie LA, et al. Cognitive dysfunction and the neurobiology of ageing in cats. J Small Anim Pract 2007;48:546–53.

36. Head E, Liu J, Hagen TM, et al. Oxidative damage increases with age in a canine model of human brain aging. J Neurochem 2002;82:375–81.

37. Landsberg GM, Nichol J, Araujo JA. Cognitive dysfunction syndrome. A disease of canine and feline brain aging. Vet Clin North Am Small Anim Pract 2012;42: 749–68.

38. Rème CA, Dramard V, Kern L, et al. Effect of S-adenosylmethionine tablets on the reduction of age-related mental decline in dogs: a double-blinded, placebo-controlled trial. Vet Ther Res Appl Vet Med 2007;9:69–82.

39. Araujo JA, Faubert ML, Brooks M, et al. NOVIFIT (NoviSAMe) Tablets improve executive function in aged dogs and cats: implications for treatment of cognitive dysfunction syndrome. Int J Appl Res Vet Med 2012;10:90–8.

40. Heath SE, Barabas S, Craze PG. Nutritional supplementation in cases of canine cognitive dysfunction-A clinical trial. Appl Anim Behav Sci 2007;105:284–96.

41. Araujo JA, Landsberg GM, Milgram NW, et al. Improvement of short-term memory performance in aged beagles by a nutraceutical supplement containing phosphatidylserine, Ginkgo biloba, vitamin E, and pyridoxine. Can Vet J 2008;49: 379–85.

42. Houpt K, Levine E, Landsberg G, et al. Antioxidant fortified food improves owner perceived behaviour in the aging cat. In: Proceedings of the ESFM Conference. Prague, Czech Republic, September 21-23, 2007.

43. Pan Y, Araujo JA, Burrows J, et al. Cognitive enhancement in middle-aged and old cats with dietary supplementation with a nutrient blend containing fish oil, B vitamins, antioxidants and arginine. Br J Nutr 2013;110:40–9.

44. Head E. Combining an antioxidant-fortified diet with behavioral enrichment leads to cognitive improvement and reduced brain pathology in aging canines: strategies for healthy aging. Ann N Y Acad Sci 2007;1114:398–406.

45. Landsberg GM, DePorter T, Araujo JA. Management of anxiety, sleeplessness and cognitive dysfunction in the senior pet. Vet Clin North Am Small Anim Pract 2011;41:565–90.

46. Ruehl WW, Bruyette DS, DePaoli A, et al. Canine cognitive dysfunction as a model for human age-related cognitive decline, dementia, and Alzheimer's disease: clinical presentation, cognitive testing, pathology and response to l-deprenyl therapy. Prog Brain Res 1995;106:217–25.

47. Landsberg GM, Denenberg S, Araujo JA. Cognitive dysfunction in cats: a syndrome we used to dismiss as 'old age'. J Feline Med Surg 2010;12:837–48.

48. Acierno MJ, Brown S, Coleman AE, et al. ACVIM consensus statement: guidelines for the identification, evaluation, and management of systemic hypertension in dogs and cats. J Vet Intern Med 2018;32:1803–22.

49. Syme HM, Barber PJ, Markwell PJ, et al. Prevalence of systolic hypertension in cats with chronic renal failure at initial evaluation. J Am Vet Med Assoc 2002; 220:1799–804.

50. Kobayashi DL, Peterson ME, Graves TK, et al. Hypertension in Cats With Chronic Renal Failure or Hyperthyroidism. J Vet Intern Med 1990;4:58–62.

51. Belew AM, Barlett T, Brown SA. Evaluation of the white-coat effect in cats. J Vet Intern Med 1999;13:134–42.

52. Bijsmans ES, Jepson RE, Chang YM, et al. Changes in Systolic Blood Pressure over Time in Healthy Cats and Cats with Chronic Kidney Disease. J Vet Intern Med 2015;29:855–61.

53. Payne JR, Brodbelt DC, Luis Fuentes V. Blood Pressure Measurements in 780 Apparently Healthy Cats. J Vet Intern Med 2017;31:15–21.

54. Pittari J, Rodan I, Beekman G, et al. AAFP Senior Care Guidelines. J Feline Med Surg 2009;11:763–78.

55. Carney HC, Little S, Brownlee-Tomasso D, et al. AAFP and ISFM feline-friendly nursing care guidelines. J Feline Med Surg 2012;14:337–49.

56. Sandhas E, Merle R, Eule JC. Consider the eye in preventive healthcare—ocular findings, intraocular pressure and Schirmer tear test in ageing cats. J Feline Med Surg 2018;20:1063–71.

57. Milgram NW, Head E, Zicher SC, et al. Learning ability in aged Beagle dogs is preserved by behavioural enrichment and dietary fortification: a two year longitudinal study. Neurobiol Aging 2005;26:77–90.

58. Ramsey I. BSAVA small animal formulary 8th edition. BSAVA British Small Animal Veterinary Association; 2014. Available at: https://beta.vin.com/members/cms/project/defaultadv1.aspx?id=4353471&pid=286&. Accessed January 30, 2020.

59. Verdon DR. Banfield releases major veterinary study showing spike in diabetes, dental disease and otitis externa. 2011. Available at: www.dvm360.com/view/banfield-releases-major-veterinary-study-showing-spike-diabetes-dental-disease-and-otitis-externa. Accessed April 14, 2016.

60. Marino CL, Lascelles BDX, Vaden SL, et al. Prevalence and classification of chronic kidney disease in cats randomly selected from four age groups and in cats recruited for degenerative joint disease studies. J Feline Med Surg 2014; 16:465–72.

61. Landsberg GM. Behavior problems of older cats. In: Schaumburg I, editor. Proceedings of the 135th Annual Meeting of the American Veterinary Medical Association. San Diego, CA, July 25-29, 1998. pp. 317–320.

62. Köhler I, Hartmann K, Wehner A, et al. Prevalence of and risk factors for feline hyperthyroidism among a clinic population in Southern Germany. Tierarztl Prax Ausg K Kleintiere Heimtiere 2016;44:149–57.

63. McLean JL, Lobetti RG, Schoeman JP. Worldwide prevalence and risk factors for feline hyperthyroidism: a review. J S Afr Vet Assoc 2014;85:1097.

64. Öhlund M, Fall T, Ström Holst B, et al. Incidence of Diabetes Mellitus in Insured Swedish Cats in Relation to Age, Breed and Sex. J Vet Intern Med 2015;29:1342–7.

65. McCann TM, Simpson KE, Shaw DJ, et al. Feline diabetes mellitus in the UK: the prevalence within an insured cat population and a questionnaire-based putative risk factor analysis. J Feline Med Surg 2007;9:289–99.

66. Pereira JS, Fragoso S, Beck A, et al. Improving the feline veterinary consultation: the usefulness of Feliway spray in reducing cats' stress. J Feline Med Surg 2016;18:959–64.

67. van Haaften KA, Eichstadt Forsythe LR, Stelow EA, et al. Effects of a single pre-appointment dose of gabapentin on signs of stress in cats during transportation and veterinary examination. J Am Vet Med Assoc 2017;251:1175–81.

68. Stevens BJ, Frantz EM, Orlando JM, et al. Efficacy of a single dose of trazodone hydrochloride given to cats prior to veterinary visits to reduce signs of transport- and examination-related anxiety. J Am Vet Med Assoc 2016;249:202–7.

Analgesia
What Makes Cats Different/Challenging and What Is Critical for Cats?

Paulo V. Steagall, MV, MSc, PhD

KEYWORDS

- Analgesia • Antiinflammatory drugs • Feline • Opioid • Pain • Pain assessment
- Pharmacology • Toxicity

KEY POINTS

- The advent of pain scoring systems, novel analgesic drugs and techniques, and species-specific pharmacokinetics and pharmacodynamics of analgesics have been crucial in the improvement of feline pain management.
- Cats have unique anatomic and physiologic considerations that may affect analgesia. Dosage regimens and analgesic techniques should not be extrapolated from dogs.
- Pain can only be treated after appropriate pain assessment. An overview of pain scoring tools for acute pain assessment is described in this article.
- The principles of pain management include not only preventive analgesia and multimodal analgesia but also nonpharmaceutical options and nursing care. Adjuvant analgesics should be also considered in the therapeutic analgesic plan, which should be tailored to each individual and its needs.
- Use of opioids, nonsteroidal antiinflammatory drugs, local anesthetics, ketamine, tramadol, and gabapentin for feline pain management is discussed in this article.

INTRODUCTION

Pain affects feline health and welfare. As the fourth vital sign, it must always be assessed in every physical examination. Knowledge of feline pain management has grown greatly. The advent of pain scoring systems/instruments, novel analgesic techniques and drugs with market authorization for use in cats, and knowledge about the species-specific pharmacokinetic-pharmacodynamic of analgesics are examples on how our understanding of feline analgesia has advanced. Review articles on feline pain management have been recently published.[1–6] In feline practice, pain needs to be part of client communication; cat owners are concerned about how analgesia is provided in the clinical setting.[7] Mostly importantly, feline pain management no longer relies on extrapolation of canine studies.

Department of Clinical Sciences, Faculty of Veterinary Medicine, Université de Montréal, 3200 Rue Sicotte, Saint-Hyacinthe, Quebec J2S2M2, Canada
E-mail address: paulo.steagall@umontreal.ca

Vet Clin Small Anim 50 (2020) 749–767
https://doi.org/10.1016/j.cvsm.2020.02.002
0195-5616/20/© 2020 Elsevier Inc. All rights reserved.

Recent studies have shown that attitudes and perceptions of veterinarians toward feline pain management have improved. Perioperative analgesics are now more commonly administered to cats than in the past. There is no longer a major gap between analgesic administration between dogs and cats especially in the perioperative setting.[8] However, some challenges remain. Some veterinarians do not administer or prescribe analgesics after patient discharge from hospital.[9] In several countries, analgesia in cats is still suboptimal, and analgesic availability is an issue.

This article presents the most important features and unique challenges of pain management in cats. Additional information on the pathophysiology of pain, types and causes of pain, and feline chronic pain management (ie, osteoarthritis, neuropathic pain, etc.) is presented in the chapters on Feline Chronic Pain and Osteoarthritis (by Monteiro) and Feline Neuropathic Pain (by Epstein).

MAIN CONSIDERATIONS REGARDING FELINE ANATOMY, PHYSIOLOGY, AND PHARMACOLOGY RELATED TO ANALGESIA
Nervous System

The distribution, density, and number of opioid receptors in the central nervous system across mammalian species could explain differences in analgesic efficacy produced by opioid analgesics and their adverse effects in cats.[10,11] For example, in cats, opioids evoke sympathetic stimulating effects at high doses that are mediated by autonomic centers in the brain, spinal cord, and adrenal glands.[12] These responses include mydriasis and increases in blood pressure and heart rate and adrenal vein hormone levels (ie, norepinephrine, epinephrine, dopamine and met-enkephalin). Behavioral changes (eg, fear, anxiety, vocalization, dysphoria) may be observed with opioid overdose in the conscious cat. On the other hand, opioids provide excellent analgesia in cats when appropriate doses are administered especially as part of multimodal analgesia.

Lumbosacral epidural administration of opioids and local anesthetics should be considered for the treatment of feline perioperative pain. In cats, the spinal cord and dural sacs terminate at the first and third sacral vertebra, respectively, and the end of the conus medullaris is located within the sacral canal.[13] The epidural space is shallow, and there is greater risk of intrathecal drug administration[14] compared with dogs. Anatomic landmarks and techniques used to confirm epidural placement (ie, "hanging-drop" or loss of resistance) can be more difficult to identify in cats due to their small size, making epidurals more challenging to perform than in dogs. With training and practice, they can definitely be used successfully in cats. Sacrococcygeal epidural anesthesia has been used as an alternative to lumbosacral epidural injections for cats with urethral obstruction. In cats, the depth of needle insertion for sacrococcygeal epidural anesthesia is approximately 0.6 cm, whereas the distance between skin and the ligamentum flavum is 1 cm using a lumbosacral approach (https://vetgirlontherun.com/coccygeal-block-feline-urethral-obstruction-vetgirl-veterinary-ce-video-blog/).[15]

Drug Metabolism and Disposition

Differences in drug metabolism and disposition exist between cats and other species. A review article presented some molecular and genetic evidence and mechanisms behind these differences.[16] Drugs eliminated by metabolic conjugation (ie, glucuronidation, sulfation, and/or glycination) are commonly excreted more slowly in cats than in humans or dogs. For example, acetylsalicylic acid, acetaminophen, carprofen, ketoprofen, and morphine undergo metabolic conjugation and, in some cases, may produce toxicity when doses and intervals of administrations are inappropriate. Conversely, drugs metabolized primarily by oxidation are commonly eliminated faster in cats when compared with dogs. These drugs include meloxicam, piroxicam, buprenorphine, and meperidine, among others. Finally, drugs that are excreted primarily unchanged into urine and/or bile (eg, gabapentin and several antibiotics) have similar elimination half-lives between dogs and cats.[16] These changes in drug metabolism and disposition may result in changes in dosage regimens.

Acetaminophen (paracetamol) toxicity is a classic example of how feline metabolism is unique. The administration of acetaminophen causes a life-threatening methemoglobinemia due to oxidative injury to erythrocytes with consequent anemia and Heinz bodies formation. In addition, cats do not produce several uridine diphosphate glucuronosyltransferases (UGTs) (eg, UGT1A6 and UGT1A9) needed for metabolism of acetaminophen.[17]

Glucuronidation pathway differences might also explain nonsteroidal antiinflammatory drug (NSAID)-induced adverse effects with drugs that do not produce the same effects in dogs.

- Carprofen is cleared significantly more slowly in cats than in dogs; cats present much longer elimination high-life.[18]
- On the other hand, another NSAID from the oxicam group, piroxicam, has been used for the treatment of cancer with added analgesic benefit in feline medicine.[19] The latter drug has faster clearance and elimination half-life when compared with dogs.[20]
- The major route of elimination of meloxicam is fecal in this species similar to dogs. Indeed, meloxicam has similar half-lives in dogs and cats. As in other species, the main pathway of meloxicam biotransformation is oxidation. This could be an advantage with deficient glucuronidation,[21] often the reason for fear of NSAID toxicity in cats. Meloxicam is approved for daily, long-term administration in cats in the European Union.
- There is evidence showing that contemporary NSAIDs can be used safely in cats with appropriate dosage regimens even in cats with concomitant osteoarthritis (OA) and chronic kidney disease (CKD) (see Feline Chronic Pain and Osteoarthritis by Monteiro).[22]
- Deficient glucuronidation is mostly related to drug structure and cannot be generalized to all drugs undergoing glucuronidation (**Box 1**).

Drug Excretion

The prevalence of CKD is between 30% and 40% in cats older than 10 years of age and represents a significant cause of mortality. The International Society of Feline

---

Box 1
Phenolic compounds and deficient glucuronidation in cats

Phenolic compounds are the ones mostly affected by deficient glucuronidation.[16] These drugs require metabolization by several UGT1A isoforms that may be lacking in cats. The deficient UGT pathways in cats may also be responsible for differences in reduced morphine glucuronidation in cats.[23] Cats eliminate morphine at a similar rate to dogs; however they produce lower concentrations of morphine-3-glucuronide, and do not produce morphine-6-glucuronide, an active metabolite responsible for analgesia in humans.

Medicine has published consensus guidelines on diagnosis and management of CKD in cats.[24] Some important considerations for analgesia of CKD cats undergoing surgery or requiring analgesia for other reasons are described in the following section.

- The pharmacokinetics and pharmacodynamics of anesthetics and analgesics may be influenced by CKD. Drugs or metabolites that require normal kidney function for excretion may accumulate.
- Analgesic dosage regimens may require adjustment based on clinical experience and pain assessment.
- The anesthetic plan should favor drugs that can be reversed and that do not require active renal excretion.
- Azotemia and renal dysfunction decrease anesthetic and sedative requirements by changing the blood-brain barrier permeability. Doses for intraoperative analgesia should be adjusted and administered "to effect."
- Ketamine is metabolized in the liver to the active metabolite norketamine, which is renally excreted. In cats with CKD, the effect of ketamine and norketamine may be prolonged (**Box 2**).
- Fluid therapy is required not only to correct dehydration, electrolyte, and acid-base abnormalities before anesthesia but also to maintain adequate blood flow during anesthesia and to support drug excretion. Surgery will cause inflammation, tissue damage, and pain.
- The administration of a minimum effective dose of NSAID should be considered for normovolemic cats with stable renal disease once blood pressure is controlled and there is no risk of bleeding. In some cases, it may be preferable to administer an NSAID when the cat is eating and drinking after anesthetic recovery.

PAIN ASSESSMENT

Pain assessment is central to providing appropriate treatment. The cat often exhibits subtle pain behaviors, which make pain assessment a challenge in clinical practice. Recent studies have provided important advances in recognition of feline pain.

Differences Between Dogs and Cats

- Cats have evolved as solitary hunters needing a smaller repertoire of inter- and intraspecies social communication as compared with dogs, leading to differences in how they express pain.
- Cats have domesticated themselves in a process of "tolerance" of human proximity in exchange for access to rodent-infested grain storage.[25]

Box 2
The metabolism and excretion of ketamine in cats

Ketamine undergoes rapid distribution and biotransformation to form norketamine; however, cats do not produce dehydroketamine (ie, metabolite II) as other species do, which is required for further metabolism, resulting in small concentrations of ketamine and norketamine after parenteral administration. Cats with a decline in renal function are at risk of excessive levels of these products. The prolonged anesthetic effects of ketamine in cats with urethral obstruction or kidney dysfunction are likely also due to altered biodisposition of the drug caused by metabolic acidosis. The author has administered subanesthetic doses of ketamine infusions (10 μg/kg/min) for postoperative pain control after feline subcutaneous urethral bypass when renal function is improving.

- These differences in domestication result in cats hiding pain-related behaviors and humans having decreased ability to identify these behaviors, making pain assessment more challenging in this species.

Physiologic changes including heart and respiratory rates, pupil size, and neuroendocrine assays are poorly correlated with pain and should not be used on their own in assessing pain.[26] The only physiologic parameter that has been correlated with pain is blood pressure.

Acute pain assessment relies on the behavioral expression of pain (**Fig. 1**). Key behaviors following abdominal postoperative pain, dental extractions, and other painful conditions have been identified (**Table 1**).[27–30] A comprehensive review of assessing acute pain in cats is available elsewhere.[5]

Studies have shown that pain can be detected as early as 30 minutes after ovariohysterectomy, even if the cat is still sedated and recovering from general anesthesia.[31] Thus, pain assessment should be started approximately 30 min following surgery and every 1 to 2 hours afterward until at least 6 to 8 hours after an ovariohysterectomy. The frequency of pain assessment will be dictated by the type of surgery/pain condition. If a cat is comfortable and sleeping (eg, "bagel" curled-up position), it should not be disturbed for pain assessment.

Pain scales are useful for consistent, practical, and objective assessment of acute pain and provide cut-off scores to guide administration of rescue analgesia (**Table 2**). Facial expressions of pain have been identified in cats,[29,32,33] and a novel Feline Grimace Scale pain scoring tool has been published[29] (**Fig. 2**). Feline chronic pain

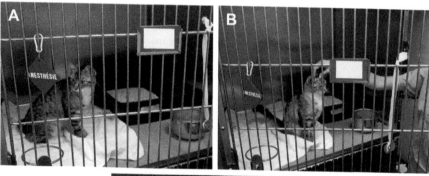

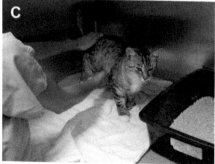

Fig. 1. A cat is evaluated for postoperative pain following ovariohysterectomy using the Unesp-Botucatu multidimensional composite pain scale. (*A*) First the cat is evaluated at a distance. (*B*) The cage is opened, and the cat is gently approached. (*C*) The flank and wound are gently palpated while observing any behavioral reactions.

Table 1
Behaviors that suggest acute pain in cats based on different categories

Type of Pain	Category	Description of Behavior
Abdominal pain and various painful conditions	Posture and activity	Crouched/hunched posture Laying in dorsolateral recumbency with pelvic limbs extended or contracted Laying down being quiet Abdominal muscle contraction (flank) Vocalization (growling, groaning, howling, hissing) Depression/dull mentation Restlessness
	Interaction with the observer and the environment	Lack of interest in the surroundings Withdrawing/hiding Facing the back of the cage Reluctance to move after stimulation Unwillingness to play or interact with the observer Attempts to hide/escape from the observer Irritation Aggression/self-defensiveness
	Other behaviors	Excessive attention to the wound (licking, biting) Reaction to palpation of the wound Decreased grooming and/or appetite
	Facial expressions	Ears are pulled apart and rotated outwards Squinted eyes Tense muzzle (elliptical shape) Straight whiskers (pointing forwards) Lowered head position (in relation to the shoulder line)
Postoperative pain, for example, following dental extractions	General behaviors	Decreased activity Reluctance to move Decreased playfulness Difficulty prehending dry food Head shaking

Data from Refs.[27–30]

assessment is described in the chapter Feline Chronic Pain and Osteoarthritis and elsewhere.[6]

Challenges in Pain Assessment and Limitations of Pain Scoring Systems in Cats

- Pain assessment can be confounded by variables including demeanor, drugs, and illness.[34]
- Stress, fear, and anxiety may affect pain assessment particularly in hospitalized cats. Strategies to reduce stress and negative emotions during transport and veterinary consultation/hospitalization should be taken in consideration to reduce the impact of stress on pain assessment.
- Differences in pain scores between evaluators of different sex using the same pain scale in different languages[35] and among evaluators with different level of training have also been reported.[36]

Table 2
Overview of feline acute pain assessment tools

Pain Scale	UNESP-Botucatu Multidimensional Composite Pain Scale (UNESP-Botucatu MCPS)	Glasgow Feline Composite Measure Pain Scale (CMPS-Feline)	Feline Grimace Scale (FGS)
Components	Pain expression • Miscellaneous behaviors • Reaction to palpation of the flank • Reaction to palpation of the surgical wound • Vocalization Psychomotor change • Posture • Comfort • Activity • Attitude Physiologic variables • Appetite • Blood pressure	• Vocalization • Posture and Activity • Attention to wound • Ear position • Shape of muzzle • Response to interaction with the observer • Palpation of painful area • Qualitative behavior	Action units • Ear position • Orbital tightening • Muzzle tension • Whisker position • Head position
How to use the tool	Each item is scored from 0–3. The sum of the scores from all 10 items is the final score of that cat. Evaluation starts by observing the undisturbed cat. Then, the cat is approached for the evaluation of remaining items.	Each item is scored (scores vary from item to item). The sum of the scores from all 8 items is the final score of that cat. Evaluation starts by observing the undisturbed cat including its facial expressions. The cat is approached for the evaluation of remaining items.	Each action unit is rated from 0–2, where 0 = action unit is absent; 1 = moderate appearance of the action unit or uncertainty over its presence or absence and 2 = obvious appearance of the action unit. Nonvisible action units are not scored. The final score is the sum of scores divided by the number of scored action units.
Validation of tool	Comprehensive validity, reliability in cats with postoperative pain following ovariohysterectomy.	Evidence of construct validity and responsiveness in cats with varied painful conditions.	Shown to be valid and reliable in cats with varied painful conditions in both real-time and image assessment.
Intervention score	$\geq 7/30$ (or $\geq 6/27$ if blood pressure is not included)	$\geq 5/20$	$>0.39/1.0$

(continued on next page)

Pain Scale	UNESP-Botucatu Multidimensional Composite Pain Scale (UNESP-Botucatu MCPS)	Glasgow Feline Composite Measure Pain Scale (CMPS-Feline)	Feline Grimace Scale (FGS)
Table 2 *(continued)*			
Comments	Developed in cats with postoperative pain following ovariohysterectomy. The original tool was developed in Brazilian Portuguese and was further translated and validated in English, Spanish, French, and Italian.	Easy and quick to use.	Reported high discriminative ability, good overall interrater reliability, excellent intrarater reliability, and excellent internal consistency. Easy and quick to use.
Source	Video-based training on feline acute pain and the use of the scale is available at http://animalpain.com.br/en-us/	http://www.newmetrica.com/acute-pain-measurement/download-pain-questionnaire-for-cats/	The training manual is available as "Supplementary information" within the original article: https://www.nature.com/articles/s41598-019-55693-8
References	Brondani et al,[27] 2013; Brondani et al,[64] 2012	Reid et al,[28] 2017; Calvo et al,[65] 2014	Evangelista et al,[29] 2019

Data from Refs.[27–29,64,65]

THE ANALGESIC PLAN

Historically, analgesics were not used in cats due to toxic and adverse effects. Davis and Donnelly provided evidence in 1968 that opioids produce an analgesic effect in cats and adverse effects were observed only after overdosing.[37] The principles of acute feline pain management are described in **Box 3**.

- Veterinarians should choose the most appropriate opioid for the condition.
- Surgery will inevitably produce some degree of inflammation. An NSAID should always be administered for pain relief. The duration of treatment should be considered as well as the palatability of the drug.
- Local anesthetic techniques for the head, thoracic, and pelvic limbs as well as for desexing procedures are available. The onset and duration of local anesthesia should be part of the plan.
- Consideration should also be given to whether adjuvant analgesics are required and which analgesics should be prescribed for hospital discharge.

Cats may need to be hospitalized for analgesic infusions and for frequent pain reassessment. Drugs that may contribute to a better experience in the hospital setting include maropitant to reduce perioperative vomiting[38] and gabapentin or trazodone to reduce anxiety.[39,40] **Table 3** provides suggested dosage regimens and routes of administration for drugs used for treating acute pain in cats.

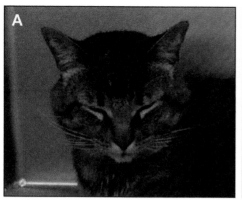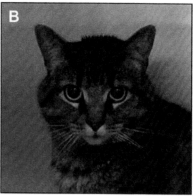

Fig. 2. The Feline Grimace Scale. This tool uses changes in facial expressions (action units) for acute pain assessment in cats (instructions are provided in **Table 2**). (A) In this painful cat, the ears are pulled apart, the eyes are squinted, the muzzle is tense and in an elliptical shape, the whiskers are straight and moving cranially, and the head is slightly below the shoulder line. (B) After the administration of analgesics, the ears are now facing forward, the eyes are opened, the muzzle is relaxed and in a round shape, the whiskers are loose, and the head is above the shoulder line.

ANALGESIC DRUGS
Opioids

Appropriate doses of opioids provide analgesia in painful cats.[1-3] At effective doses, opioids produce mydriasis and behavioral changes including purring, kneading, euphoria, and rubbing against objects or the caregiver. However, morphine, oxymorphone and hydromorphone may cause vomiting and excessive salivation, which compromises feline welfare (**Fig. 4**). These side effects are not observed after the administration of methadone, meperidine, fentanyl, buprenorphine, or butorphanol (see **Table 3**).

- Agonists of μ-opioid receptors (eg, morphine, hydromorphone, oxymorphone, methadone, fentanyl, remifentanil, meperidine) provide dose-dependent analgesia and are recommended for moderate to severe painful conditions. They are the cornerstone of acute pain management. Their side effects are easily prevented or treated.

Box 3
The analgesic plan

Acute pain is best treated with preventive and multimodal analgesia using a combination of locoregional anesthesia along with opioids and NSAIDs. These 3 classes of analgesics are often sufficient to treat mild to moderate pain produced by elective surgery. Adjuvant analgesics (eg, tramadol, gabapentin, ketamine) are usually required for invasive surgical procedures when pain is severe, especially when there is a contraindication to use of NSAIDs or when locoregional anesthesia cannot be used. Most importantly, analgesic protocols and dosage regimens should be tailored to the patient and based on objective pain reassessment. An analgesic plan should be in place for every patient. Nursing and nonpharmacological therapy are paramount in feline pain management. For example, a box or covered bed is provided for comfort and a place that they can hide and feel safe (**Fig. 3**).

Table 3
Suggested dosing and routes of administration for some analgesics used in the treatment of acute pain in cats[a]

Drug	Doses (mg/kg), or Otherwise Indicated	Route	Comments
Opioids			
Morphine	0.2–0.5 q 4–6 h	IM	Caution: Give slowly via IV route due to histamine release. May cause nausea and vomiting. Morphine (0.1 mg/kg) may be administered by the epidural route or intraarticularly as an adjuvant analgesic technique
Meperidine (pethidine)	3–5 q 1–2 h	IM	Do not administer IV due to histamine release
Methadone	0.3–0.5 q 4 h	IM, IV, buccally	Has NMDA receptor antagonist properties
Oxymorphone	0.025–0.1 q 4–6 h	IM, IV	May also produce vomiting
Hydromorphone	0.025–0.1 q 4–6 h	IM, IV	May cause hyperthermia in cats. May cause nausea and vomiting
Tramadol	2–4 q 6–8 h	IM, IV, PO	Noradrenaline (norepinephrine) and serotonin reuptake inhibitor in addition to opioid-like effects
Fentanyl injectable	Bolus 1–3 µg/kg + CRI 5–15 µg/kg/h	IV	High doses may produce dysphoria in awake patients Maximum decreases in minimum alveolar concentration are observed at 10–15 µg/kg/h
Remifentanil	4–6 µg/kg/h (analgesia) 10–20 µg/kg/h (anesthetic-sparing)	IV	Limited decreases in the minimum alveolar concentration of inhalant anesthetics in cats (15%–20%). Remifentanil does not require a bolus. See comments on fentanyl. Remifentanil is half as potent as fentanyl. Sympathetic stimulation may be observed at high doses
Butorphanol	0.2–0.4 q 1–2 h	IM, IV	Limited analgesic efficacy only suitable for mild pain or for sedation. It can be used to reverse pure opioid agonist-induced respiratory depression (0.05 mg/kg IV) It can be used as a CRI for some types of visceral pain at 0.05 mg/kg/h
Buprenorphine 0.3 mg/mL (Vetergesic, Buprenex, Temgesic)	0.02–0.04 q 4–8 h	IM, IV, buccally	Euphoria is commonly observed SC administration does not produce adequate analgesia

(continued on next page)

Table 3
(continued)

Drug	Doses (mg/kg), or Otherwise Indicated	Route	Comments
Buprenorphine 1.8 mg/mL (Simbadol)	0.24 every 24 h for up to 3 d	SC	Control of postoperative pain in cats—is designed for SC use Good analgesia especially when administered with local anesthesia and NSAIDs
Naloxone (antagonist)	0.04 q 0.5–1 h	IV	Commonly diluted and titrated to effect to reverse adverse effects. Naloxone is diluted with 5 mL of saline 0.9% and given at 0.5 mL/min until the side effects have subsided
NSAIDs[a]			
Meloxicam	0.2 or 0.3 followed by 0.05 mg/kg for 3–5 d	SC, PO	Can be administered at 0.05 mg/kg/d for control of postoperative pain
Robenacoxib	2 followed by 1–2 mg/kg for 3–5 d	SC, PO	Can be administered at 1 mg/kg/d for control of postoperative pain
Carprofen	4	SC	Single administration in cats
Tolfenamic acid	4	SC	Single administration in cats (not preoperative)
Ketoprofen	2	SC	Single administration in cats (not preoperative)
Local Anesthetics			
Bupivacaine	Doses should not exceed 2		Never administer IV due to cardiotoxicity
Lidocaine	Doses should not exceed 7		Can be administered intravenously at 1–2 mg/kg to treat ventricular dysrhythmias. CRI is not recommended due to cardiovascular depression

Abbreviations: CRI, constant rate infusion; NMDA, N-methyl D-aspartate.
[a] Suggested doses because regional label/licences vary.
Adapted from Steagall PV, Taylor PM. Treatment of acute (adaptive pain). In: Steagall PV, Robertson SA, Taylor PM, editors. Feline Anesthesia and Pain Management, 1st edition. Hoboken, NJ: Wiley; 2017. p. 221-240; with permission.

- Human transdermal patches of fentanyl have been used to provide long-term pain relief (ie, 72–96 hours) in hospitalized cats. Because there is high individual variability in drug absorption particularly in cats, they may fail to provide analgesia. Onset of analgesia takes 6 to 7 hours, and the duration of action may continue for up to 7 to 8 hours after patches are removed.[41]
- Opioid infusions also provide dose-dependent analgesia with the benefit of dose titration. However, there is a ceiling effect in terms of inhalant anesthetic sparing effect in cats. High doses of fentanyl and remifentanil only reduce anesthetic requirements by up to 20% in cats.
- Epidural opioids (eg, morphine) provide good analgesia for acute pain especially when combined with local anesthetics to reduce inhalant anesthetic

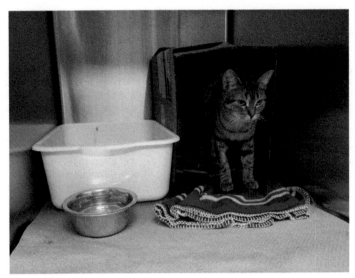

Fig. 3. A standard size hospital cage with a card box provides a hiding area and elevated surfaces on which the cat can perch. These simple measures enrich the cage and can improve the hospital experience.

requirements. The bladder should always be gently expressed before anesthetic recovery to avoid urinary retention produced by epidural morphine.

- Buprenorphine is a partial agonist of μ-opioid receptors. The drug does not produce dose-dependent analgesic effects. It is often administered for mild to moderate pain as part of multimodal analgesia.
- Methadone and buprenorphine can be administered buccally/transmucosally. There is reasonable bioavailability after buccal administration of these drugs because cats have a high oral pH favoring drug absorption. However, both the intravenous (IV) and intramuscular (IM) buprenorphine provided better analgesia in cats undergoing ovariohysterectomy.
- Nalbuphine and butorphanol are agonists of κ-opioid receptors. They provide limited analgesia and are best used for sedation in combination with agonists of $α_2$-adrenergic receptors or acepromazine.
- The route of administration affects analgesia and opioid-induced adverse effects (**Box 4**).
- Pediatric cats may require more frequent dosing because age can influence opioid-induced antinociception. One study showed that hydromorphone provided a shorter duration and smaller magnitude of antinociception in cats of 6 months of age when compared with the same cats at 9 and 12 months of age.[42]

Tramadol

Tramadol is considered a dual-action analgesic drug. It is a synthetic weak opioid agonist and a serotonin and norepinephrine reuptake inhibitor. The injectable formulation is a popular means of analgesic administration in some countries. In North America, Oceania, and other countries in Europe, tramadol is available for oral administration. However, its poor palatability and bitter taste have precluded it from becoming a popular analgesic in cats in those countries. Cats may salivate profusely after drug administration and treatment compliance can be poor. Differences in the

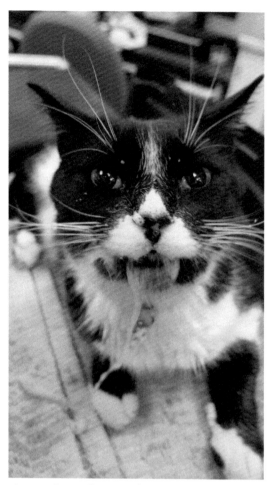

Fig. 4. A cat showing profuse salivation after the administration of hydromorphone. Morphine, oxymorphone, and hydromorphone stimulate the chemoreceptor trigger zone and dopamine receptors in the vomiting center to induce profound salivation, nausea, and vomiting. This is a concern in terms of patient welfare. The prevalence of vomiting after SC administration of hydromorphone is higher than after administration via IV or IM route.[45]

metabolism and analgesic efficacy of tramadol between dogs and cats are presented in the chapter Feline Neuropathic Pain (by Epstein), but tramadol is considered a better analgesic agent in cats than in dogs.

There is substantial intersubject variability regarding the analgesic efficacy and adverse effects of tramadol in cats. Use of tramadol in cats is summarized as follows:

- Tramadol is often administered for the treatment of acute and chronic pain, especially when other analgesic drugs are not available or contraindicated.
- Injectable tramadol (2–4 mg/kg IM) is often used in combination with acepromazine or dexmedetomidine for premedication.[47,48] Doses of 4 mg/kg every 6 hours PO are recommended for multimodal analgesia.[49] Lower doses have been used in the treatment of feline OA (2–4 mg/kg PO every 12 hours).[50,51] However, palatability limits the usefulness of the oral form.

Box 4
The influence of route of administration in opioid-induced analgesia and adverse effects

The route of administration has been shown to influence the onset, magnitude, and duration of analgesic effects following administration of buprenorphine and hydromorphone in cats. A review article has explored this issue in more detail.[3] The SC route is often used for drug administration because it produces less pain at injection than the IM route; however, SC administration of some opioids have not provided analgesia/antinociception when compared with IV and IM[43–45] so should not be used with standard formulations of these drugs. Analgesia is often of shorter duration, and the prevalence of vomiting was higher after SC hydromorphone when compared with the IM or IV routes.[45] However, readers should not confuse standard formulations of buprenorphine with the Food and Drug Administration–approved high-concentration formulation of buprenorphine (1.8 mg/mL; Simbadol). This formulation produces sustained antinociception (24 hours) after one subcutaneous injection of 0.24 mg/kg[46] and can be administered for up to 3 consecutive days.

Data from Refs.[3,43–46]

- Gastrointestinal adverse effects and sedation are observed in some cats when tramadol is administered orally for long-term pain management.[51]
- The risk of serotonin toxicity is a concern after the administration of tramadol in combination with other serotonin inhibitors (eg, fluoxetine and trazodone), monoamine oxidase inhibitors (ie, selegiline), and tricyclic antidepressants (ie, clomipramine). In a case report, clinical signs include increased neuromuscular activity, tachycardia, fever, tachypnea, and agitation.[52]
- Tramadol may fail to produce clinical analgesia, and pain should be monitored.[47]

Nonsteroidal Antiinflammatory Drugs

NSAIDs are widely used for their antiinflammatory, antipyretic, and analgesic effects (see **Table 3**). Adverse effects are observed when doses or intervals of administration are not adhered to or if given in combination with corticosteroids. Adverse effects include gastrointestinal irritation, protein-losing enteropathy, and renal damage. However, NSAID-induced acute kidney injury in healthy cats receiving NSAIDs is a myth. These drugs are palatable and facilitate treatment compliance. Injectable formulations are important in the perioperative period and can be administered IV or subcutaneously (SC) depending on the label.

- NSAIDs are similar in terms of analgesic efficacy in the postoperative period after a single injection. However, some NSAIDs may not be tolerated for long-term use such as for treatment of chronic pain.
- Variable doses of meloxicam and robenacoxib have been shown to be safe in cats and are licensed for long-term use in some countries.[53,54]
- The timing of NSAID delivery is a controversial subject. They can be administered preoperatively for routine neutering in healthy cats especially if blood pressure is monitored and cats are normovolemic, fluid therapy is administered, and contraindications have been excluded.
- Veterinarians should not fear NSAID-induced adverse effects if contraindications do not exist and if dosage regimens are adhered to. Dosing should be based on lean body weight, and cats should ideally be normovolemic before administration. These drugs are key players in control of inflammation and perioperative pain.

Local Anesthetics

Using local anesthetics decreases perioperative analgesic requirements and the prevalence of anesthetic-related death (see **Table 3**).

- Contraindications are rare. Adverse effects have been reported from human error (ie, miscalculation of maximum doses and concentrations resulting in toxicity, poor technique, and nerve damage during drug administration) and accidental IV administration of local anesthetic with high cardiotoxicity (eg, bupivacaine).
- They provide excellent perioperative analgesia, muscle relaxation, and anesthetic and opioid sparing effect. They can prevent central sensitization. Anesthetic maintenance and recoveries are usually calm when locoregional anesthesia is incorporated in the analgesic plan.
- Several locoregional techniques have been reported in cats recently, providing better descriptions into terms of anatomic landmarks, safety, and efficacy, especially with the advent of ultrasound-guided techniques.[15]
- Simple and cost-effective techniques can now be included in routine desexing surgery including intraperitoneal, incisional, and intratesticular techniques.

Ketamine

There is renewed interest in the use of ketamine as an analgesic, antihyperalgesic therapy for its noncompetitive and nonspecific antagonism of the N-methyl D-aspartate receptors.[55] These receptors are activated during excitatory neurotransmission after sustained nociception in the dorsal horn of the spinal cord and are involved in central sensitization and cumulative depolarization ("wind-up") (**Box 5**)[56] (see also Feline Neuropathic Pain by Epstein). Studies on ketamine in cats as an analgesic drug are lacking.

Agonists of Alpha-2 Adrenergic Receptors

Medetomidine and dexmedetomidine are used for premedication/sedation and provide muscle relaxation and analgesia. They are not commonly used for pain

---

Box 5
The clinical use of ketamine infusion in cats

- Ketamine has been used as an adjunctive analgesic agent within multimodal analgesia protocols in 3 cats with major injury.[57] The drug should never be used as a stand-alone analgesic.

- Ketamine is given by the intravenous route of administration with appropriate pain assessment and monitoring during hospitalization.

- Administer an intravenous loading dose (0.15–0.7 mg/kg) followed by a CRI (2–10 µg/kg/min). The administration of a single bolus without an infusion is uncommon due to the rapid clearance of ketamine.

- The author uses ketamine in cats undergoing major surgery or after major trauma to prevent or treat hyperalgesia and allodynia commonly associated with central sensitization. These cats are often transferred to an intermediate or intensive care unit after surgery where the infusion is continued for 24 to 72 hours postoperatively.[55]

- The administration of intravenous remifentanil and ketamine (bolus of 0.5 mg/kg followed by 30 µg/kg/min infusions) provided greater reductions in isoflurane requirements when compared with a control group or remifentanil alone after ovariohysterectomy in cats.[58]

Data from Refs.[55,57,58]

management as first choice but are incorporated into multimodal protocols. They enhance opioid analgesia while reducing anesthetic requirements in a dose-dependent manner. Sedation is also important in reducing the "pain experience". However, their use should be reserved to cats with stable cardiovascular function.

Gabapentin

Gabapentin acts primarily by binding to voltage-gated calcium channels,[59] as well as the descending noradrenergic inhibitory system. In feline medicine, the drug is used for managing acute[31] and chronic pain.[60]

- Postoperative analgesia produced by gabapentin (using 50 mg, PO, at 12 and 1 hour before surgery) and buprenorphine was similar to combining meloxicam with buprenorphine in cats undergoing ovariohysterectomy.[31]
- Cats with OA receiving gabapentin (10 mg/kg, PO, every 12 hours) showed improvement in owner-identified impaired activities. Sedation was recorded by objective measures of activity levels.[60]
- Gabapentin (50 or 100 mg, PO) has also been shown to attenuate stress and fear response in client-owned and cage-trap community cats undergoing transportation and veterinary consultation.[39,61]
- Pharmacokinetic data revealed high bioavailability in cats (90%–95%)[62,63] following administration of 10 mg/kg. Peak plasma concentrations were recorded between 45 minutes and 2 hours,[62,63] and elimination half-lives were recorded between 3 and 4 hours.[62,63]

DISCLOSURE

Dr P.V. Steagall has provided consultancy services and received honorarium from Boehringer Ingelheim, Dechra, Elanco, Vetoquinol, and Zoetis.

REFERENCES

1. Steagall PVM, Monteiro-Steagall BP, Taylor PM. A review of the studies using buprenorphine in cats. J Vet Intern Med 2014;28(3):762–70.
2. Bortolami E, Love EJ. Practical use of opioids in cats: a state-of-the-art, evidence-based review. J Feline Med Surg 2015;17(4):283–311.
3. Simon BT, Steagall PV. The present and future of opioid analgesics in small animal practice. J Vet Pharmacol Ther 2017;40(4):315–26.
4. Adrian D, Papich M, Baynes R, et al. Chronic maladaptive pain in cats: a review of current and future drug treatment options. Vet J 2017;230:52–61.
5. Steagall PV, Monteiro BP. Acute pain in cats: recent advances in clinical assessment. J Feline Med Surg 2019;21(1):25–34.
6. Monteiro BP, Steagall PV. Chronic pain in cats: Recent advances in clinical assessment. J Feline Med Surg 2019;21(7):601–14.
7. Steagall PV, Monteiro BP, Ruel HLM, et al. Perceptions and opinions of Canadian pet owners about anaesthesia, pain and surgery in small animals. J Small Anim Pract 2017;58(7):380–8.
8. Hunt JR, Knowles TG, Lascelles BDX, et al. Prescription of perioperative analgesics by UK small animal veterinary surgeons in 2013. Vet Rec 2015;176(19):493.
9. Simon BT, Scallan EM, Carroll G, et al. The lack of analgesic use (oligoanalgesia) in small animal practice. J Small Anim Pract 2017;58(10):543–54.
10. Walker JM, Bowen WD, Thompson LA, et al. Distribution of opiate receptors within visual structures of the cat brain. Exp Brain Res 1988;73(3):523–32.

11. Billet O, Billaud JN, Phillips TR. Partial characterization and tissue distribution of the feline μ opiate receptor. Drug Alcohol Depend 2001;62(2):125–9.
12. Gaumann DM, Yaksh TL, Tyce GM, et al. Sympathetic stimulating effects of sufentanil in the cat are mediated centrally. Neurosci Lett 1988;91(1):30–5.
13. Maierl J, Liebich HG. Investigations on the postnatal development of the macroscopic proportions and the topographic anatomy of the feline spinal cord. Anat Histol Embryol 1998;27(6):375–9.
14. O'Hearn AK, Wright BD. Coccygeal epidural with local anesthetic for catheterization and pain management in the treatment of feline urethral obstruction. J Vet Emerg Crit Care (San Antonio) 2011;21(1):50–2.
15. Credie L, Luna S. The use of ultrasound to evaluate sacrococcygeal epidural injections in cats. Can Vet J 2018;59(2):143–6.
16. Court MH. Feline drug metabolism and disposition: pharmacokinetic evidence for species differences and molecular mechanisms. Vet Clin North Am Small Anim Pract 2013;43(5):1039–54.
17. Court MH, Greenblatt DJ. Molecular genetic basis for deficient acetaminophen glucuronidation by cats: UGT1A6 is a pseudogene, and evidence for reduced diversity of expressed hepatic UGT1A isoforms. Pharmacogenetics 2000;10(4):355–69.
18. Taylor PM, Delatour P, Landoni FM, et al. Pharmacodynamics and enantioselective pharmacokinetics of carprofen in the cat. Res Vet Sci 1996;60(2):144–51.
19. Bulman-Fleming JC, Turner TR, Rosenberg MP. Evaluation of adverse events in cats receiving long-term piroxicam therapy for various neoplasms. J Feline Med Surg 2010;12(4):262–8.
20. Heeb HL, Chun R, Koch DE, et al. Multiple dose pharmacokinetics and acute safety of piroxicam and cimetidine in the cat. J Vet Pharmacol Ther 2005;28(5):447–52.
21. Grudé P, Guittard J, Garcia C, et al. Excretion mass balance evaluation, metabolite profile analysis and metabolite identification in plasma and excreta after oral administration of [14C]-meloxicam to the male cat: preliminary study. J Vet Pharmacol Ther 2010;33(4):396–407.
22. Monteiro B, Steagall PVM, Lascelles BDX, et al. Long-term use of non-steroidal anti-inflammatory drugs in cats with chronic kidney disease: from controversy to optimism. J Small Anim Pract 2019;60(8):459–62.
23. Taylor P, Robertson S, Dixon M, et al. Morphine, pethidine and buprenorphine disposition in the cat. J Vet Pharmacol Ther 2001;24(6):391–8.
24. Sparkes AH, Caney S, Chalhoub S, et al. ISFM consensus guidelines on the diagnosis and management of feline chronic kidney disease. J Feline Med Surg 2016;18(3):219–39.
25. Serpell J. Domestication and history of the cat. In: Turner D, Bateson P, editors. The domestic cat: the biology of its behaviour. Cambridge, UK: Cambridge University Press; 2013. p. 83–100.
26. Cambridge AJ, Tobias KM, Newberry RC, et al. Subjective and objective measurements of postoperative pain in cats. J Am Vet Med Assoc 2000;217(5):685–90.
27. Brondani JT, Mama KR, Luna SPL, et al. Validation of the English version of the UNESP-Botucatu multidimensional composite pain scale for assessing postoperative pain in cats. BMC Vet Res 2013;9(1):1.
28. Reid J, Scott EM, Calvo G, et al. Definitive Glasgow acute pain scale for cats: validation and intervention level. Vet Rec 2017;180(18):449.

29. Evangelista MC, Watanabe R, Leung VSY, et al. Facial expressions of pain in cats: the development and validation of a Feline Grimace Scale. Sci Rep 2019; 9(1):19128.

30. Merola I, Mills DS. Behavioural signs of pain in cats: an expert consensus. PLoS One 2016;11(2):1–15.

31. Steagall PV, Benito J, Monteiro BP, et al. Analgesic effects of gabapentin and buprenorphine in cats undergoing ovariohysterectomy using two pain-scoring systems: a randomized clinical trial. J Feline Med Surg 2018;20(8):741–8.

32. Holden E, Calvo G, Collins M, et al. Evaluation of facial expression in acute pain in cats. J Small Anim Pract 2014;55(12):615–21.

33. Finka LR, Luna SP, Brondani JT, et al. Geometric morphometrics for the study of facial expressions in non-human animals, using the domestic cat as an exemplar. Sci Rep 2019;9(1):9883.

34. Dawson L, Cheal J, Niel L, et al. Humans can identify cats' affective states from subtle facial expressions. Anim Welf 2019;28(4):519–31.

35. Benito J, Monteiro BP, Beauchamp G, et al. Evaluation of interobserver agreement for postoperative pain and sedation assessment in cats. J Am Vet Med Assoc 2017;251(5):544–51.

36. Doodnaught GM, Benito J, Monteiro BP, et al. Agreement among undergraduate and graduate veterinary students and veterinary anesthesiologists on pain assessment in cats and dogs: A preliminary study. Can Vet J 2017;58(8):805–8.

37. Davis LE, Donnelly EJ. Analgesic drugs in the cat. J Am Vet Med Assoc 1968; 153(9):1161–7.

38. Hickman MA, Cox SR, Mahabir S, et al. Safety, pharmacokinetics and use of the novel NK-1 receptor antagonist maropitant (Cerenia) for the prevention of emesis and motion sickness in cats. J Vet Pharmacol Ther 2008;31(3):220–9.

39. van Haaften KA, Forsythe LRE, Stelow EA, et al. Effects of a single preappointment dose of gabapentin on signs of stress in cats during transportation and veterinary examination. J Am Vet Med Assoc 2017;251(10):1175–81.

40. Stevens BJ, Frantz EM, Orlando JM, et al. Efficacy of a single dose of trazodone hydrochloride given to cats prior to veterinary visits to reduce signs of transport- and examination-related anxiety. J Am Vet Med Assoc 2016;249(2):202–7.

41. Hofmeister EH, Egger CM. Transdermal fentanyl patches in small animals. J Am Anim Hosp Assoc 2004;40(6):468–78.

42. Simon BT, Scallan EM, Monteiro BP, et al. The effects of aging on hydromorphone-induced thermal antinociception in healthy female cats. Pain Rep 2019;4(2):e722.

43. Giordano T, Steagall PVM, Ferreira TH, et al. Postoperative analgesic effects of intravenous, intramuscular, subcutaneous or oral transmucosal buprenorphine administered to cats undergoing ovariohysterectomy. Vet Anaesth Analg 2010; 37(4):357–66.

44. Steagall PVM, Pelligand L, Giordano T, et al. Pharmacokinetic and pharmacodynamic modelling of intravenous, intramuscular and subcutaneous buprenorphine in conscious cats. Vet Anaesth Analg 2013;40(1):83–95.

45. Robertson SA, Wegner K, Lascelles BDX. Antinociceptive and side-effects of hydromorphone after subcutaneous administration in cats. J Feline Med Surg 2009; 11(2):76–81.

46. Doodnaught GM, Monteiro BP, Benito J, et al. Pharmacokinetic and pharmacodynamic modelling after subcutaneous, intravenous and buccal administration of a highconcentration formulation of buprenorphine in conscious cats. PLoS One 2017;12(4):e0176443.

47. Brondani JT, Loureiro Luna SP, Beier SL, et al. Analgesic efficacy of perioperative use of vedaprofen, tramadol or their combination in cats undergoing ovariohysterectomy. J Feline Med Surg 2009;11(6):420–9.

48. Steagall PVM, Taylor PM, Brondani JT, et al. Antinociceptive effects of tramadol and acepromazine in cats. J Feline Med Surg 2008;10(1):24–31.

49. Pypendop BH, Ilkiw JE. Pharmacokinetics of tramadol, and its metabolite O-desmethyl-tramadol, in cats. J Vet Pharmacol Ther 2008;31:52–9.

50. Monteiro BP, Klinck MP, Moreau M, et al. Analgesic efficacy of tramadol in cats with naturally occurring osteoarthritis. PLoS One 2017;12(4):1–13.

51. Guedes AGP, Meadows JM, Pypendop BH, et al. Evaluation of tramadol for treatment of osteoarthritis in geriatric cats. J Am Vet Med Assoc 2018;252: 565–71.

52. Indrawirawan Y, McAlees T. Tramadol toxicity in a cat: case report and literature review of serotonin syndrome. J Feline Med Surg 2014;16(7):572–8.

53. King JN, Hot R, Reagan EL, et al. Safety of oral robenacoxib in the cat. J Vet Pharmacol Ther 2012;35(3):290–300.

54. Gunew MN, Menrath VH, Marshall RD. Long-term safety, efficacy and palatability of oral meloxicam at 0.01-0.03 mg/kg for treatment of osteoarthritic pain in cats. J Feline Med Surg 2008;10(3):235–41.

55. Ruel HLM, Steagall PV. Adjuvant analgesics in acute pain management. Vet Clin North Am Small Anim Pract 2019;49(6):1127–41.

56. Pozzi A, Muir WW, Traverso F. Prevention of central sensitization and pain by N-methyl-D-aspartate receptor antagonists. J Am Vet Med Assoc 2006;228(1): 53–60.

57. Steagall PVM, Monteiro-Steagall BP. Multimodal analgesia for perioperative pain in three cats. J Feline Med Surg 2013;15(8):737–43.

58. Steagall PVM, Aucoin M, Monteiro BP, et al. Clinical effects of a constant rate infusion of remifentanil, alone or in combination with ketamine, in cats anesthetized with isoflurane. J Am Vet Med Assoc 2015;246(9):976–81.

59. Cheng JK, Chiou LC. Mechanisms of the antinociceptive action of gabapentin. J Pharmacol Sci 2006;100(5):471–86.

60. Guedes AGP, Meadows JM, Pypendop BH, et al. Assessment of the effects of gabapentin on activity levels and owner-perceived mobility impairment and quality of life in osteoarthritic geriatric cats. J Am Vet Med Assoc 2018;253(5): 579–85.

61. Pankratz KE, Ferris KK, Griffith EH, et al. Use of single-dose oral gabapentin to attenuate fear responses in cage-trap confined community cats: a double-blind, placebo-controlled field trial. J Feline Med Surg 2018;20(6):535–43.

62. Siao KT, Pypendop BH, Ilkiw JE. Pharmacokinetics of gabapentin in cats. Am J Vet Res 2010;71(7):817–21.

63. Adrian D, Papich MG, Baynes R, et al. The pharmacokinetics of gabapentin in cats. J Vet Intern Med 2018;32(6):1996–2002.

64. Brondani JT, Luna SPL, Minto BW, et al. Validity and responsiveness of a multidimensional composite scale to assess postoperative pain in cats e. Arq Bras Med Vet Zootec 2012;64(6):1529–38.

65. Calvo G, Holden E, Reid J, et al. Development of a behaviour-based measurement tool with defined intervention level for assessing acute pain in cats. J Small Anim Pract 2014;55(12):622–9.

Feline Chronic Pain and Osteoarthritis

Beatriz P. Monteiro, DVM, PhD

KEYWORDS

- Affective • Analgesia • Cat • Feline • Chronic pain • Osteoarthritis
- Pain management • Welfare

KEY POINTS

- Perception of pain involves complex sensory and affective mechanisms that are influenced by emotions, past experiences, and social and environmental context.
- Chronic pain should be viewed as maladaptive, occurring in conditions including, but not restricted to, osteoarthritis.
- Clinical assessment of pain relies mainly on the use of clinical metrology instruments (ie, pain scoring tools) and quality-of-life questionnaires.
- Meloxicam, robenacoxib, tramadol, and gabapentin have been studied in cats with osteoarthritis-related pain. Amitriptyline and amantadine are potential therapies, although scientific evidence is poor. Emerging therapies include anti-nerve growth factor antibody, piprants, cannabinoids, and mesenchymal stem cell therapy.
- Emotions affect pain perception. Strategies to provide positive emotions, increase physical and mental activity, and reinforce the owner-cat bond are of utmost importance in the management of chronic painful conditions.

INTRODUCTION

Pain is a personal, complex, and multidimensional experience involving sensory and emotional components. The intensity of pain does not correlate linearly with the severity of the pathology; rather, it involves stress response and cognitive functions of the brain including fear, memory, anxiety, and distraction (**Fig. 1**). Genetics and neuro-hormonal mechanisms of stress are considered equally important in pain perception as the neural mechanisms of sensory transmission.[1,2]

Feline patients can be affected by a multitude of chronic painful conditions (**Box 1**). Chronic pain negatively affects quality of life (QoL), causes changes in behavior, and impacts health and welfare as well as the owner-companion animal bond.[3,4] Pain management is a significant ethical and economic component in the modern practice of veterinary medicine. It is considered to be the fourth vital sign.[3]

Department of Clinical Sciences, Faculty of Veterinary Medicine, Université de Montréal, 3200 Rue Sicotte, Saint Hyacinthe, Quebec J2S 2M2, Canada
E-mail address: beatrizpmonteiro@gmail.com

Vet Clin Small Anim 50 (2020) 769–788
https://doi.org/10.1016/j.cvsm.2020.02.003
0195-5616/20/© 2020 Elsevier Inc. All rights reserved.

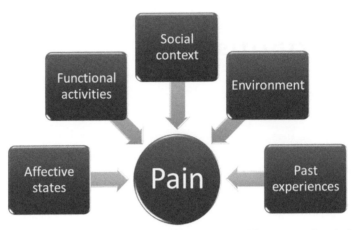

Fig. 1. Pain perception is influenced by internal and external factors associated with neuro-hormonal modulation of pain.

Most research in feline chronic pain relates to osteoarthritis (OA). This article reviews the recent advances in the assessment and treatment of OA in cats as a structure in which to discuss feline chronic pain.

RELEVANT CONCEPTS IN THE PATHOPHYSIOLOGY OF PAIN

Nociceptors are highly specialized structures in the skin, muscles, joints, and viscera.[5] Their activation by noxious stimuli results in the generation of an action potential that is then transmitted to the dorsal horn of the spinal cord where signal modulation occurs (ie, the nociceptive input can be inhibited [pain inhibition] or enhanced [pain

---

Box 1
Examples of chronic painful conditions in cats

- Degenerative joint disease and OA
- Cancer (including primary tumor, metastasis, diagnostic procedures, and therapy-related adverse-effects such as chemotherapy-induced neuropathy and radiation-induced skin burns)
- Orofacial conditions including feline orofacial pain syndrome (see the article in this issue by Epstein titled Feline Neuropathic Pain)
- Persistent postoperative pain (eg, onychectomy, other amputations, or thoracotomy)
- Trauma
- Skin conditions (eg, chronic dermatitis, chronic wounds)
- Otitis
- Ocular conditions (eg, corneal disease, ulcers, uveitis, and glaucoma)
- Gastrointestinal conditions (eg, inflammatory bowel disease, megacolon, and constipation)
- Idiopathic cystitis
- Feline hyperesthesia syndrome
- Diabetes-induced neuropathy

facilitation]). This signal is transmitted to the cerebral cortex, where pain is perceived, resulting in a series of autonomic, motor, and affective responses.

For most chronic painful conditions, inflammation is an important triggering factor. In OA, chronic tissue damage and low-grade inflammation produce and release inflammatory mediators. This process activates nociceptors and promotes a cycle of further joint destruction.[6]

When joint inflammation develops, the release of inflammatory mediators such as prostaglandins and nerve growth factor (NGF) render peripheral nociceptors hyperexcitable,[7] resulting in peripheral sensitization.

The sustained nociceptive input from the periphery to the spinal cord contributes to development of central sensitization, characterized by increased membrane excitability, facilitated synaptic strength, and decreased inhibitory mechanisms, resulting in neuroplasticity and wind-up.[5] These mechanisms are generally short lived and reversible; nevertheless, they can become pathologic in the face of sustained inflammation and/or nerve injury (see article titled Feline Neuropathic Pain by Epstein in this issue).

Chronic pain results from a mixture of inflammatory, neuropathic, and functional components (**Boxes 2** and **3**), resulting in a multitude of clinical presentations and response to therapy within a same clinical condition.

Clinically, patients develop hyperalgesia (ie, increased pain from a stimulus that normally provokes pain) and allodynia (ie, pain caused by a stimulus that does not normally provoke pain). (See Epstein, Feline Neuropathic Pain)

OSTEOARTHRITIS IN CATS

The pathophysiology of OA involves inflammatory, biomechanical, and metabolic components, resulting in degeneration of synovial joints. It causes long-term pain and physical dysfunction.[8,9] Age, obesity, metabolic disease, sex, lifestyle, joint trauma, and genetics are major risk factors for the development of OA in people[6] and likely the same is true in companion animals.

The prevalence of chronic pain or OA-related pain is unknown, but it is believed to affect a large number of cats. Evidence of radiographic OA is highest in older cats (however changes may be seen in cats as young as 1 year of age),[10] with 90% of cats older

---

Box 2
Characteristics of chronic pain

- Should be thought of as maladaptive pain (vs adaptive pain, which subsides once the primary lesion has healed)
- Outlasts the normal healing time of an acute disease process
- Serves no biological purpose
- Pain severity does not correlate with severity of the disease
- Can be associated with a primary condition (eg, OA) or it can exist by itself (ie, with no detectable primary condition such as in functional pain)
- Can have acute episodes within a relatively stable chronic manifestation (so-called acute on chronic)
- Can be spontaneous, constant, or induced by movement and can manifest as different sensations (eg, sharp, burning, tingling, or numbness)
- Has large individual variability in terms of clinical presentation and response to treatment

---

Box 3
Types of pain

- Nociceptive pain: physiologic pain that serves a purpose and usually subsides once the potential or actual tissue damage is no longer present (ie, adaptive pain)

- Inflammatory pain: involves the release of inflammatory mediators

- Neuropathic pain: pain caused by a lesion or disease of the somatosensory nervous system

- (Dys)Functional pain: pain disorders for which no pathology or organic disease is found after comprehensive search to explain the pain

- Cancer pain: some authors claim that cancer pain should be regarded as a fifth entity because of complex interactions between cancers and the somatosensory system

---

than 12 year old being affected.[11] Although some differences exist among studies, the thoracic vertebral column (T7-T10) is most frequently affected, whereas the lumbar or lumbosacral regions show the most severe lesions.[10–13] In the appendicular skeleton, the elbow and hips are most commonly affected, followed by the stifle and tarsus.[10–14]

ASSESSMENT OF OSTEOARTHRITIS-RELATED CHRONIC PAIN

Identifying chronic pain in cats can be challenging. Cats with OA frequently have bilateral disease, and lameness is not seen as commonly as in dogs.[8,9,15] Interactions with cats are different than with dogs: cats move when and if they want to rather than being taken for walks, runs, or to play catch. Coupled with their small body size and frequent stress response during examination, clinical signs of OA are difficult to diagnose.[16] The sensory component of pain is assessed using quantitative sensory testing (QST) and physical examination in the research and clinical settings, respectively. The affective component of pain is assessed with the goal of understanding how much the pain affects the cat's life in terms of physical function and emotional state. Gait analysis and accelerometer-based activity monitoring are used as objective measures of limb function and mobility, respectively, and as indirect markers of functional disability particularly in the research setting. Clinical metrology instruments (CMIs) are used as subjective measures of pain and QoL. A summary of these assessment tools in cats is presented.

Quantitative Sensory Testing

In QST, calibrated devices are used to induce a noxious stimulus (eg, mechanical, thermal, electrical) against the skin of the animal until a behavioral reaction is observed. The end point is objectively recorded (eg, value in Newtons, grams, °C, seconds, number of repetitions) (**Fig. 2**). Quantification of sensory sensitivity allows researchers to compare animals with and without disease, as well as the effects of treatment.

The recent use of QST in cats (**Table 1**) has provided information to show that cats with OA present with hyperalgesia, allodynia and facilitated temporal summation of pain when compared with healthy cats, reflecting peripheral and central sensitization mechanisms of pain, similar to what is reported in people and dogs.[17,18]

Gait Analysis

Gait analysis provides information on the ground reaction forces produced by each paw during the gait cycle.[19] Using peak vertical force (PVF), studies have shown that cats with OA have lower PVF when compared with healthy individuals.[20–22]

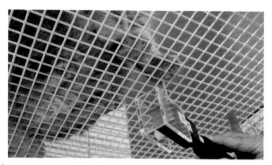

Fig. 2. Example of quantitative sensory testing. The cat is gently placed on a cage with mesh floor. The observer pushes the probe against the metacarpal pad of the cat until a behavior response (eg, paw withdrawal). The maximum amount of force used to elicit this response is defined as the punctate mechanical threshold of that individual.

However, when PVF was used to study the effects of analgesics in comparison with placebo, most cats seem to improve regardless of treatment.[22,23] This could be a result of increased physical activity, muscle mass and joint stability, and increased cognitive stimulus that are acquired by cats during training and acclimation for PVF testing.

The feasibility and repeatability of PVF in untrained client-owned cats have been investigated in a few studies.[24,25] In general, the test was not feasible in a large portion of cats, resulting in decreased test sensitivity for discriminating healthy from osteoarthritic cats.[24,25]

Accelerometer-Based Activity Monitoring

Activity is assessed using collar-attached accelerometer devices that continuously record changes in acceleration (**Fig. 3**).[20,21,23,26–28] Collected data have been correlated with distance moved using simultaneous video analysis,[27] as well as with scores from clinical metrology instruments (CMIs).[22,28–31]

In studies assessing analgesic treatments, motor activity generally increased after treatment in research and client-owned cats with OA.[20,22,28,31,32] However, its ability to differentiate healthy from cats with OA is not evident, with conflicting results among studies.[20–22,33] This might be explained by the large variability in mobility among cats and by the approach to data analysis.

Recently, actimetry data from client-owned cats were evaluated using functional data analysis. Marked intercat variability was detected, and activity was not always lower in osteoarthritic cats; however, peaks and troughs of activity were less extreme than those of healthy cats.[26] Cats exhibited a bimodal pattern of activity, with a sharp peak in the morning and broader peak in the evening. Additionally, there were differences between activity patterns during weekdays and weekends, reflecting the influence of human activity.[34]

Clinical Metrology Instruments

In the clinical setting, owner-reported behavioral signs remain the best assessment tool of feline chronic pain. Yet, perceived efficacy of a treatment by proxy (ie, owners) seems to be largely overinflated. A recent study reported that up to 70% of cats given a placebo treatment might be assessed as successful treatment as measured by improved ability to perform activities.[35]

Specific behaviors are collected using CMIs, QoL or health-related QoL (HRQoL) questionnaires (**Table 2**). These instruments are constructed based on rigorous

Table 1
Studies using quantitative sensory testing in healthy cats and those with osteoarthritis

Population	Quantitative Sensory Testing	Body Location	Main Findings	Reference
Research cats: • 39 cats with spontaneous OA • 6 healthy cats	PMT using electronic von Frey	Palmar or plantar aspect of the metacarpal or metatarsal pad	• Cats with OA had significantly lower values • Test had good repeatability over time • Around 30% of cats were classified as having allodynia according to pre-established threshold • No change in threshold after treatment with meloxicam, but improvement in function using motor activity and kinetics	22
Research cats: • 10 cats with spontaneous OA • 4 healthy cats	PMT using electronic von Frey MTS[a]	PMT: palmar or plantar aspect of the metacarpal or metatarsal pad MTS: Cranial to the midradius	• PMT: cats with OA had significantly lower values • MTS: cats with OA responded earlier to the repetitive mechanical stimulus when compared with healthy cats • PMT was positively correlated with MTS	21
Research cats: • 15 cats with spontaneous OA • 5 healthy cats	MTS[a]	Cranial to the midradius	• Cats with OA responded earlier to the repetitive mechanical stimulus when compared with healthy cats • MTS improved in cats after tramadol, but not after placebo treatment	20
Research cats: • 15 cats with spontaneous OA	MTS[a]	Cranial to the midradius	• MTS only improved in cats receiving meloxicam-tramadol, and not in cats receiving meloxicam only	23
Client-owned cats: • 7 cats with spontaneous OA • 14 healthy cats	PMT using electronic and manual von Frey Thermal latency using a hot and a cold plate	PMT: palmar or plantar aspect of the metacarpal or metatarsal pad Thermal latency: plantar and palmar surface	• All QST were considered moderately repeatable • PMT using manual or electronic von Frey was different between osteoarthritic and healthy cats • Thermal latency to cold stimulus was different between osteoarthritic and healthy cats • Thermal latency to hot stimulus was not different between healthy and osteoarthritic cats	25

Population	Method	Location	Findings	
Client-owned cats: • 15 healthy cats	PMT using electronic and manual von Frey	Upper lip and medial aspect of the stifle	• Cats were evaluated twice on two consecutive days and they were much less cooperative on the second day • Cats evaluated in the presence of the owners were considered more cooperative • Agreement between manual and electronic von Frey was fair	66
Client-owned cats: • 13 healthy cats	PMT using electronic von Frey and SMALGO	Medial aspect of stifle and lumbosacral joint	• Cats were evaluated by 2 observers twice (45-min interval) and were less cooperative on the second round of testing, with consistently decreased thresholds • Inter-rater reliability was fair, and interdevice reliability was good	67

Abbreviations: MTS, mechanical temporal summation; PMT, punctate mechanical threshold; SMALGO, small animal algometer.

[a] MTS is considered as a measure of spinal-wind up, which is in turn, interpreted as central sensitization.

Data from Refs.[20–23,25,66,67]

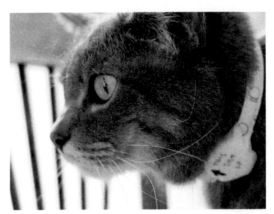

Fig. 3. A cat wearing a collar-attached accelerometer-based activity monitor.

research to identify and validate key behaviors that are indicative of pain or QoL. They generally include questions pertaining to mobility, ability and willingness to perform activities, sociability, and self-care (eg, eating or grooming).

A checklist was recently developed in an effort to increase awareness of OA in cats and to provide an easy, quick and practical tool for screening of cats with OA-associated pain.[36] The Feline Musculoskeletal Pain Screening Checklist (Feline MiPSC) is used as a starting point for discussion of feline OA with owners and to check the need of further veterinary investigation.[36] Briefly, the Feline MiPSC is comprised of six items asking if a specific activity can be performed normally or not. If any of the items is scored as 'no' (ie, the activity is not normal), this should prompt further evaluation with a more detailed screening.[36]

Based on the current literature, the following approach is suggested. The Feline MiPSC is used as a screening tool, whereas other tools such as the FMPI, CSOM or MI-CAT might be used for monitoring treatment efficacy.[36]

Quality of Life and Health-Related Quality of Life

Although studies generally lack a definition, QoL and HRQoL questionnaires measure different things. Assessment of QoL takes in consideration all aspects of a pet's life,[37] whereas HRQoL refers to the effect of a medical condition on the physical and emotional health of the individual (see **Table 2**).[38]

To date there is no single instrument that has been thoroughly validated and is freely available for use in clinical practice. Nevertheless, the clinician should attempt to use what is available to assess QoL in cats with chronic pain, particularly in advanced disease and end-of-life decisions. Research on this topic is advancing, and hopefully these instruments will be incorporated into everyday practice in the near future.

Clinical Signs

Clinical signs of chronic pain are generally subtle and progress slowly (**Table 3**). Recognition relies mostly on owner-reported changes in behaviors (expression of new behaviors and disappearance of old behaviors).

In cats with OA, pain and loss of function are the main clinical signs (eg, decreased activity, decreased ability to perform routine behaviors [eg, grooming, using the litter box, exploring elevated surfaces], and decreased socialization) (**Fig. 4**).

Cats with OA show significant differences in responses during orthopedic examination when compared with sound cats[36] and are less friendly.[39] These behaviors might

Table 2
Summary of published clinical metrology instruments, quality of life, and health-related quality of life questionnaires for use in cats with chronic painful conditions (alphabetical order)

Type	Condition	Name or Description	Comments	References
HRQoL	Cancer	Cancer Treatment Form	Only a preliminary assessment (face validity) of the instrument has been performed; available within the published article	68
HRQoL	Any	Cat Health and Wellbeing (CHEW)	Preliminary validation has been performed; available as supplementary file within the original article	69
CMI	OA	Client-specific outcome measure (CSOM)	One of the most extensively studied and valid instruments; available at: www.cvm.ncsu.edu/research/labs/clinical-sciences/comparative-pain-research/clinical-metrology-instruments	28,32,52,70
CMI	OA	Feline musculoskeletal pain index (FMPI)	One of the most extensively studied and valid instruments; available at: www.cvm.ncsu.edu/research/labs/clinical-sciences/comparative-pain-research/clinical-metrology-instruments	30,32,35,36,52,70–72
Checklist	OA	Feline Musculoskeletal Pain Screening Checklist (Feline MiPSC)	Developed and tested to screen for cats with OA-associated pain and also used to increase owner awareness of OA in cats; available within the published article	36
HRQoL	Any	Feline QoL measure	Preliminary validation has been performed; its comprising items are described in the original article	73
CMI	OA	Montreal Instrument for Cat Arthritis Testing for use by caretakers (MICAT(C))	Preliminary validation has been performed; available as a supplementary file within the original article	31

(continued on next page)

Table 2
(continued)

Type	Condition	Name or Description	Comments	References
CMI	OA	Montreal Instrument for Cat Arthritis Testing for use by veterinarians (MICAT(V))	Preliminary validation and refinement have been performed; available as a supplementary file within the original articles	46,74
CMI	OA	Owner Behavior Watch (OBW)	Preliminary validation has been performed; its comprising items are described in the original article	8
HRQoL	Any	VetMetrica HRQL for cats	Preliminary validation and reliability testing have been performed; available as a Web-based instrument via paid subscription. There is initial evidence suggesting that this tool can differentiate between healthy cats and cats with mild and moderate/severe OA; further validation of this instrument may prove it useful in the staging of cats with OA	75,76
CMI	OA	Zamprogno Question Bank	The items identified in this instrument were later used to construct the FMPI	71

Note that the definitions of QoL and HRQoL are not uniformly described among studies.
Data from Refs.[8,30–32,35,36,46,52,68–76]

be indicative of negative emotions related with long-standing pain and consequent poor animal welfare states.

Radiographic signs of OA do not correlate well with clinical signs of pain (**Box 4**). This is well documented in human medicine[40] and a common finding in feline practice.[39]

TREATMENT OF CHRONIC PAIN IN CATS

Treatment of chronic pain relies on the use of pharmacologic and nonpharmacologic approaches. Ideally, only nonpharmacological therapy is used in early disease with mild pain. As disease progresses and pain increases, analgesics are added to the treatment protocol. A summary of the available evidence from the most commonly used therapies is described.

Current and Emerging Drug Therapies

Ideally, analgesic treatment of chronic pain should be mechanism-based. This means that the mechanism of action of the chosen agent should target the pain mechanisms

Table 3
Owner-reported and clinician-observed changes in behavior and clinical signs of chronic pain in cats

Category	Description of Behavioral and Clinical Sign
Mobility and ability to perform activities	Peaks and troughs of activity are less extreme Movement seems stiffer and less fluid Daily distance moved is decreased Difficulty in getting up after sleeping/long rest Hesitation to, or avoidance of, jumping up or down Use of steps to reach high or low surfaces instead of jumping up or down Difficulty in getting up or down the stairs Decreased or loss of interest in play and exploratory activities
Social interactions	Decreased interaction with owners and other animals Seems less friendly and more irritable Isolation Loss of interest toward activities that used to interest the cat such as novelties (eg, new object or new person), toys, or distractions through a window Adverse reaction when picked up
Self-care	Greasy hair coat and dirty nails Excessive grooming and or self-plucking leading to areas of alopecia Decreased scratching and stretching behavior Changes in food and water intake (quantity and behaviors) Difficulty with food prehension/mastication while eating (ie, drops kibble while chewing; takes longer to eat) Eliminating habits are affected – misuse of litter box because of difficulty in getting into or out of the litter box
Hypersensitivity reactions	Aversive response to pain during orthopedic examination Resents being touched, petted or brushed Sudden episodes of vocalization and running away without any apparent reason Sudden episodes of looking at a region of the body (usually mid to lower back or tail) followed by licking, hair plucking or biting (self-mutilation) without any apparent reason

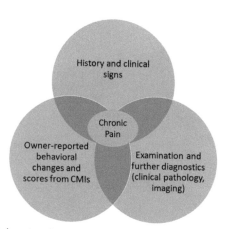

Fig. 4. Components of chronic pain assessment. CMIs: clinical metrology instruments. (*Adapted from* Bergadano A. Diagnosis of chronic pain in small animals. *EJCAP.* 2010;20(1):55-60.)

> **Box 4**
> **Are radiographs useful in the diagnosis of OA-related pain?**
>
> A cat may present with normal radiographs yet have joint pain, or vice versa. In 1 study, 34% of painful joints lacked radiographic signs of OA.[12] Another study found that the correlation between radiographic findings and pain on palpation is influenced by the joint in question.[39] Regardless, a behavioral reaction elicited during joint palpation should be interpreted as possible evidence of OA,[36] indicating the need of further diagnostics (although the absence of radiographic changes does not rule out OA).
>
> The lack of correlation between radiographic and clinical signs could be because of the lack of detail in radiographs that would enable detection of early changes of the joint. MRI provides superior sensitivity to detect early joint lesions,[33] but its use is limited by cost, need for general anesthesia, and availability. Another explanation for this discrepancy in correlation is that joint pain is influenced by many factors other than joint lesions (**Fig. 5**). For example, a neuropathic pain component may predominate in individuals with minor joint changes yet high levels of pain refractory to analgesic treatment.

affecting that patient. For example, nonsteroidal anti-inflammatories drugs (NSAIDs) are administered when there is predominantly inflammatory pain; antidepressants acting on serotonin pathways are administered when there is predominantly pain disinhibition. This approach has been published in people,[41,42] and some data also exist in cats with OA.[20,22] The main challenge is that clinical pain is normally a mixture of different pain mechanisms (see **Box 3**). Thus, clinically, individual treatment protocols are based on therapeutic trial. It is believed that an analgesic agent should be administered for at least 4 weeks before deciding on treatment efficacy (provided

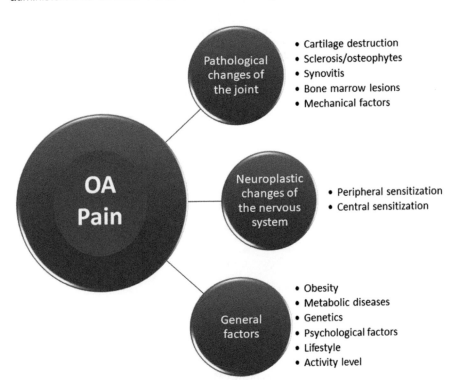

Fig. 5. Factors contributing to joint pain in patients with OA.

there are no adverse effects). Drugs labeled for use in cats should be the first choice because of safety and efficacy data, and they are generally more palatable and easier to administer long term. The most commonly used analgesics in the treatment of chronic pain are detailed in **Table 4**.

NSAIDs inhibit the expression of cyclooxygenase enzymes in cell membranes, decreasing the release of inflammatory mediators. They are widely used in the treatment of chronic pain in cats, and enough data exist to support long-term use in cats with OA. Particularly, meloxicam and robenacoxib have been shown to be safe when administered to cats with concomitant OA and stable chronic kidney disease. Recent reviews on this topic provide further information.[43,44]

Table 4		
Commonly used analgesics for the management of feline chronic pain		
Analgesic	**Dosing Recommendations**	**Comments**
Amantadine	3–5 mg/kg, orally, every 12–24 h	• Should be used as an adjuvant drug in combination with other analgesics • Scientific information on its efficacy or safety for long-term treatment in cats is not yet available
Amitriptyline	1–4 mg/kg, orally, every 12–24 h	• Reported sedation, weight gain, and decreased grooming after 12 mo of treatment • Should not be administered in combination with other serotoninergic drugs because of the risk of serotonin toxicity • Little scientific information available in cats with idiopathic cystitis
Gabapentin	5–10 mg/kg, orally, every 8–12 h	• Sedation and ataxia may be observed • Much higher doses have been anecdotally reported • Reported efficacy in cats with OA; sedation is a possible adverse-effect
Meloxicam	Loading dose of 0.1 mg/kg, orally, once followed by 0.05 mg/kg, orally, every 24 h	• Most common adverse-effects are gastrointestinal (GI) signs (vomiting, diarrhea, anorexia) • No evidence of renal or hepatic toxicity after long-term treatment. • Seems to be safe when administered to cats with stable chronic kidney disease [CKD] (especially IRIS I and II cats with normal drinking and eating habits) • Efficacy is dose-dependent; administration of the minimum effective dose (0.01–0.03 mg/kg) should be attempted if there are concerns with potential adverse-effects
		(continued on next page)

Table 4 (continued)		
Analgesic	**Dosing Recommendations**	**Comments**
Robenacoxib	1–2.4 mg/kg, orally, every 24 h	• Most common adverse-effects are GI signs (vomiting, diarrhea, anorexia) • No evidence of renal or hepatic toxicity after long-term treatment. • Seems to be safe when administered to cats with stable CKD (especially IRIS I and II cats with normal drinking and eating habits) • Efficacy has not yet been reported • Administration of the minimum effective dose should be attempted to decrease the risk of adverse-effects
Tramadol	2–5 mg/kg, orally, every 8–12 h	• Sedation or euphoria, vomiting, and constipation may be observed • Salivation may be observed after administration because of the bitter taste • Treatment is unacceptable to some cats when palatability is an issue; forced pilling could impair owner-cat bond and compromise feline welfare • Should not be administered in combination with other serotoninergic drugs because of the risk of serotonin toxicity • Reported efficacy in cats with osteoarthritis

Tramadol acts mainly by binding to μ-opioid receptors and the reuptake of serotonin and norepinephrine. It has been shown to decrease central sensitization and to improve motor activity and global QoL in cats with OA (2–4 mg/kg every 12 h, for 5–19 days).[20,23,45] Although it seems to be safe and provide analgesia, oral tramadol is bitter, making it unsuitable for many cats.

Gabapentin is a calcium channel blocker that reduces neuronal excitability. It decreased hypersensitivity in research cats with OA when administered at 10 mg/kg, every 8 hours, for 30 days.[46] In client-owned cats, treatment with gabapentin (10 mg/kg, every 12 h for 2 weeks) was compared with placebo; cats receiving gabapentin showed improved owner-identified impaired activities (CSOM), but decreased motor activity, likely because of sedation.[47] Because of the large safety margin and robust evidence of efficacy in human neuropathic pain, gabapentin is currently recommended in the management of feline chronic and neuropathic pain.

Amitriptyline is a tricyclic antidepressant acting mainly via inhibition of serotonin and norepinephrine reuptake, thus reinforcing inhibitory mechanisms of pain. It improved clinical signs in most cats with severe recurrent idiopathic cystitis when administered at 10 mg/d for 12 months.[48] In other studies using 5 or 10 mg/d for 7 days, no efficacy was observed.[49,50] This was likely because of the short duration of treatment, especially considering that an analgesic trial of a minimum of 4 weeks is recommended in people.[51]

Amantadine is an antagonist of N-methyl D-aspartate (NMDA) receptors and is used to treat central sensitization. Although studies on its efficacy are lacking, amantadine is anecdotally administered as an adjuvant to cats with chronic pain that are refractory to NSAIDs.

Feline-specific anti-NGF antibody is a promising therapy in management of chronic pain. Nerve growth factor contributes to peripheral and central sensitization, and its concentrations are increased in chronic painful conditions including OA and neoplasia. In a pilot study in cats with OA, a single treatment with feline-specific anti-NGF antibody administered subcutaneously increased motor activity and improved CSOM scores for 3 to 6 weeks.[52]

Grapiprant is a prostaglandin E4 receptor antagonist with analgesic and anti-inflammatory effects through selectively inhibiting a single prostanoid receptor without inhibiting other homeostatic functions of prostaglandins. It is labeled for use in dogs with OA. Although it has a good safety profile, its efficacy in feline chronic pain is unknown.[53]

Mesenchymal stem cell therapy has immunomodulatory and anti-inflammatory effects. Although not evaluated for OA, a small recent study reported complete remission or substantial clinical improvement in cats with severe refractory gingivostomatitis after 2 monthly intravenous injections of autologous adipose-derived mesenchymal stem cells.[54]

Cannabinoids bind to cannabinoid receptors and modulate the release of neurotransmitters. Analgesic effects observed in people with chronic pain might be primarily related to a reduction in the affective, but not sensory, perception of pain.[55] Robust efficacy data are not yet available in veterinary medicine. Veterinarians should remember that dose-response studies and dosage regimens for potential clinical use in cats are lacking. Formulations of oil-based products are variable, and little is known on the safety and efficacy of such compounds. A recent study showed clear differences in the pharmacokinetic profile after administration of a single dose of CBD-infused fish oil (2 mg/kg orally) between dogs and cats, so extrapolation between species is not viable.[56] Furthermore, in 8 cats administered the CBD oil twice daily, serum biochemistries and complete blood count were evaluated before and every 4 weeks for 12 weeks. No clinically significant changes were noted. Excessive licking and head shaking during oil administration were frequently observed.[56] Larger safety and pharmacodynamic studies are still needed.

Bisphosphonates are used to manage bone cancer pain; they decrease bone resorption and tumor-associated osteolytic lesions. Although no adverse effects were seen in cats with bone-invasive tumors,[57] efficacy remains unknown.

Nonpharmacological Treatments

The potential benefits of nondrug therapies in the management of chronic pain are enormous but underappreciated, particularly as one better understands the role of affective states on pain perception.[1,2] Work in this aspect of pain management is lacking in veterinary medicine, and an awareness of potential benefits is needed. It is generally accepted that a positive emotional and mental state decreases pain and vice versa. Therefore, promoting a positive emotional state can potentially provide analgesia and improve feline welfare.

Sedentary lifestyle and obesity are common findings in domestic cats, and both factors are known to contribute to chronic pain. Physical therapy and weight control play an important part in preventing and managing chronic pain.

Environmental enrichment to promote the expression of species-specific behaviors provides physical and mental stimulation (**Fig. 6**). This modality decreases pain and

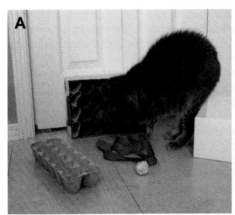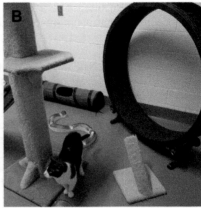

Fig. 6. Examples of (A) home-made and (B) commercially available environmental enrichment options.

stress and increases activity and mobility. Many resources are available, particularly for indoor-housed cats.[58–60]

Psychological treatments including cognitive behavioral therapy are used in human medicine for the treatment of chronic pain with strong evidence for reducing pain, disability, and anxiety.[61,62] Similarly, cognitive enrichment of shelter cats improved measures of affect and health.[63] Although data are lacking on the effects of cognitive enrichment on chronic pain in cats, strategies to provide mental stimulation such as environmental enrichment and play sessions (eg, 10 minutes, 2–3 times/d) are strongly recommended. The clinician could include these treatments on the discharge form to enhance owner compliance.

Acupuncture is believed to produce analgesia via neuromodulatory effects. Although it is a recognized pain management modality in people with chronic pain, data are not available in cats. In cats undergoing ovariohysterectomy, laser acupuncture decreased the postoperative analgesic requirement.[64]

Massage reduces stress, pain, tension, and discomfort in pediatric chronic pain patients.[65] Owners can be trained to perform massage and passive range of motion exercises in their cats. This might further reinforce the owner-pet bond.

Transcutaneous electrical nerve stimulation, photobiomodulation therapy, and targeted pulse electromagnetic field therapy have the potential to reduce pain and inflammation. No data are available in cats.

Euthanasia should be regarded as a final treatment strategy in cases of severe pain that is refractory to treatment or when pain cannot be managed because of financial or time commitment restraints.

DISCLOSURE

Dr. Monteiro has provided consultancy services to Zoetis and Vetoquinol.

REFERENCES

1. Roy M, Piche M, Chen J-I, et al. Cerebral and spinal modulation of pain by emotions. Proc Natl Acad Sci U S A 2009;106(49):20900–5.

2. Melzack R, Katz J. Pain. Wiley Interdiscip Rev Cogn Sci 2013;4:1–15.

3. Mathews K, Kronen P, Lascelles D, et al. Guidelines for recognition, assessment and treatment of pain: WSAVA Global Pain Council. J Small Anim Pract 2014;55: E10–68.

4. Monteiro B, Lascelles BDX. Assessment and recognition of chronic (maladaptive) pain. In: Steagall PVM, Robertson SA, Taylor PM, editors. Feline anesthesia and pain management. 1st edition. Hoboken (NJ): Wiley/Blackwell; 2017. p. 241–56.

5. Klinck MP, Troncy E. The physiology and pathophysiology of pain. In: Duke-Novakovski T, de Vries M, Seymour C, editors. BSAVA manual of canine and feline anaesthesia and analgesia. Gloucester, UK: BSAVA; 2016. p. 97–112.

6. Mobasheri A, Batt M. An update on the pathophysiology of osteoarthritis. Ann Phys Rehabil Med 2016;59(5–6):333–9.

7. Enomoto M, Mantyh PW, Murrell J, et al. Antinerve growth factor monoclonal antibodies for the control of pain in dogs and cats. Vet Rec 2019;184(1):23.

8. Bennett D, Morton C. A study of owner observed behavioural and lifestyle changes in cats with musculoskeletal disease before and after analgesic therapy. J Feline Med Surg 2009;11:997–1004.

9. Lascelles BDX. Feline degenerative joint disease. Vet Surg 2010;39(1):2–13.

10. Lascelles BDX, Henry JB, Brown J, et al. Cross-sectional study of the prevalence of radiographic degenerative joint disease in domesticated cats. Vet Surg 2010; 39(5):535–44.

11. Hardie EM, Roe SC, Martin FR. Radiographic evidence of degenerative joint disease in geriatric cats: 100 cases (1994-1997). J Am Vet Med Assoc 2002;220(5): 628–32.

12. Clarke SP, Bennett D. Feline osteoarthritis: a prospective study of 28 cases. J Small Anim Pract 2006;47:439–45.

13. Clarke SP, Mellor D, Clements DN, et al. Prevalence of radiographic signs of degenerative joint disease in a hospital population of cats. Vet Rec 2005;157: 793–9.

14. Godfrey DR. Osteoarthritis in cats: a retrospective radiological study. J Small Anim Pract 2005;46(9):425–9.

15. Slingerland LI, Hazewinkel HAW, Meij BP, et al. Cross-sectional study of the prevalence and clinical features of osteoarthritis in 100 cats. Vet J 2011;187(3):304–9.

16. Monteiro BP, Steagall PV. Chronic pain in cats: Recent advances in clinical assessment. J Feline Med Surg 2019;21(7):601–14.

17. Arendt-Nielsen L, Nie H, Laursen MB, et al. Sensitization in patients with painful knee osteoarthritis. Pain 2010;149(3):573–81.

18. Knazovicky D, Helgeson ES, Case B, et al. Widespread somatosensory sensitivity in naturally occurring canine model of osteoarthritis. Pain 2016;157(6):1325–32.

19. Schnabl E, Bockstahler B. Systematic review of ground reaction force measurements in cats. Vet J 2015;206(1):83–90.

20. Monteiro BP, Klinck MP, Moreau M, et al. Analgesic efficacy of tramadol in cats with naturally occurring osteoarthritis. PLoS One 2017;12(4):1–13.

21. Guillot M, Taylor PM, Rialland P, et al. Evoked temporal summation in cats to highlight central sensitization related to osteoarthritis-associated chronic pain: A preliminary study. PLoS One 2014;9(5):e97347.

22. Guillot M, Moreau M, Heit M, et al. Characterization of osteoarthritis in cats and meloxicam efficacy using objective chronic pain evaluation tools. Vet J 2013; 196(3):360–7.

23. Monteiro BP, Klinck MP, Moreau M, et al. Analgesic efficacy of an oral transmucosal spray formulation of meloxicam alone or in combination with tramadol in cats with naturally occurring osteoarthritis. Vet Anaesth Analg 2016;43(6):643–51.

24. Lascelles BDX, Findley K, Correa M, et al. Kinetic evaluation of normal walking and jumping in cats, using a pressure-sensitive walkway. Vet Rec 2007; 160(15):512–6.

25. Addison ES, Clements DN. Repeatability of quantitative sensory testing in healthy cats in a clinical setting with comparison to cats with osteoarthritis. J Feline Med Surg 2017;19(12):1274–82.

26. Gruen ME, Alfaro-Córdoba M, Thomson AE, et al. The use of functional data analysis to evaluate activity in a spontaneous model of degenerative joint disease associated pain in cats. PLoS One 2017;12(1):1–23.

27. Lascelles BDX, Hansen BD, Thomson A, et al. Evaluation of a digitally integrated accelerometer-based activity monitor for the measurement of activity in cats. Vet Anaesth Analg 2008;35(2):173–83.

28. Lascelles BDX, Hansen BD, Roe S, et al. Evaluation of client-specific outcome measures and activity monitoring to measure pain relief in cats with osteoarthritis. J Vet Intern Med 2007;21(3):410–6.

29. Klinck M, Rialland P, Guillot M, et al. Preliminary validation and reliability testing of the Montreal Instrument for Cat Arthritis Testing, for use by veterinarians, in a colony of laboratory cats. Animals 2015;5(4):1252–67.

30. Benito J, Hansen B, Depuy V, et al. Feline musculoskeletal pain index: responsiveness and testing of criterion validity. J Vet Intern Med 2013;27(3):474–82.

31. Klinck MP, Gruen ME, del Castillo JRE, et al. Development and preliminary validity and reliability of the montreal instrument for cat arthritis testing, for use by caretaker/owner, MI-CAT(C), via a randomised clinical trial. Appl Anim Behav Sci 2018;200:96–105.

32. Gruen ME, Griffith EH, Thomson AE, et al. Criterion validation testing of clinical metrology instruments for measuring degenerative joint disease associated mobility impairment in cats. PLoS One 2015;10(7):e0131839.

33. Guillot M, Moreau M, D'Anjou M-A, et al. Evaluation of osteoarthritis in cats: novel information from a pilot study. Vet Surg 2012;41(3):328–35.

34. Piccione G, Marafioti S, Giannetto C, et al. Comparison of daily distribution of rest/activity in companion cats and dogs. Biol Rhythm Res 2014;45(4):615–23.

35. Gruen ME, Dorman DC, Lascelles BDX. Caregiver placebo effect in analgesic clinical trials for cats with naturally occurring degenerative joint disease-associated pain. Vet Rec 2017;180(19):473.

36. Enomoto M, Lascelles BDX, Gruen ME, et al. Development of a checklist for the detection of degenerative joint disease-associated pain in cats. J Fel Med Surg 2020. https://doi.org/10.1177/1098612X20907424.

37. McMillan FD. Quality of life in animals. J Am Vet Med Assoc 2000;216(12): 1904–10.

38. Freeman LM, Rush JE, Oyama Ma, et al. Development and evaluation of a questionnaire for assessment of health-related quality of life in cats with cardiac disease. J Am Vet Med Assoc 2012;240(10):1188–93.

39. Lascelles BDX, Dong YH, Marcellin-Little DJ, et al. Relationship of orthopedic examination, goniometric measurements, and radiographic signs of degenerative joint disease in cats. BMC Vet Res 2012;8. https://doi.org/10.1186/1746-6148-8-10.

40. Finan PH, Buenaver LF, Bounds SC, et al. Discordance between pain and radiographic severity in knee osteoarthritis. Arthritis Rheum 2013;65(2):363–72.

41. Yarnitsky D, Granot M, Nahman-Averbuch H, et al. Conditioned pain modulation predicts duloxetine efficacy in painful diabetic neuropathy. Pain 2012;153(6): 1193–8.

42. Edwards RR, Dolman AJ, Martel MO, et al. Variability in conditioned pain modulation predicts response to NSAID treatment in patients with knee osteoarthritis. BMC Musculoskelet Disord 2016;17(1):284.

43. Monteiro B, Steagall PVM, Lascelles BDX, et al. Long-term use of non-steroidal anti-inflammatory drugs in cats with chronic kidney disease: from controversy to optimism. J Small Anim Pract 2019;1–4. https://doi.org/10.1111/jsap.13012.

44. Monteiro B, Steagall PV. Antiinflammatory drugs. Vet Clin North Am Small Anim Pract 2019;49(6):993–1011.

45. Guedes AGP, Meadows JM, Pypendop BH, et al. Evaluation of tramadol for treatment of osteoarthritis in geriatric cats. J Am Vet Med Assoc 2018;252:565–71.

46. Klinck MP, Monteiro BP, Lussier B, et al. Refinement of the Montreal instrument for cat arthritis testing, for use by veterinarians: detection of naturally occurring osteoarthritis in laboratory cats. J Feline Med Surg 2018;20(8):728–40.

47. Guedes AGP, Meadows JM, Pypendop BH, et al. Assessment of the effects of gabapentin on activity levels and owner-perceived mobility impairment and quality of life in osteoarthritic geriatric cats. J Am Vet Med Assoc 2018;253(5):579–85.

48. Chew DJ, Buffington CAT, Kendall MS, et al. Amitriptyline treatment for severe recurrent idiopathic cystitis in cats. J Am Vet Med Assoc 1998;213(9):1282–6.

49. Kruger JM, Conway TS, Kaneene JB, et al. Randomized controlled trial of the efficacy of short-term amitriptyline administration for treatment of acute, nonobstructive, idiopathic lower urinary tract disease in cats. J Am Vet Med Assoc 2003;222(6):749–58.

50. Kraijer M, Fink-Gremmels J, Nickel RF. The short-term clinical efficacy of amitriptyline in the management of idiopathic feline lower urinary tract disease: a controlled clinical study. J Feline Med Surg 2003;5(3):191–6.

51. Kremer M, Salvat E, Muller A, et al. Antidepressants and gabapentinoids in neuropathic pain: Mechanistic insights. Neuroscience 2016;338:183–206.

52. Gruen ME, Thomson AE, Griffith EH, et al. A feline-specific anti-nerve growth factor antibody improves mobility in cats with degenerative joint disease-associated pain: a pilot proof of concept study. J Vet Intern Med 2016;30(4):1138–48.

53. Rausch-Derra LC, Rhodes L. Safety and toxicokinetic profiles associated with daily oral administration of grapiprant, a selective antagonist of the prostaglandin E2EP4 receptor, to cats. Am J Vet Res 2016;77(7):688–92.

54. Arzi B, Mills-Ko E, Verstraete FJM, et al. Therapeutic efficacy of fresh, autologous mesenchymal stem cells for severe refractory gingivostomatitis in cats. Stem Cells Transl Med 2016;5(1):75–86.

55. Lötsch J, Weyer-Menkhoff I, Tegeder I. Current evidence of cannabinoid-based analgesia obtained in preclinical and human experimental settings. Eur J Pain 2018;22(3):471–84.

56. Deabold KA, Schwark WS, Wolf L, et al. Single-dose pharmacokinetics and preliminary safety assessment with use of cbd-rich hemp nutraceutical in healthy dogs and cats. Animals 2019;9(10). https://doi.org/10.3390/ani9100832.

57. Wypij JM, Heller DA. Pamidronate disodium for palliative therapy of feline bone-invasive tumors. Vet Med Int 2014;2014. https://doi.org/10.1155/2014/675172.

58. Ellis SLH, Rodan I, Carney HC, et al. AAFP and ISFM feline environmental needs guidelines. J Feline Med Surg 2013;15(3):219–30.

59. Dantas LMS, Delgado MM, Johnson I, et al. Food puzzles for cats: Feeding for physical and emotional wellbeing. J Feline Med Surg 2016;18(9):723–32.

60. Heath S, Wilson C. Canine and feline enrichment in the home and kennel: A guide for practitioners. Vet Clin North Am Small Anim Pract 2014;44(3):427–49.

61. Eccleston C, Palermo TM, Williams AC, et al. Psychological therapies for the management of chronic and recurrent pain in children and adolescents. Cochrane Database Syst Rev 2014. https://doi.org/10.1002/14651858.CD003968.pub4.

62. Kroon Van Diest AM, Powers SW. Cognitive behavioral therapy for pediatric headache and migraine: why to prescribe and what new research is critical for advancing integrated biobehavioral care. Headache 2019;59(2):289–97.

63. Gourkow N, Phillips CJC. Effect of cognitive enrichment on behavior, mucosal immunity and upper respiratory disease of shelter cats rated as frustrated on arrival. Prev Vet Med 2016. https://doi.org/10.1016/j.prevetmed.2016.07.012.

64. Marques VI, Cassu RN, Nascimento FF, et al. Laser acupuncture for postoperative pain management in cats. Evid Based Complement Alternat Med 2015; 2015. https://doi.org/10.1155/2015/653270.

65. Suresh S, Wang S, Porfyris S, et al. Massage therapy in outpatient pediatric chronic pain patients: do they facilitate significant reductions in levels of distress, pain, tension, discomfort, and mood alterations? Paediatr Anaesth 2008;18(9): 884–7.

66. Machin H, Kato E, Adami C. Quantitative sensory testing with Electronic von Frey Anaesthesiometer and von Frey filaments in nonpainful cats: a pilot study. Vet Anaesth Analg 2019;46(2):251–4.

67. Adami C, Lardone E, Monticelli P. Inter-rater and inter-device reliability of mechanical thresholds measurement with the Electronic von Frey Anaesthesiometer and the SMALGO in healthy cats. J Feline Med Surg 2018. https://doi.org/10. 1177/1098612X18813426. 1098612X1881342.

68. Lynch S, Savary-Bataille K, Leeuw B, et al. Development of a questionnaire assessing health-related quality-of-life in dogs and cats with cancer. Vet Comp Oncol 2011;9(3):172–82.

69. Freeman LM, Rodenberg C, Narayanan A, et al. Development and initial validation of the Cat HEalth and Wellbeing (CHEW) questionnaire: a generic health-related quality of life instrument for cats. J Feline Med Surg 2016;18(9):689–701.

70. Gruen ME, Griffith E, Thomson A, et al. Detection of clinically relevant pain relief in cats with degenerative joint disease associated pain. J Vet Intern Med 2014; 28(2):346–50.

71. Zamprogno H, Hansen BD, Bondell HD, et al. Item generation and design testing of a questionnaire to assess degenerative joint disease-associated pain in cats. Am J Vet Res 2010;71(12):1417–24.

72. Benito J, DePuy V, Hardie E, et al. Reliability and discriminatory testing of a client-based metrology instrument, feline musculoskeletal pain index (FMPI) for the evaluation of degenerative joint disease-associated pain in cats. Vet J 2013; 196(3):368–73.

73. Tatlock S, Gober M, Williamson N, et al. Development and preliminary psychometric evaluation of an owner-completed measure of feline quality of life. Vet J 2017;228:22–32.

74. Klinck MP, Frank D, Guillot M, et al. Owner-perceived signs and veterinary diagnosis in 50 cases of Feline osteoarthritis. Can Vet J 2012;53(11):1181–6.

75. Noble CE, Wiseman-Orr LM, Scott ME, et al. Development, initial validation and reliability testing of a web-based, generic feline health-related quality-of-life instrument. J Feline Med Surg 2019;21(2):84–94.

76. Noble C, Scott E, Nolan AM, et al. Initial evidence to support the use of a generic health-related quality of life instrument to measure chronic pain in cats with osteoarthritis. Vet Comp Orthop Traumatol 2018;31:A0012.

Feline Neuropathic Pain

Mark E. Epstein, DVM*

KEYWORDS

- Feline • Neuropathic pain • Maladaptive • Peripheral/Central nervous system
- Sensitization • Hypersensitization • Windup • Neuroplasticity

KEY POINTS

- Neuropathic pain is likely under-recognized and underdiagnosed in cats.
- Aggressive perioperative multimodal analgesic approaches (including local anesthetics, ketamine infusions, and anticonvulsants) can mitigate the likelihood and severity of post-surgical maladaptive pain.
- Cats with suspected neuropathic pain are candidates to receive a variety of antihypersensitization therapeutics.

INTRODUCTION

Pain itself is an unpleasant multidimensional (sensory and emotional) experience associated with actual or potential tissue damage. Neuropathic pain is the extreme aberration of pain processing in which normal, protective, functional, adaptive, and reversible pain has transformed into a debilitating, maladaptive, nonprotective disease state. The International Association for the Study of Pain has defined neuropathic pain as "that pain arising from a primary lesion *or disease* of the somatosensory nervous system."[1] "Lesion" generally refers to nerve or spinal cord damage that can be grossly appreciated. Somatosensory "disease" is more problematic to diagnose or even define because it involves molecular, cellular, microanatomic, phenotypic and even genotypic changes to the central nervous system (CNS) and peripheral nervous system (PNS). Regardless of the etiology, onset, or duration, neuropathic pain is a disease in which pain has become exaggerated in some combination of scope, severity, character, field, duration, and spontaneity, with attendant impacts on patient morbidity and quality of life.

CLINICAL FEATURES AND DEFINITIONS OF NEUROPATHIC PAIN STATE

- Hyperesthesia: exaggerated pain out of proportion to a noxious stimulus
- Allodynia: pain from a non-noxious stimulus (eg, touch, pressure)
- Extended duration: pain persisting past the time of expected tissue inflammation and healing
- Expanded field: increased tactile sensitivity and/or pain at site(s) distant to the damaged tissue

TotalBond Veterinary Hospital, c/o Forestbrook, 3200 Union Road, Gastonia, NC 28056, USA
* Corresponding author: 2138 Winterlake Drive, Gastonia, NC 28054.
E-mail address: mark.epstein@totalbondvets.com

Vet Clin Small Anim 50 (2020) 789–809
https://doi.org/10.1016/j.cvsm.2020.02.004
0195-5616/20/© 2020 Elsevier Inc. All rights reserved.

- Spontaneous pain: in the absence of known tissue injury
- Dysesthesias: pain with other sensations, including itch, tingling, and even numbness
- Exaggerated character of pain: stabbing, "lancinating" (cutting, piercing), radiating, pulsing, burning
- Sympathetic signs: pain that worsens with stress, or the painful site exhibits autonomic signs (vasodilation, edema, vasoconstriction, etc)

WHAT MIGHT THIS LOOK LIKE IN A CAT?

Think of the cat that:

- No longer wishes to be stroked or petted, or have feet touched
- Grooms less
- Conversely, abruptly grooms, perhaps radiating down to the distal extremity, or chronically overgrooms a region
- Newly dislikes being held, objects to restraint
- Increasingly objects to nail trims and/or venipuncture
- Progressively interacts less with owners
- Increasingly grouchy/self-defensive
- Spontaneously rubs its mouth
- Reacts to (runs from) an invisible stimulus
- Spontaneous panniculus
- Exhibits avoidance behavior

DIAGNOSIS

Confirming neuropathic pain in humans involves validated self-reporting questionnaires and Quantitative Sensory Testing (QST). Some patients may be assumed to have neuropathic pain if diagnosed with certain conditions such as postherpetic neuralgia (shingles) or diabetic neuropathy.

A grading system in humans defines criteria for neuropathic pain on a probability spectrum (**Fig. 1**).[2] In this schema, history and clinical observations are enough to speculate that a patient has possible neuropathic pain. Additional examination may reveal signs consistent with probable neuropathic pain, and confirmatory testing (often advanced diagnostics not available to the clinical generalist) can lend a diagnosis of definite neuropathic pain; however (and importantly), known direct nerve damage qualifies as a confirmatory test. Because it exists along a spectrum, it may be described as pain with a neuropathic component (PNC).

In dogs and cats, validated clinical metrology instruments exist for postoperative and chronic osteoarthritis-related pain (See Analgesia: What Makes Cats Different/Challenging and What is Critical for Cats? Steagall or Feline Chronic Pain and Osteoarthritis, Monteiro). However, none of these specifically address the presence or absence of a neuropathic pain component. A semiobjective sensory testing rubric for hyperalgesia and allodynia in dogs and cats has been proposed (**Table 1**).

Although not a pain measurement mechanism per se, the QST evaluates sensory changes (gain or loss of function) elicited in, and contributing to, a pain state with central and/or peripheral sensitization. The QST modalities include mechanical and thermal threshold analyses among others. Current work with the QST is beset by a lack of standardization of instruments, modalities, methods, and outcome measures used. Such standardization in veterinary patients must be established before the QST can become a clinical cage-side tool.

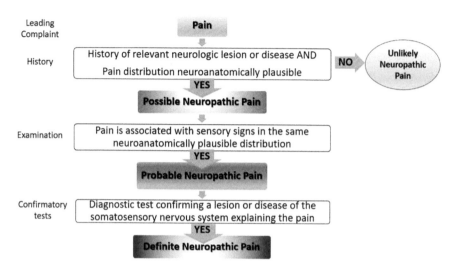

Fig. 1. Updated grading system for neuropathic pain in humans. (*From* Finnerup NB, Haroutounian S, Kamerman P, et al. Neuropathic pain: an updated grading system for research and clinical practice. Pain. 2016;157(8):1599-606.)

PREVALENCE OF NEUROPATHIC PAIN IN CATS

A study conducted in a teaching hospital evaluated cats for the presence of pain with neuropathic features. Among outpatients, 92 of 652 cats (14%) exhibited pain, and one-half of these (7%) had a neuropathic component, with most all experiencing pain lasting 1 to 12 months (1% experienced pain for >1 year).[3] This represents a somewhat similar prevalence as found in the general human population (6.9%–10.0%),[4] although some specific subpopulations have much higher rates. In the emergency setting, 23% of cats experienced a combination of inflammatory and neuropathic pain.[5]

NEUROPHYSIOLOGY AND NEUROPHARMACOLOGY OF NEUROPATHIC PAIN

The continuum through which pain transforms into a neuropathic state occurs along a spectrum of peripheral and central hypersensitization. "Wind up" is often used to describe this amplification of pain signaling. The neuromolecular changes of sensitization and maladaptive signaling are summarized in **Box 1**. Complicating matters,

Table 1
Semiobjective sensory testing in dogs and cats

Hyperalgesia: Produces an exaggerated response in affected area compared with an unaffected area	Allodynia: Normally nonpainful, but elicits pain in affected area compared with an unaffected area
Manual pinprick with a needle	Manual light pressure
Thermal cold (acetone, cold metal 0°C)	Light manual prick (sharpened wooden stick, stiff von Frey hair)
Thermal heat (object at 46°C)	
Algometry: lowered threshold and tolerance	Stroking (brush, gauze, cotton applicator)
	Thermal cool (objects at 20°C)
	Thermal warm (objects at 40°C)

Data from Mathews KA. Neuropathic pain in dogs and cats: if only they could tell us if they hurt. Vet Clin North Am Small Anim Pract. 2008 Nov;38(6):1365-414, vii-viii.

Box 1
Neuromolecular changes involved with sensitization and maladaptive signaling[1]

- Decreased (and/or reversed) inhibitory control
- Postsynaptic NMDA channel activation, with calcium influx resulting in increased membrane excitability and decreased firing threshold (nociceptor hypopolarization)
- Upregulation of receptor ion channel production in the DRG, then trafficked up and down the axon, increasing dendritic termini expression.
- Upregulation of endogenous neuronal agonists, including nerve growth factor, calcitonin gene-related peptide, substance P–neurokin-1 binding, protein kinase C, proinflammatory mediators and cytokines (eg, Interleukin-1)
- Spinal cord glial activation
- Antidromic signaling (efferent action potential from dorsal horn to periphery)
- Nociceptor cross-talk in peripheral tissue, DRG, and spinal cord; recruitment and activation of normally quiescent bystanding neurons from noninjured tissue (nociceptors and non-nociceptors; eg, touch fibers, sympathetic neurons)
- Phenotypic changes of neuron; gene expressions transcribe aberrant proteins, producing permanent microstructural changes of the neuron resulting in hyposensitization and activation by non-noxious stimuli

Abbreviation: DRG, dorsal root ganglia.
Data from Treede RD, Jensen TS, Campbell JN, et al. J. Neuropathic pain: redefinition and a grading system for clinical and research purposes. Neurology. 2008 Apr 29;70(18):1630-5.

---

sensitization may, but need not, have an gross inflammatory component. It can occur acutely (as in the case of nerve injury), chronically, or as acute-on-chronic (eg, surgery in a patient with preexisting chronic inflammation). What differentiates neuropathic pain from other sorts of pathologic pain processing, including "mere" chronic pain with or without inflammation, is that the CNS and PNS have undergone damage, and pain emanates directly from it. The terms neuroplasticity, algoplasticity, and noci-plasticity have been suggested to describe the ability of the CNS and PNS to remodel and reorganize into a neuropathic pain state.

RECOGNIZED OR SUSPECT NEUROPATHIC PAIN CONDITIONS IN CATS
Feline Orofacial Pain Syndrome

First described in 1994, affected cats exhibit episodic, spontaneous unilateral paw-ing at the mouth; excessive and exaggerated licking movements; growling when eating, drinking, or grooming; and food aversion or anorexia.[6] More severe cases involve self-mutilation of tongue, lips, and buccal mucosa. In the UK, there seems to be genetic disposition (Burmese cats, <1 year old). In the United States, it has been observed in many breeds (excluding Burmese cats, the median age of onset is 9 years of age), and a majority (63%) were associated with erupting teeth or oral pathology such as odontoclastic resorptive lesions, periodontal disease, lympho-plasmacytic gingivitis/stomatitis, or postextraction surgery. Environmental stress may precipitate episodes. Current understanding suggests a condition analogous to trigeminal neuralgia and/or glossodynia in humans, with involvement of the sym-pathetic nervous system. Many different therapies, often multimodal in the same cat, been reported in the treatment of feline orofacial pain syndrome. Because of the retrospective, uncontrolled nature of these reports, conclusions regarding treatment efficacy are difficult to draw. However, it seems that anticonvulsant medications (gabapentin, phenobarbital, diazepam, and carbamazepine) seem to be more effective than anti-inflammatory drugs, opioids, or other therapies (See Newly Recognized Neurological Entities [FOPS, Auditory Seizures] in the next issue).

Feline Hyperesthesia Syndrome

First described in 1980, feline hyperesthesia syndrome is an idiopathic condition characterized by skin twitching and muscle spasm in the lumbar area; licking of lumbar, flank, and tail regions; tail chasing; exaggerated response to a non-noxious stimulus (eg, stroking); and reactive (including vocalization) avoidance behavior to a nonapparent stimulus.[7] In extreme cases, a non-noxious stimulus can elicit a seizure-like tetany response or self-mutilation (especially of the tail). Affected cats are generally younger (median age, 1 year; range, 1–7 years) and male cats (both intact and altered) may be overrepresented. Episodes are intermittent, ranging from several times per day or per week. Proposed etiologies include idiopathic focal epilepsy, primary (and idiopathic) neuropathic pain disorders, displacement behavior, and infectious agents (eg, toxoplasmosis). In a recent case series,[8] 7 cats responded variably to a variety of single or multimodal therapies, including gabapentinoids and other anticonvulsant medications (eg, phenobarbital, topiramate), TCAs (eg, amitriptyline), anti-inflammatories (eg, nonsteroidal anti-inflammatory drugs [NSAIDs], glucocorticoids), immunomodulators (eg, cyclosporin), and less often, tramadol, fluoxetine, and clomipramine. The cats represented in this case series may represent subset of feline hyperesthesia syndrome because they had been referred to a specialty center.

Feline Idiopathic, Interstitial, and Sterile Cystitis

Under variable names, including Pandora syndrome for its complex (and evil) nature,[9,10] this condition mirrors an analogous syndrome in women (interstitial cystitis) more broadly called bladder pain syndrome or pelvic pain syndrome. Indeed, the term cystitis is inappropriate, because significant inflammation is not a feature of the condition in cats or humans.[9] In both species, there are similar clinical signs and abnormalities of afferent sensory neurons (lowered firing threshold, recruitment of otherwise silent mechanoreceptors, and increased norepinephrine [NE] content, and activity in bladder wall,[11] increased PNS and CNS excitability,[12] enhanced sympathetic efferent neuronal function, and upregulation of bladder mucosal substance P and neurokinin-1 receptors).[13] The result of this cascade represents peripheral and central hypersensitization along with disrupted epithelial excretion of glycosaminoglycans. Several subtypes of lower urinary tract disease are described in both cats and women, but both species almost always express a type 1, nonulcerative form that is considered neuropathic in origin.[14]

The complex etiology seems to include early life (both prenatal and postnatal) stressors, presumptively contributing to a strong sympathetic response on the developing pituitary-adrenal axis and high plasticity of the developing CNS. Later in life, with chronic activation of the central threat response system, the condition becomes a clinical entity and can involve other extra-bladder comorbidities in addition to their lower urinary tract signs.[15] Fundamentally, feline idiopathic cystitis, and interstitial cystitis seem to represent a neuropathic phenomenon whereby the sympathetic nervous system is wired into nociceptive pathways. Treatment is variable, but should always involve stress reduction summarized as multimodal environmental modification, which is covered in detail elsewhere (see also C.A. Tony Buffington and Melissa Bain's article, "Stress and Feline Health"; and "Environment and Feline Health: At Home and in the Clinic," in this issue).

Long-term amitriptyline has modest usefulness for severe and recurrent forms of feline idiopathic cystitis,[16] but is only recommended when multimodal environmental modification has failed.[9] Originally described for its antianxiety effect, amitriptyline may elicit significant antihypersensitization effects through its serotoninergic mechanisms. It may take weeks before an effect is seen, and abrupt withdrawal should be avoided. Given the absence of significant inflammation, it is not surprising that corticosteroids and NSAID are not indicated. Consideration might be given to gabapentinoids for their antihypersensitivity effect.

Feline Herpesvirus-1

Postherpetic neuralgia (shingles) is an extremely common and painful neuropathic pain condition in humans. Herpes zoster virus infects and damages peripheral nerve endings, creating the cascade of sensitization events characteristic of peripheral nerve injury. Viral activation elicits painful erupting skin lesions most often on the back, neck, and face; however, the hyperalgesia and allodynia of postherpetic neuralgia can be present without the dermatologic lesions.

Cats are infected by a different virus, feline herpesvirus 1, but it also results in a latent infection and dermatoses.[17] These lesions are often mistaken for miliary dermatitis, eosinophilic granuloma complex, dermatophytosis, or squamous cell carcinoma. Biopsy, dermatohistopathology, and polymerase chain reaction can correctly identify lesions that are herpetic in origin.[18] Treatment focuses on antiviral therapy and managing secondary bacterial infections. Although the degree of discomfort cannot be known with certainty, it is most likely not minor and analgesic strategies should be considered. In humans, amitriptyline is among the most effective medications for postherpetic neuralgia, but, owing to adverse effects, is not as popular as gabapentinoids[19] (see Kimberly Coyner's article, Distinguishing Between Dermatologic Disorders of the Face, Nasal Planum, and Ears: Great Lookalikes in Feline Dermatology, in this issue).

Feline Chronic Gingivostomatitis

Feline chronic gingivostomatitis (FCGS) is a common, often severe and refractory disorder of uncertain etiology but thought to involve an immune-mediated response to dental plaque and a variety of organisms of indeterminate causality.[20] FCGS can be exquisitely painful, and peripheral and central sensitization processes may be involved (including an antidromic, efferent neurogenic component contributing to the inflammation). Although there are numerous treatments, full mouth extraction is the most successful. Antihypersensitization agents should be considered. Anecdotal experience supports using gabapentin as an adjunctive medical treatment for FCGS, and as part of transoperative antisensitization strategies for full mouth extraction, including subanesthetic ketamine at a constant rate infusion and a long-acting orofacial, locoregional nerve blockade. It is possible that cats with feline chronic gingivostomatitis undergoing any type of oral surgery may be at higher risk for developing persistent postsurgical pain including Orofacial Pain Syndrome (See An Update on Feline Chronic Gingivostomatitis in Part II Arzi).

Osteoarthritis

See Beatriz Monteiro's article, "Feline Chronic Pain and Osteoarthritis," in this issue for a comprehensive discussion on the assessment and management of feline osteoarthritis. Many experimental models demonstrate that osteoarthritis can be accompanied by peripheral[21] and central[22] sensitization, consistent with a neuropathic component. In humans with osteoarthritis, approximately 25% have a neuropathic component to their pain.[23] A study of cats with *hip* osteoarthritis identified temporal summation and a lower mechanical threshold in the *feet* of 25% of patients.[24] This study illustrates 2 classic features of peripheral and central sensitization: increased tactile sensitivity and an expanded field (distant from the affected site). The potential usefulness of gabapentin as an adjunctive pain-modifying medication for feline osteoarthritis is further evidenced by a small case series,[25] and a study demonstrating improved activity levels, owner-perceived mobility, and quality of life.[26] Gabapentin is in fact the most commonly prescribed therapeutic by US veterinarians (71% of respondents) for chronic feline musculoskeletal pain.[27]

Inflammatory Bowel Disease

Inflammatory bowel disease produces an ongoing afferent barrage of visceral nociceptors producing changes in the dorsal horn consistent with central sensitization. Furthermore, intestinal high- and low-threshold mechanoreceptors can undergo a phenotypic alteration into nociceptive function, with normal motility eliciting visceral pain.[28] An antidromic, efferent neurogenic component may enhance inflammation. In humans, inflammatory bowel diseases are characterized by debilitating, painful flare-ups (including stress-related sympathetic nervous system coupling), and are comorbid with other hyperalgesic syndromes.[28] The extent to which cats with inflammatory bowel disease experience visceral pain, cramping, and/or hyperalgesia may be difficult to discern, but, if suspected, therapeutic trials of antihypersensitization modalities are indicated and anecdotal benefits are reported.[29]

Pancreatitis (Acute and Chronic)

Abdominal pain is a classic feature of acute and chronic pancreatitis but may be difficult to appreciate in cats. In humans the neuroimmune response is especially robust in pancreatitis (and pancreatic cancer), leading to remarkable visceral discomfort. Inflammatory cells and a unique brew of local neurotrophins and neuropeptides activate pancreatic afferent nociceptors, leading to central changes consistent with hypersensitization and somatic neuropathic pain disorders. Owing to the diffuse projections of afferent nociceptors in the spinal cord, pain may not be confined to the upper/cranial right abdominal quadrant; humans with pancreatitis (and cholecystitis; perhaps similar to feline triaditis) report pain in the back and even the shoulder.[30] Additionally, as with other inflammatory states, a neurogenic component may additionally contribute to the pathophysiology of pancreatitis (See Is it being over diagnosed? Feline pancreatitis, Bazelle and Watson in the next issue).

Diabetic Neuropathy

In humans, diabetic neuropathy is so prevalent and debilitating that several drugs are labeled specifically for this indication. Reported sensations include walking on glass shards or barbed wire, and spontaneous tingling and itch without evoked stimulus; these signs are also reported in the hands (diabetic hand and foot syndrome). In cats, diabetes mellitus is associated with motor neuropathy and a classic plantigrade stance in the rear legs (less often paresis in the forelimbs and tail). However, classic sensory neuropathic changes in the peripheral nociceptors and spinal cord have been found in cats like those in humans,[31] including endoneural microvascular pathology.[32] This state may account for anecdotal observations in diabetic cats objecting to handling of paws, being held or stroked, and/or objecting increasingly to their insulin injections. Drugs in humans approved to treat diabetic neuropathy include duloxetine (Cymbalta), pregabalin (Lyrica), and tapentadol (Nucytna); generic gabapentin is commonly used. If sensory diabetic neuropathy is suspected in a cat, treatment suggestions have included gabapentin and amitriptyline[29]; in humans, gabapentin was shown to be more effective and better tolerated than amitriptyline.[33] (See Updates in Feline Diabetes Mellitus and Hypersomatotropism in Part II Fleeman in the next issue).

Gross Nerve Injury: Entrapment or Transection

Nerve injury so reliably produces central and peripheral sensitization that it serves as a model for neuropathic pain. One case report describes neuropathic pain in a cat whose sciatic nerve had inadvertently been ligated during rear limb amputation.[34] This patient experienced both hyperalgesia and hypoesthesia (numbness) in different aspects of the stump region. Any amputation requires severing of major nerves and in humans, postamputation neuropathic pain signs occur in a high proportion of patients (45% -85%). Most cases are managed medically and resolve, but the condition persists in 5% to 10% of patients.[35] In cats, manifestations of postamputation neuropathic pain may also include persistent tactile sensitivity and constant grooming at the stump site (possibly owing to dysesthesia [tingling or itch]). Cats experiencing chronic lameness months or years after onychectomy may be experiencing neuropathic pain in their feet.[36] Pathophysiology of postamputation neuropathic pain, including phantom limb pain, may include microscopic or macroscopic neuroma formation and/or sprouting of nerve endings at the transaction site into a bundle of hyperexcitable, cross-linking neurons, typical of peripheral sensitization. Changes are also detectable in peripheral axons, the dorsal root ganglia, spinal cord, and even the cerebral cortex. Applicable strategies in humans to minimize postamputation pain include perioperative gabapentinoids, a ketamine constant rate infusion, locoregional anesthesia, and serotonin–NE reuptake inhibitors, which can also be used for treatment when postamputation pain is suspected.

Spinal Cord Injury

In a majority of humans, hyperalgesia and tactile allodynia follow a spinal cord injury. In cats, blunt force trauma, sacrococcygeal tail avulsion, intervertebral disc herniation, lumbosacral stenosis (LSS), neoplasia, congenital malformations, infectious disease, and iatrogenic injury from epidural injection may cause a spinal cord injury. Although intervertebral disc disease is uncommon in cats (affecting <0.3%), both cervical and thoracolumbar intervertebral disc diseases are reported, with a possible pure-bred breed disposition (Persians, British Shorthairs) in the latter.[37] Clinically relevant LSS may be more common than currently recognized and is based on either suggestive radiographic changes or advanced imaging (specifically MRI) to identify lesions not apparent radiographically. Affected cats may present with low tail carriage, hyperalgesia of the lumbosacral region and/or upon dorsoflexion of the tail, reluctance to jump and/or ambulate, elimination outside the litter box, pelvic–limb paresis, urinary incontinence, and constipation.[38] Humans with LSS may have pudendal nerve entrapment with neuropathic pain, resulting in chronic disabling perineal discomfort (anorectal, urogenital) especially upon sitting, or urgency to urinate or defecate;[39] in cats, this might result in more vigorous objections to insertion of a rectal thermometer than expected.

The presence of transitional lumbosacral vertebrae is a risk factor for LSS, with affected cats having a 9-fold increased risk of developing the condition over cats without transitional vertebrae (54% vs 6% in the general population).[40] Management for intervertebral disc disease and LSS includes anti-inflammatory and analgesic agents, nonpharmacologic modalities such as acupuncture, and surgical correction. Analgesics for both medical and perisurgical management should include antisensitization agents such as gabapentin, amitriptyline, possibly a serotonin–NE reuptake inhibitor, and transoperatively, a subanesthetic ketamine constant rate infusion and locoregional blockade (eg, caudal epidural technique).

Central Nervous System Infection and Neoplasia

Any disease of the cerebral cortex, meninges, or spinal cord involving inflammation, vascular changes, ischemia, or necrosis can potentially cause pain with a neuropathic component. This pain may include a profound headache with migraine-like features. Migraines themselves, whether primary idiopathic or comorbid to another disorder, are essentially a neuropathic pain condition that involves blood vessels in addition to afferent and efferent neurons.[41] Head pressing associated with intracranial disease, including brain tumor, may be in part from severe debilitating headache. Infectious agents known to cause encephalitis and/or myelitis in cats include viruses (feline infectious peritonitis, rabies, feline leukemia virus, and feline immunodeficiency virus), protozoa (toxoplasmosis), systemic fungi (most commonly *Cryptococcus neoformans*), and parasites (*Cuterebra myiasis*). Feline nonsuppurative meningoencephalomyelitis and eosinophilic meningoencephalitis are idiopathic, but likely involve an as-yet-unidentified infectious agent.[42,43]

Vascular Disorders

Aortic thromboembolism elicits sudden, massive ischemic myopathy and neuropathy and induces neuropathic pain. A central part of the initial management should be aggressive analgesia along with other care described for this disease.[44]

Persistent Postsurgical Pain

Persistent postsurgical pain is a significant and well-described neuropathic phenomenon in humans, with up to one-half of patients developing chronic pain after surgery (even common outpatient procedures), and signs of neuropathic pain in 35% to 57%. Overall, 11.8% of patients still experienced moderate to severe pain 12 months postoperatively.[45] Veterinary metrics are not available, but if persistent postsurgical pain exists in even a fraction of cats as reported in humans, it would represent a potentially significant unrecognized clinical problem.

In humans, the degree of trauma (surgical and otherwise) and the degree of acute postoperative pain[46] are predictive factors for chronic pain with a neuropathic component. In humans, every 10% increase in the time spent in severe postoperative pain was associated with a 30% increase in chronic pain 12 months after surgery.[47]

Aggressive multimodal analgesic approaches (including local anesthetics, ketamine infusions, anticonvulsants, etc) can mitigate the likelihood and severity of subsequent maladaptive pain.[45]

Bone Disease

Trabecular bone and the periosteum are richly innervated. Fracture, infection, or neoplasia cause damage to periosteal and intrinsic mechanosensitive neurons, followed by massive release of excitatory neuropeptides that activate and sensitize neurons and promote ectopic nerve sprouting (including sympathetic fibers) at the callous. With proper healing, these factors return to baseline and pain subsides, but if proper healing does not occur, chronic bone pain results.[48] Complex regional pain syndrome is a poorly understood sympathomimetic neuropathic pain syndrome reported as a complication of fracture (and other trauma) in humans and many animal species (but not as of yet in cats). Pelvic fractures are especially prone to severe and chronic maladaptive pain complications.[49]

Osteosarcoma and any metastatic bone cancer can elicit neuropathic pain through similar mechanisms, but also central glial hypertrophy, peripheral upregulation of cyclo-oxygenase (occurring in multiple neoplasms found in cats[50]), and a unique proalgesic neurochemical signature from osteoclastic activity.[51] Palliative bisphosphonate infusions to freeze osteoclastic activity have been shown to improve pain scores in about two-thirds of dogs with osteosarcoma, with a durable effect (>4 months) in 28%.[52] The pain parameters of feline osteosarcoma are poorly described, and bisphosphonates have not been studied in this species.

Allergic Inflammation

Allergic inflammation has been established as potential cause of neuropathic pain in mice,[53] and implications for this in cats (as established in mice) include well-recognized syndromes such as feline asthma, flea allergy dermatitis, atopic and flood allergy dermatitis, and possibly eosinophilic granuloma complex. In the extreme, the phenomenon of neuropathic itch is well-described in humans and animal models.[54]

TREATMENT OF NEUROPATHIC PAIN

Although there is considerable experience in treating humans and rodent models of neuropathic pain, there are few feline case series; caution is always warranted when attempting to extrapolate across species lines. Pharmacokinetic data are available in cats for several drugs, but dose titration, safety, toxicity, and pharmacodynamic data are sorely lacking. Case series of neuropathic pain must be interpreted cautiously owing to the multimodal approach generally taken, and the very high (85%) caregiver placebo effect observed in treating cats with osteoarthritis.[55] The task is made more difficult by the lack of validated clinical metrology instruments or clinical, cage-side QST tools to detect specifically neuropathic pain. A summary of possible therapeutics and their possible clinical usefulness can be found in **Table 2**.

Nonsteroidal Anti-inflammatory Drugs

Neuropathic pain is generally poorly responsive to NSAIDs, unsurprising since NP generally lacks a gross inflammatory component. However, if chronic inflammation (eg, osteoarthritis) contributes to peripheral and central sensitization, then NSAIDs may have potential benefit by abating that underlying component on a sustained basis. See Feline Chronic Pain and Osteoarthritis, Monteiro for a more complete discussion of long-term NSAIDs in cats.

Gabapentinoids

Gabapentinoids downregulate calcium channels at the terminal endings of nociceptors (and other neurons). With less intracellular calcium, the release of excitatory neurotransmitters across synapses in the dorsal horn is dampened, and sensitized second- and third-order neurons are hyperpolarized (providing an anticonvulsant action as well). Case series suggest the usefulness of gabapentin in various maladaptive, probably neuropathic pain states, including feline orofacial pain syndrome,[6] feline hyperesthesia syndrome,[8] and osteoarthritis.[24,26]

The pharmacokinetics of gabapentin have been described in cats after a single 10 m/kg dose.[56] Bioavailability ranged from 50% to 100% possibly dependent on food intake, with a half-life of 3 hours. Based on murine and human pharmacokinetic–pharmacodynamic modeling, the authors recommended a dose of 8 mg/kg every 6 hours for antihyperalgesia. A more recent pharmacokinetic study[57] evaluated serial oral administration in cats (10 mg/kg 2 times per day for 2 weeks)

Table 2
Suggested doses for treating feline neuropathic pain

	Feline	
	Perioperative	Chronic
Amantadine	N/A	Consider 3–5 mg/kg PO SID–BID
		No toxicity, safety, dose titration, or clinical studies in cats
Amitriptyline	N/A	0.5–2.0 mg/kg PO SID[a]
Gabapentin	10 mg/kg PO every 8 h (ideally 1 dose evening before, 1 dose morning of surgery; followed by 1–3+ days as may be needed)	Initiate 3–5 mg/kg PO BID, gradual taper upwards as needed to target of 8–10 mg/kg. Suggested dosing modifications in cats with chronic kidney disease
Ketamine	Loading dose 0.25–0.5 mg/kg IV (lower induction agent doses accordingly) 5–10 μg/kg/min[a] intraoperatively followed by 2 μg/kg/min 1–24 h postoperatively. Administered at customary surgical fluid rate of 5–10 mL/kg/h (depending on blood and/or insensible fluid loss) = 5–10 μg/kg/min. Maintenance rate of 2 mL/kg/h = 2 μg/kg/min	Many protocols described in human literature; none standardized for humans or cats. Consider: 2–5 μg/kg/min[b] constant rate infusion 4 h daily for 4 d; 2 μg/kg/min[b] constant rate infusion for 3 d
Maropitant	1 mg/kg IV, SC, PO[c]	1 mg/kg PO SID[d]
Pregabalin	1–2 mg/kg PO BID	1–2 mg/kg PO BID
Tapentadol	5–10 mg/kg PO BID[e]	5–10 mg/kg PO BID[e]
Tramadol	1–3 mg/kg PO BID[f]	1–3 mg/kg PO BID[f]

Gabapentin dosing modifications in cats with chronic kidney disease:

IRIS Stage	Creatinine mg/dL	μmol/L	Gabapentin dose, frequency
IRIS 1	<1.6	<141	5 mg/kg BID
IRIS 2	1.6–2.8	142–247	3 mg/kg BID
IRIS 3	2.8–5.0	248–442	2 mg/kg SID
IRIS 4	>5.0	>442	1 mg/kg SID-EOD

Investigational or Limited Data Therapeutics for Neuropathic Pain in Cats

Anti-nerve growth factor monoclonal antibody	0.4–0.8 mg/kg SC once monthly

(continued on next page)

Table 2 (continued)	
	Investigational or Limited Data Therapeutics for Neuropathic Pain in Cats
Cannabinoid	Species differences may be significant and there are currently no pharmacokintenics, safety, toxicity, or clinical cannabinoid data in cats. Additionally, quality control, regulatory, and potential impurity toxicity concerns are significant at present. Presently no recommendations can be made for these products.
Duloxetine, venlafaxine and other selective serotonin–NE reuptake inhibitors	Pharmacokintenics, dose titration, and clinical studies of selective serotonin–NE reuptake inhibitors are needed before treatment recommendations can be made. Should not be given with other serotoninergic or noradrenergic drugs, for example, amitriptyline, tapentadol, tramadol.

Abbreviations: BID, 2 times per day; EOD, every other day IRIS, International Renal Interest Society; IV, intravenous; N/A, not applicable; PO, by mouth; SC, subcutaneous; SID, once daily.

a Safety, pharmacokinetic, toxicity, and dose titration data for amitriptyline are lacking for cats; should not be given with other serotoninergic or noradrenergic drugs for example, tramadol, tapentadol, and selective serotonin–NE reuptake inhibitors.

b At 60 mg (0.6 mL of 100 mg/mL product) and added to 1 L of crystalloid fluids 5 60 mg/L.

c Limited data to support postoperative analgesia at this time.

d Anecdotal only for chronic visceral pain; generally amounts to 4 mg (one-fourth of a 16-mg tablet) per cat daily.

e No clinical data; drug is bitter, which may limit use. Should not be given with other serotoninergic or noradrenergic drugs for example, amitriptyline, tramadol, or an selective serotonin–NE reuptake inhibitor.

f Oral formulation is bitter, which may limit use; IV formulations exist outside the United States. Higher doses are reported but may increase risk of ADE; transdermal formulations are available but there are no data to support favorable pharmacokintenics and its molecular features make it unlikely that this route is useful. Should not be given with other serotoninergic or noradrenergic drugs for example, amitriptyline, tapentadol, and selective serotonin–NE reuptake inhibitors.

and found very high bioavailability (95%; range, 82.46%–122.83%), a half-life of 4 hours (range, 3.12–4.51 hours), and, in apparent contradistinction to humans and dogs, no decrease in maximum serum concentration was detected over the duration of the study. This finding implies that dose escalations recommended in other species are not required in cats. The same study found that a transdermal preparation had very low bioavailability and was inappropriate choice for cats. Dose adjustments are recommended in cats with chronic kidney disease because gabapentin undergoes renal clearance.[58]

Pregabalin is a gabapentin-like analogue and is believed to have similar mechanisms of action as gabapentin. In the United States, pregabalin (class IV) is labeled for pain associated with diabetic neuropathy, fibromyalgia, and postherpetic neuralgia in humans. Pharmacokinetics have been established in cats after a single 4 mg/kg oral dose, with 4 of 6 cats experiencing sedation.[59] There are anecdotal reports of successful use of pregabalin in cats with neuropathic pain of traumatic origin.[60]

Tramadol

Tramadol's mechanism of action in cats and humans is through 2 metabolites, one with mu-agonist activity (M1, O-desmethyltramadol, ODM) and another that enhances the inhibitory neurotransmitters NE and serotonin. It has high bioavailability in cats (93% ± 7%) after a single oral dose of 5 mg/kg, with a half-life of about 5 hours (4.82 ± 0.32 hours). Recent studies illustrate improvement in cats with osteoarthritis receiving oral tramadol,[61] and that tramadol specifically diminishes central sensitization in this species.[62] The drug is bitter, which is a limiting factor in oral use, but 1 small case series describes successful compounding for cats.[63] A parenteral form is approved outside the United States (see also Paulo V. Steagall's article, "Analgesia: What Makes Cats Different/Challenging and What Is Critical for Cats?" in this issue). There are no safety, toxicity, or dose titration data for tramadol in cats. Reported adverse effects include hypersalivation and other gastrointestinal signs, depression, behavioral changes including altered mentation, ataxia, and 1 case report of serotonin syndrome.[64] Although transdermal preparations of tramadol are available, there are no data and its molecular features make it unlikely that this route is effective (Dawn Boothe, DACVP, 2017, Personal communication).

Tapentadol (Nucytna) is a tramadol-like drug in which the parent molecule is a mu-agonist. Bioavailability in cats is high (>90%) via parenteral routes, but it has a relatively short half-life of 2 to 3 hours.[65] Pharmacokinetics of oral tapentadol in cats have not been established. A study of oral tapentadol in cats revealed a dose-dependent increase (25 and 50 mg per adult cat; mean, 5.7 mg/kg and 11.4 mg/kg, respectively) in the thermal threshold in cats, lasting 1 to 2 hours (the thermal threshold is a model validated for opioid-induced analgesia, but not for central sensitization). As with tramadol, the oral form of tapentadol is bitter; different formulations may be necessary before this drug can be used in feline practice.[66]

Opioids

The usefulness of opioids for neuropathic pain remains controversial. In humans, vigorous systematic reviews fail to demonstrate convincing evidence of benefit in short- and long-term neuropathic pain states,[67] and are only recommended as a third-line agent to treat neuropathic pain. Long-term opioid use is not commonplace in veterinary medicine, is beset by regulatory issues, and because there are no data to support the pharmacokinetics, clinical usefulness, and safety in cats, they cannot be recommended for the treatment of neuropathic pain in this species.

Ketamine

A phencyclidine dissociative anesthetic, ketamine's pain-modifying effects have been known for decades. As a potent N-methyl-D-aspartate (NMDA)-receptor antagonist, it decreases the channel's opening time and frequency, thus reducing Ca[+] ion influx and secondary intracellular signaling cascades. The NMDA receptor has been well-established for its role in central sensitization, and subanesthetic ketamine constant rate infusion has been shown convincingly in humans to have pain-preventive, antihyperalgesic, and antiallodynic effects.[68] Studies support a similar clinical effect in cats.[69] It is recommended perioperatively in humans.[70] Veterinary guidelines advise ketamine constant rate infusion for patients with risk factors for maladaptive pain and for its opioid-sparing ability.[71]

Human guidelines also describe the role of ketamine in the management of chronic neuropathic pain, without a consensus on exact protocol.[72] Anecdotal veterinary use with chronic refractory osteoarthritis-related pain is reported (Jamie Gaynor, Lindsey Fry, personal communication, 2019). Ketamine is a promising therapeutic agent for cats with neuropathic pain and pilot trials are under development; however, until more data are available, recommendations cannot yet be made for use in feline chronic pain.

Amantadine and Other N-Methyl-D-Aspartate Receptor Antagonists

Amantadine is an antiviral, anti-Parkinson's (dopaminergic) agent that exerts a pain-modifying effect through blockade of spinal postsynaptic NMDA receptors.[73] Oral NMDA antagonists have been investigated for their potential to treat neuropathic pain in humans,[74] and there are clinical data to support use in chronic maladaptive pain in dogs[75] and other species. Feline data are more limited, confined to anecdotal reports,[76] and show a possible opioid-sparing effect in some cats when administered as a constant rate infusion.[77]

Pharmacokinetics of amantadine in cats after a single 5 mg/kg oral dose showed 100% bioavailability with a terminal half-life of 5.7 hours, suggesting a 2 times per day dose schedule.[78] There are no toxicity, safety, efficacy, or dose titration studies in cats.

Amitriptyline and Other Tricyclic Antidepressants

Tricyclic Antidepressants (TCAs) are a complex drug class, with serotoninergic, noradrenergic, antihistamine, anticholinergic, antimuscarinic, NMDA receptor antagonistic, and sodium channel blocking actions. Amitriptyline has a balanced NE and serotonin effect, and is among the more sedating, anticholinergic, and effective TCAs in humans.[79] In humans, TCAs are the most effective medications for classic neuropathic pain conditions.[19] In cats, use and clinical studies of amitriptyline are in house soiling and feline idiopathic cystitis.[16] Owing to the lack of cystoscopic changes in cats receiving amitriptyline, clinical improvement is attributed to antisensitization and pain modification, although a benefit may also occur from anxiolytic effects as well. Adverse effects include bitter taste, weight gain, sedation, and decreased grooming.[16]

Pharmacokinetic data for amitriptyline in cats is limited, with one study showing a plasma half-life of 2 hours, and poor transdermal absorption.[80] Safety, toxicity, and dose-titration data are lacking altogether in cats. Additional feline studies are required to understand how to use it safely and effectively for neuropathic pain. Amitriptyline should not be given with other serotoninergic or noradrenergic drugs (such as tramadol and a selective serotonin–NE reuptake inhibitor, discussed elsewhere in this article).

Selective Serotonin–Norepinephrine Reuptake Inhibitors

Selective serotonin-NE reuptake inhibitors enhance the concentration and duration of these inhibitory neurotransmitters in the dorsal horn synaptic cleft. Fluoxetine, used for behavior disorders in cats—a strictly serotonin reuptake inhibitor—is not known to have a significant pain-modifying effect in humans or rodent models. Duloxetine, on the other hand, with both selective serotonin *and* NE reuptake inhibitor activity, has a neuropathic pain indication in humans (including osteoarthritis and low back pain, fibromyalgia and diabetic neuropathy). Toxicologic data are available,[81] with most (76%) cats known to have ingested at least a human dose of an selective serotonin–NE reuptake inhibitor remaining nonsymptomatic. In 8 affected cats, one-half experienced gastrointestinal signs with one each showing CNS stimulation, cardiovascular signs, and hyperthermia. Affected cats were treated symptomatically and all survived.

Selective serotonin-NE reuptake inhibitors may be a safe class of analgesic for cats if pharmacokinetic, dose titration, and efficacy data can be established for neuropathic pain in this species However, many drugs and compounds enhance monoamines and/or serotonin and NE, so caution is warranted when used in combination with other drugs such as tramadol, TCAs (amitriptyline and clomipramine), amantadine, metoclopramide, selegiline, amitraz, and mirtazapine.

Cannabinoids

The cannabinoid (CB) system facilitates pain modulation, although the exact mechanisms remain an area of intense study. CB1 receptors are located in the brain and spinal cord, but also in viscera and adipose tissue modulating opioid, NMDA, and gamma-aminobutyric acid receptors on the postsynaptic side. CB2 receptors are found in highest concentrations on immunoregulatory cells, including microglia. They are G-protein coupled and when activated decrease the release of excitatory neurotransmitters into the synaptic cleft, resulting in hyperpolarization of the postsynaptic neuron. CB receptors are generally downregulated in a healthy state, but upregulate in both neurons and microglia with injury or inflammation.[82] Pharmacologically, the goal is to selectively activate this aspect of the CB system in a sustained way, without activation of other effects including psychotropic activity.

Species differences may be significant and there are currently no pharmacokinetics, safety, toxicity, or clinical CB data in cats. Additionally, quality control, regulatory, and potential impurity toxicity concerns are significant at present. Presently no recommendations can be made for these products.

Maropitant

Maropitant is a central antiemetic that acts through blockade of substance P to the neurokinin-1 receptor in the midbrain. Because this same substance P–neurokinin-1 interaction has been identified as a part of inflammatory pathways and central sensitization, a pain-modifying effect has been postulated. The true pain-modifying effect in animals remains uncertain; maropitant performed poorly in development as an analgesic agent in humans. Intravenous maropitant has been shown to elicit an anesthetic-sparing effect in cats,[83] suggesting, but not confirming, analgesia (eg, midazolam is anesthetic sparing but not analgesic). A recent study in cats undergoing ovariohysterectomy demonstrated an apparent dose-dependent analgesic effect of maropitant.[84] However, postovariohysterectomy pain ought not have a maladaptive component, and more studies are required to understand maropitant's potential in treating neuropathic pain. It is possible that anecdotal reports of improved clinical status in cats with inflammatory bowel disease receiving daily oral maropitant are due to decreased nausea, visceral pain, or both.

Anti-Nerve Growth Factor Monoclonal Antibody

Nerve growth factor (NGF) is produced and used by many cell types including epithelium, endothelium, immunoreactive cells, and CNS glia. It is found in abundance during neonatal and infant development, gradually decreasing over time.[85] However, it is upregulated with chronic inflammation (including osteoarthritis) in both spinal and peripheral tissue.

NGF binding to Trk-A receptors elicits several aberrations of pain processing, including an increase in nociceptor excitability, degranulation of mast cells, and the release of proinflammatory and proalgesic mediators, as well as sprouting of terminal nerve endings (promoting nociceptor and non-nociceptor neuronal cross-talk). These sensitization effects contribute to hyperalgesia and an expanded field of pain.

Multiple investigations are being pursued in humans, dogs, and cats toward an anti-NGF product for treatment of osteoarthritis pain. A veterinary therapeutic anti-NGF monoclonal antibody product has been felinized (frunevetmab)[86] from a murine protein with favorable pharmacokinetics in cats: the time to maximum effect is 3 days (range, 1.9–4.3 days), the plasma half-life is 9 days (range, 7–15 days), and the plasma concentrations were still detected at 42 days. Safety was also established at up to 14 times the therapeutic dose. In a subsequent pilot study, efficacy of frunevetmab was demonstrated in cats lasting from 2 to 6 weeks after a single subcutaneous injection with greater improvement than observed with meloxicam during the first 3 weeks.[87] Notably, for the first time in the published literature, owners were able to differentiate treatment from placebo in a parallel group design. Data from an unpublished, randomized, placebo-controlled, blinded pilot field study (Gearing and others, 2016) supports efficacy and safety of frunevetmab for 6 weeks following intravenous and subcutaneous administration, and a pivotal trial using 3 monthly subcutaneous injections is currently under review by the US Food and Drug Administration for the treatment of pain associated with the osteoarthritis in cats. If approved, veterinarians will have to radically accept the novel mechanisms involved: it targets peripheral sensitization rather than inflammation directly.

SUMMARY

Neuropathic pain in cats is underappreciated and exists in a wide variety of presentations, conditions, and circumstances. Recognition, assessment, prevention, and treatment options are available, but more research is necessary to determine those that are most effective.

DISCLOSURE

The author has advisory and honoraria relationships with Zoetis Animal Health, Elanco Animal Health, Virbac North America, and PetPace.

REFERENCES

1. Treede RD, Jensen TS, Campbell JN, et al. J. Neuropathic pain: redefinition and a grading system for clinical and research purposes. Neurology 2008;70(18):1630–5.
2. Finnerup NB, Haroutounian S, Kamerman P, et al. Neuropathic pain: an updated grading system for research and clinical practice. Pain 2016;157(8):1599–606.

3. Muir WW III, Weise AJ, Wittum TE. Prevalence and characteristics of pain in dogs and cats examined as outpatients at a veterinary teaching hospital. J Am Vet Med Assoc 2004;224:1459–63.

4. van Hecke O, Austin SK, Khan RA, et al. Neuropathic pain in the general population: a systematic review of epidemiological studies. Pain 2014;155(4):654–62.

5. Wiese AJ, Muir WWW III, Wittum TE, et al. Characteristics of pain and response to analgesic treatment in dos and cats examined at a veterinary teaching hospital emergency service. J Am Vet Med Assoc 2005;226:2004–9.

6. Rusbridge C, Heath S, Gunn-Moore DA, et al. Feline orofacial pain syndrome (FOPS): a retrospective study of 113 cases. J Feline Med Surg 2010;12(6): 498–508.

7. Ciribassi J. Understanding behavior: feline hyperesthesia syndrome. Compend Contin Educ Vet 2009;31(3):E10.

8. Amengual Batle P, Rusbridge C, Nuttall T, et al. Feline hyperaesthesia syndrome with self-trauma to the tail: retrospective study of seven cases and proposal for an integrated multidisciplinary diagnostic approach. J Feline Med Surg 2019;21(2): 178–85.

9. Westropp JL, Delgado M, Buffington CAT. Chronic lower urinary tract signs in cats: current understanding of pathophysiology and management. Vet Clin North Am Small Anim Pract 2019;49(2):187–209.

10. Buffington CAT. Idiopathic cystitis in domestic cats—beyond the lower urinary tract. J Vet Intern Med 2011;25:784–96.

11. Buffington CA, Teng B, Somogyi GT. Norepinephrine content and adrenoceptor function in the bladder of cats with feline interstitial cystitis. J Urol 2002;167(4): 1876–80.

12. Sculptoreanu A, de Groat WC, Buffington CA, et al. Abnormal excitability in capsaicin-responsive DRG neurons from cats with feline interstitial cystitis. Exp Neurol 2005;193:437–43.

13. Buffington CAT, Wofle SA. High affinity binding sites for [3H] substance P in urinary bladders of cats with interstitial cystitis. J Urol 2000;163:1112–5.

14. Potts JM, Payne CK. Urologic chronic pelvic pain. Pain 2012;153(4):755–8.

15. Stella JL, Lord LK, Buffington CA. Sickness behaviors in response to unusual external events in healthy cats and cats with feline interstitial cystitis. J Am Vet Med Assoc 2011;238:67–73.

16. Chew DJ, Buffington CA, Kendell MS, et al. Amitriptyline treatment for severe recurrent idiopathic cystitis in cats. J Am Vet Med Assoc 1998;213:1282–96.

17. Persico P, Roccabianca P, Corona A, et al. Detection of F-HV1 via PCR and IHC in cats with ulcerative facial dermatitis. Vet Dermatol 2011;22(6):521–7.

18. Mazzei M, Vascellari M, Zanardello C, et al. Quantitative real time polymerase chain reaction (qRT-PCR) and RNAscope in situ hybridization (RNA-ISH) as effective tools to diagnose feline herpesvirus-1-associated dermatitis. Vet Dermatol 2019;30(6):491-e147.

19. Finnerup NB, Otto M, McQuay HJ, et al. Algorithm for neuropathic pain treatment: an evidence based proposal. Pain 2005;118(3):289–305.

20. Rolim VM, Pavarini SP, Campos FS, et al. Clinical, pathological, immunohistochemical and molecular characterization of feline chronic gingivostomatitis. J Feline Med Surg 2017;19(4):403–9.

21. Thakur M, Rahman W, Hobbs C, et al. Characterisation of a peripheral neuropathic component of the rat monoiodoacetate model of osteoarthritis. PLoS One 2012;7(3):e33730.

22. Havelin J, Imbert I, Cormier J, et al. Central sensitization and neuropathic features of ongoing pain in a rat model of advanced osteoarthritis. J Pain 2016;17(3): 374–82.

23. Hochman JR. Neuropathic pain symptoms in a community knee OA cohort. Osteoarthritis Cartilage 2011;19(6):647–54.

24. Guillot M, Taylor PM, Rialland P, et al. Evoked temporal summation in cats to highlight central sensitization related to osteoarthritis-associated chronic pain: a preliminary study. PLoS One 2014;9(5):e97347.

25. Lorenz ND, Comerford EJ, Iff I. Long-term use of gabapentin for musculoskeletal disease and trauma in three cats. J Feline Med Surg 2013;15(6):507–12.

26. Guedes AGP, Meadows JM, Pypendop BH, et al. Assessment of the effects of gabapentin on activity levels and owner-perceived mobility impairment and quality of life in osteoarthritic geriatric cats. J Am Vet Med Assoc 2018;253(5):579–85.

27. Adrian DE, Rishniw M, Scherk M, et al. Prescribing practices of veterinarians in the treatment of chronic musculoskeletal pain in cats. J Feline Med Surg 2019; 21(6):495–506.

28. Bielefeldt K, Davis B, Binion DG. Pain and inflammatory bowel disease. Inflamm Bowel Dis 2009;15(5):778–88.

29. Mathews KA. Neuropathic pain in dogs and cats: if only they could tell us if they hurt. Vet Clin North Am Small Anim Pract 2008 Nov;38(6):1365–414, vii-viii.

30. Goulden MR. The pain of chronic pancreatitis: a persistent clinical challenge. Br J Pain 2013;7(1):8–22.

31. Mizisin AP, Nelson RW, Sturges BK, et al. Comparable myelinated nerve pathology in feline and human diabetes mellitus. Acta Neuropathol 2007;113(4):431–42.

32. Estrella JS, Nelson RN, Sturges BK, et al. Endoneurial microvascular pathology in feline diabetic neuropathy. Microvasc Res 2008;75(3):403–10.

33. Dallocchio C, Buffa C, Mazzarello P, et al. Gabapentin vs. amitriptyline in painful diabetic neuropathy. an open-label pilot study. J Pain Symptom Manag 2000; 20(4):280–5.

34. O'Hagan BJ. Neuropathic pain in a cat post-amputation. Aust Vet J 2006;84:83–6.

35. Kuffler DP. Origins of Phantom Limb Pain. Mol Neurobiol 2018;55(1):60–9.

36. Gaynor JS. Chronic pain syndrome of feline onychectomy. NAVC Clinician's Brief 2005;63:11–3.

37. De Decker S, Warner AS, Volk HA. Prevalence and breed predisposition for thoracolumbar intervertebral disc disease in cats. J Feline Med Surg 2017;19(4):419–23.

38. Harris JE, Dhupa S. Lumbosacral intervertebral disk disease in six cats. J Am Anim Hosp Assoc 2008;44(3):109–15.

39. Popeny C, Ansell A, Renny K. Pudendal entrapment as an etiology of chronic perineal pain: diagnosis and treatment. Neurol Urodyn 2007;26(6):820–7.

40. Harris G, Ball J, De Decker S. Lumbosacral transitional vertebrae in cats and its relationship to lumbosacral vertebral canal stenosis. J Feline Med Surg 2019; 21(4):286–92.

41. Chakravarty A, Sen A. Migraine, neuropathic pain and nociceptive pain: towards a unifying concept. Med Hypotheses 2010;74(2):225–31.

42. Nowotny N, Weissenböck H. Description of feline nonsuppurative meningoencephalomyelitis ("staggering disease") and studies of its etiology. J Clin Microbiol 1995;33(6):1668–9.

43. Williams JH, Köster LS, Naidoo V, et al. Review of idiopathic eosinophilic meningitis in dogs and cats, with a detailed description of two recent cases in dogs. J S Afr Vet Assoc 2008;79(4):194–204.

44. Fuentes LV. Arterial thromboembolism: risks, realities and a rational first-line approach. J Feline Med Surg 2012;14(7):459–70.
45. Richebé P, Capdevila X, Rivat C. Persistent postsurgical pain: pathophysiology and preventative pharmacologic considerations. Anesthesiology 2018;129(3):590–607.
46. Powelson EB, Mills B, Henderson-Drager W, et al. Predicting chronic pain after major traumatic injury. Scand J Pain 2019;19(3):453–64.
47. Fletcher D, Stamer UM, Pogatzki-Zahn E, et al. euCPSP group for the Clinical Trial Network group of the European Society of Anaesthesiology: chronic postsurgical pain in Europe: an observational study. Eur J Anaesthesiol 2015;32:725–34.
48. Mitchell SAT, Majuta LA, Mantyh PW. New insights in understanding and treating bone fracture pain. Curr Osteoporos Rep 2018;16(4):325–32.
49. Meyhoff CS, Thomsen CH, Rasmussen LS, et al. High incidence of chronic pain following surgery for pelvic fracture. Clin J Pain 2006;22(2):167–72.
50. Beam S, Rassnick KM, Moore AS, et al. An immunohistochemical study of cyclooxygenase-2 expression in various feline neoplasms. Vet Pathol 2003; 40(5):496–500.
51. Schwei MJ, Honore P. Neurochemical and cellular reorganization of the spinal cord in a murine model of bone cancer pain. J Neurosci 1999;19(24):10886–97.
52. Fan TM, de Lorimier LP, O'Dell-Anderson K, et al. Single-agent pamidronate for palliative therapy of canine appendicular osteosarcoma bone pain. J Vet Intern Med 2007;21(3):431–9.
53. Yamasaki R, Fujii T, Wang B, et al. Allergic Inflammation Leads to Neuropathic Pain via Glial Cell Activation. J Neurosci 2016;36(47):11929–45.
54. Hachisuka J, Chiang MC, Ross SE. Itch and neuropathic itch. Pain 2018;159(3): 603–9.
55. Gruen ME, Dorman DC, Lascelles BDX. Caregiver placebo effect in analgesic clinical trials for cats with naturally occurring degenerative joint disease-associated pain. Vet Rec 2017;180(19):473.
56. Siao KT, Pypendop BH, Ilkiw JE. Pharmacokinetics of gabapentin in cats. Am J Vet Res 2010;71(7):817–21.
57. Adrian D, Papich MG, Baynes R, et al. The pharmacokinetics of gabapentin in cats. J Vet Intern Med 2018;32(6):1996–2002.
58. Trepanier LA. Applying pharmacokinetics to veterinary clinical practice. Vet Clin North Am Small Anim Pract 2013;43(5):1013–26.
59. Esteban MA, Dewey CW, Schwark WS, et al. Pharmacokinetics of Single-Dose Oral Pregabalin Administration in Normal Cats. Front Vet Sci 2018;5:136.
60. Goich M, Bascuñán A, Faúndez P, et al. Multimodal analgesia for treatment of allodynia and hyperalgesia after major trauma in a cat. JFMS Open Rep 2019;5(1). 2055116919855809.
61. Monteiro BP, Klinck MP, Moreau M, et al. Analgesic efficacy of tramadol in cats with naturally occurring osteoarthritis. PLoS One 2017;12(4):e0175565.
62. Monteiro BP, Klinck MP, Moreau M, et al. Analgesic efficacy of an oral transmucosal spray formulation of meloxicam alone or in combination with tramadol in cats with naturally occurring osteoarthritis. Vet Anaesth Analg 2016;43(6):643–51.
63. Ray J, Jordan D, Pinelli C, et al. Case studies of compounded Tramadol use in cats. Int J Pharm Compd 2012;16(1):44–9.
64. Indrawirawan Y, McAlees T. Tramadol toxicity in a cat: case report and literature review of serotonin syndrome. J Feline Med Surg 2014;16(7):572–8.
65. Lee HK, Lebkowska-Wieruszewska B, Kim TW, et al. Pharmacokinetics of the novel atypical opioid tapentadol after intravenous, intramuscular and subcutaneous administration in cats. Vet J 2013;198(3):620–4.

66. Doodnaught GM, Evangelista MC, Steagall PVM. Thermal antinociception following oral administration of tapentadol in conscious cats. Vet Anaesth Analg 2017;44(2):364–9.

67. McNicol ED, Midbari A, Eisenberg E. Opioids for neuropathic pain. Cochrane Database Syst Rev 2013;(8):CD006146.

68. Carr DB. Ketamine: does life begin at 40?. In: Carr DB, editor. IASP pain clinical updates, vol. XV 2007;. p. 3.

69. Ambros B, Duke T. Effect of low dose rate ketamine infusions on thermal and mechanical thresholds in conscious cats. Vet Anaesth Analg 2013 Nov;40(6): e76–82.

70. Schwenk ES, Viscusi ER, Buvanendran A, et al. Consensus guidelines on the use of intravenous ketamine infusions for acute pain management from the American Society of Regional Anesthesia and Pain Medicine, the American Academy of Pain Medicine, and the American Society of Anesthesiologists. Reg Anesth Pain Med 2018;43(5):456–66.

71. Epstein ME, Rodan I, Griffenhagen G, et al. 2015 AAHA/AAFP pain management guidelines for dogs and cats. J Feline Med Surg 2015;17(3):251–72.

72. Cohen SP, Bhatia A, Buvanendran A, et al. Consensus guidelines on the use of intravenous ketamine infusions for chronic pain from the American Society of Regional Anesthesia and Pain Medicine, the American Academy of Pain Medicine, and the American Society of Anesthesiologists. Reg Anesth Pain Med 2018;43(5):521–46.

73. Banpied TA, Clarke RJ, Johnson JW. Amantadine. J Neurosci 2005;25:3312–22.

74. Aiyer R A, Mehta N, Gungor S, et al. Systematic review of NMDA receptor antagonists for treatment of neuropathic pain in clinical practice. Clin J Pain 2018;34(5): 450–67.

75. Madden M, Gurney M, Bright S. Amantadine, an N-Methyl-D-Aspartate antagonist, for treatment of chronic neuropathic pain in a dog. Vet Anaesth Analg 2014;41(4):440–1.

76. Robertson SA. Managing pain in feline patients. Vet Clin North Am Small Anim Pract 2008;38:1267–90.

77. Siao KT, Pypendop BH, Escobar A, et al. Effect of amantadine on oxymorphone-induced thermal antinociception in cats. J Vet Pharmacol Ther 2012;35(2): 169–74.

78. Siao KT, Pypendop BH, Stanley SD, et al. Pharmacokinetics of amantadine in cats. J Vet Pharmacol Ther 2011;34(6):599–604.

79. Longmire DR, Jay GW, Boswell MV. Neuropathic pain. In: Boswell MV, Cole BE, editors. Weiner's pain management, A practical guide for clinicians. 7th edition. Boca Raton (FL): Taylor & Francis; 2006. p. 306–7.

80. Mealey KL, Peck KE, Bennett BS, et al. Systemic absorption of amitriptyline and buspirone after oral and transdermal administration to healthy cats. J Vet Intern Med 2004;18(1):43–6.

81. Pugh CM, Sweeney JT, Bloch CP, et al. Selective serotonin reuptake inhibitor (SSRI) toxicosis in cats: 33 cases (2004-2010). J Vet Emerg Crit Care (San Antonio) 2013;23(5):565–70.

82. Tauben D. Nonopioid medications for pain. Phys Med Rehabil Clin N Am 2015; 26(2):219–48.

83. Niyom S, Boscan P, Twedt DC, et al. Effect of maropitant, a neurokinin-1 receptor antagonist, on the minimum alveolar concentration of sevoflurane during stimulation of the ovarian ligament in cats. Vet Anaesth Analg 2013;40(4):425–31.

84. Corrêa JMX, Soares PCLR, Niella RV, et al. Evaluation of the antinociceptive effect of maropitant, a neurokinin-1 receptor antagonist, in cats undergoing ovariohysterectomy. Vet Med Int 2019;2019:9352528.
85. Aloe L, Rocco ML, Balzamino BO, et al. Nerve growth factor: a focus on neuroscience and therapy. Cur Neuropharmacol 2015;13(3):294–303.
86. Gearing DP, Huebner M, Virtue ER, et al. In vitro and in vivo characterization of a fully felinized therapeutic anti-nerve growth factor monoclonal antibody for the treatment of pain in cats. J Vet Intern Med 2016;30(4):1129–37.
87. Gruen ME, Thomson AE, Griffith EH, et al. A feline-specific anti-nerve growth factor antibody improves mobility in cats with degenerative joint disease-associated pain: a pilot proof of concept study. J Vet Intern Med 2016;30(4):1138–48.

Complex Disease Management: Managing a Cat with Comorbidities

Margie Scherk, DVM

KEYWORDS

- Comorbidities • Multiple conditions • Chronic kidney disease • Hypertension
- Hyperthyroidism • Diabetes mellitus • Degenerative joint disease

KEY POINTS

- When treating a cat with apparently conflicting comorbidities, focus on the common concerns.
- Optimize hydration and nutrition, while ensuring comfort through providing analgesia and making changes to the environment that support species-specific and individual-specific behaviors.
- Additional needs that are specific to each condition can be added to those common to all conditions.

INTRODUCTION

Elderly cats often present with multiple concurrent conditions. "Age-associated" or "age-appropriate" illnesses that we expect to see in older cats include problems related to the urinary tract (chronic kidney disease [CKD], pyelonephritis, calcium oxalate ureteronephroliths, bacterial cystitis), endocrine system (hyperthyroidism, diabetes mellitus, hyperaldosteronism), degenerative joint disease (DJD) and other musculoskeletal conditions, dental diseases, and neoplasia. Constipation, a result of dehydration and senescent motility, may become an ongoing concern. A decline in functioning of the special senses occurs frequently, and behavior changes suggestive of cognitive dysfunction may be seen in some individuals.

Making management recommendations may be challenging, as treatments for different diseases, at first glance, may appear to be in conflict. However, all body systems communicate and interact with each other. Identifying the common issues allows development of a logical treatment plan. The 4 most important therapeutic considerations that must be incorporated in caring for every patient, especially those that are older, are optimizing hydration, nutrition, comfort through analgesia, and

catsINK, Vancouver BC, Canada
E-mail address: hypurr@aol.com

Vet Clin Small Anim 50 (2020) 811–822
https://doi.org/10.1016/j.cvsm.2020.03.006
0195-5616/20/© 2020 Elsevier Inc. All rights reserved.

vetsmall.theclinics.com

ensuring that the environmental needs are met so they can perform normal behaviors.

To illustrate an approach to such a problem, a case of a cat with CKD, hypertension, hyperthyroidism, diabetes mellitus, and DJD is discussed.

IDENTIFYING THERAPEUTIC CHALLENGES

In the case of a patient with International Renal Interest Society (IRIS) Stage 2 to 3 CKD, hypertension, hyperthyroidism, diabetes, and DJD, the therapeutic goals for each condition are as follows:

- *Chronic kidney disease:* optimize hydration and feed a diet that will manage serum phosphorus levels and benefit renal health to minimize uremic episodes, manage hypertension and proteinuria, and enhance quality of life (QoL).
- *Hypertension:* reduce the risk for target organ damage (TOD), which may affect survival.
- *Hyperthyroidism:* modulate serum T3 and T4 levels to reduce metabolic rate, and normalize cardiac output, blood pressure, and renal perfusion.
- *Diabetes mellitus:* regulate blood glucose through insulin therapy and diet to reduce glucose toxicity, achieve glycemic control, and provide nutrients to cells.
- *DJD:* improve comfort through nonsteroidal antiinflammatory drugs (NSAIDs), optimize mobility, and ensure ready access to key resources.

MEETING NEEDS COMMON TO ALL CONDITIONS

The foundation for any treatment plan is achieving patient hydration, nutrition, freedom from pain, and meeting behavioral and environmental needs. The pet parent also affects outcome: in a study evaluating which factors influence decision making in clients considering the use of chemotherapy in terminally ill pets, "vomiting was considered an acceptable side effect but inappetence, weight loss and depression were considered unacceptable."[1]

Successful maintenance of euvolemia will be reflected in coat and stool character as well as subjective measures of well-being, including grooming, interaction, and posture. Feeding canned foods and improving desirability of water (bowls, location, freshness) should be considered to increase water consumption. Daily subcutaneous fluids (given with treats and warmed to body temperature) may be appropriate. A client handout is found as **Box 1**. Recently "nutrient-enriched" water supplements have become available that increase liquid intake, educe urine specific gravity, and improve measures of hydration in healthy cats.[2,3] However, studies are required to determine whether these products are beneficial in patients requiring more water.

Undoubtedly, meeting nutritional needs is important. Appetite may be negatively affected by renal disease from uremic toxins. Nausea associated with uremia may be alleviated with famotidine 5 mg orally every 24 hours or another H2 antagonist. However, the proton pump inhibitor omeprazole has been shown to provide better acid suppression than famotidine in cats.[4] In addition, twice-daily omeprazole (1 mg/kg orally twice a day) is more efficacious at suppressing acid production than once-daily dosing or ranitidine therapy.[5] Regardless, acid-suppression should be used judiciously, as the long-term use of proton pump inhibitors is not without potential negative adverse effects.[6] Antiemetics (eg, maropitant, mirtazapine, dolasetron, ondansetron), are unlikely to be required for this patient.

Appetite stimulants, including cyproheptadine (1 mg/cat orally twice a day), mirtazapine (1 to 2 mg/cat orally every 48 hours for cats with CKD)[7] may help to stimulate

Box 1
Client handout describing how to administer subcutaneous fluids

HOW TO GIVE SUBCUTANEOUS FLUIDS

To warm the fluids to body temperature:
1. Using an unopened bag:
   a. Remove the outside protective bag
   b. Microwave the bag for 2 to 3 minutes (depending on microwave)
   c. Massage the warmed bag to distribute the heat evenly.
   d. Test the bag on your wrist. It should feel comfortably warm, just about body temperature.
2. If the bag has already been used and has the line attached, do not microwave it, as the line will melt and seal shut.
   a. Boil water in a kettle or pot
   b. Put the bag into a vase or tall upright container with the bulb portion up so it will remain above the water
   c. Pour the hot water into the vase taking care to not reach the bulb
   d. Set the timer for approximately 5 minutes (depends on how much is remaining in used bag)
   e. Massage the warmed bag to distribute the heat evenly.
   f. Test the bag on your wrist. It should feel comfortably warm, just about body temperature

To connect a new line to a bag:
1. Prepare the line by rolling the wheel to a closed position
2. Take the cap off the line being careful not to touch the end of the line
3. Remove the end from the port on the bag
4. Insert the pointed end of the intravenous (IV) line into the port
5. Squeeze the bulb of the IV line to fill the bulb half full
6. Open the line by rolling the wheel to the open position and fill the line with fluids

To give your kitty fluids
1. Hang the bag of fluids on a curtain rod or shower rod with the still capped line hanging down
2. Place an unused, covered needle on the line and place the sterile cap (from the end of the line) close by
3. Sit somewhere comfortable. I prefer the floor so that kitty feels secure.
4. If you want, you can wrap your kitty in a towel, leaving head and shoulders exposed and cradle him/her
5. Remove the cover on the needle
6. With kitty facing away from you, holding the needle, rest your dominant hand on your kitty's back with the needle facing toward the kitty's head
7. Lift and make a tent with the skin between the kitty's shoulders using your nondominant hand
8. Exhale and firmly pull that skin tent over the needle
9. Open the IV line wheel and administer the volume of fluids as directed by your doctor
10. Once the needle is in place, because the fluids are warmed, kitty should be comfortable. Giving treats and praise doesn't hurt either!
11. Once you've given one-half of the fluid volume, back the needle out partially (but remain under the skin), so you can redirect it over the other shoulder and insert it fully again. This helps with weight distribution.
12. Close the IV line, remove and discard the needle, safely recapping the line with the sterile cap
13. Pinch the skin together with your nondominant hand when you remove the needle

CONGRATULATIONS! YOU'VE DONE IT!

Notes:

1. While you are getting used to this procedure, it may help to have the fur shaved over 2 places at the back of the neck. That way you can be sure the needle is getting under the skin. The fur will grow back.

2. Your kitty will look like she/he is wearing shoulder pads. The fluids will droop to one side down a leg, even to the paw. These will be absorbed over 12 to 24 hours. If the fluids have NOT been absorbed, a smaller volume is needed. Contact your veterinarian.

3. If some of the fluids or even a bit of blood leak from the injection site, there is no need to worry.

appetite. A transdermal formulation of mirtazapine has recently been licensed for cats; it may be more effective than any other appetite stimulant, including oral mirtazapine. In addition, it should be noted that mirtazapine and cyproheptadine should be used together only if serotonin syndrome occurs, as their mechanisms of action counter each other. Mirtazapine and maropitant can be administered concurrently; however, although effective in palliating vomiting, the antiemetic maropitant did not significantly improve appetite or support weight gain in cats with stage II and III CKD.[8] Although capromorelin has been shown to be effective in cats, the safe and efficacious dose has yet to be determined.

It is important to calculate caloric requirement, note it in the medical record, communicate the equivalent quantity of food to clients, and ask them to monitor the amount of food consumed.

Cats with untreated hyperthyroidism and diabetes may have an increased appetite, yet, because increased metabolism, lose weight and muscle. Once euthyroid and normoglycemic, their appetites generally normalize.

Some loss of muscle is part of normal aging and is not caused by apparent illness. Nutrition offers the possibility to improve longevity as well as QoL. Sarcopenia, the age-related loss of lean body mass (LBM), is a gradual process: initially it is unapparent because increases in body fat persist; however, the loss of weight precedes the diagnosis of CKD and has profound effects on survival.[9] Studies have identified decreased survival associated with thin body condition.[10–12] Although not yet shown in prospective studies, preservation of body weight and LBM may enhance survival and QoL in aging cats and those with CKD.

The dietary strategy must take body weight, body condition score (BCS), and muscle condition score (MCS) into consideration. When MCS is poor, protein supplementation should be considered. Rather than waiting for malnutrition to develop, early nutritional intervention is recommended if a patient

- Is hypo or anorexic for >3 to 5 days
- Has a low BCS or MCS and is unwilling or unable to consume a sufficient number of calories to achieve and maintain an ideal BCS
- Is dysrexic and is unwilling to eat a diet appropriate for its medical condition[13]

Intervention includes ensuring an appropriate, low-stress environment, use of appetite stimulants, low-stress oral-assisted (syringe) feeding, and placement of medium-term feeding tubes. Large-bore esophagostomy tubes are quick and easy to place and use.

NEEDS SPECIFIC TO EACH GIVEN CONDITION
Chronic Kidney Disease

In most cases, the initiating cause for the CKD is not known, thus management is directed toward attenuating the rate of the deterioration of function by controlling proteinuria, hypertension, and hyperphosphatemia. As 40% to 75% of cats with CKD present with dehydration, cachexia, and weight loss, rehydration, with the goal of maintaining hydration, and improving nutritional plane are important goals.[14] Indeed, as already mentioned, weight loss begins 3 years before the diagnosis of CKD is made.[9]

It is generally recommended to feed cats with IRIS Stage 2 and onward CKD, a renal diet.[15,16] Renal diets provide increased potassium, are alkalinizing, have reduced phosphorus, and are restricted in protein. Data that clearly define what nutritional requirements a cat with CKD has are lacking and most information is extrapolated from other species or from renal ablation studies. A review of the literature revealed that restricting dietary phosphorus in an alkalinizing diet supplemented with potassium appears to be beneficial to cats with CKD.[17] Many questions remain regarding the optimal composition of a renal diet; however, the previous dogma that renal diets should be restricted in protein regardless of underlying renal pathology or body condition has been challenged. Creatinine and urea are results of muscle and protein metabolism. These are, however, only 2 of more than 60 recognized uremic toxins. In addition, protein degradation products are not very toxic. In human studies, it has become apparent that tissue breakdown, rather than breakdown of nutritional protein, generates toxins. So, although uremic toxins can result in malnutrition, malnutrition itself results in inflammation, morbidity, and mortality in human patients with CKD, therefore ensuring that an individual patient is thriving on a given diet is essential.[18] It is critical to ensure that an individual is eating a sufficient amount of the renal, or any, diet to meet their protein calorie needs.

The rate of progression or decreased survival time are affected by the aforementioned proteinuria, hypertension, and hyperphosphatemia, as well as anemia, azotemia, and metabolic acidosis.[14] Correcting dehydration results in improvements in azotemia, metabolic acidosis, and hyperphosphatemia. In addition, because inadequate protein may result in poor muscle condition, with increased morbidity and mortality, other means of restricting phosphorus may need to be considered. In 2018, new renal diets were introduced with increased levels of protein while still restricted in phosphorus. In some cats, using intestinal phosphate binders along with a diet that the individual cat eats with enthusiasm may be desirable. Some cats will benefit through augmenting their diet with a low-phosphorus protein supplement.

Reassessment should include evaluating not just body weight to look for trends, but also percent weight changes, body condition, and muscle condition scoring (see Body Condition Score: https://wsava.org/wp-content/uploads/2020/01/Cat-Body-Condition-Scoring-2017.pdf; see Muscle Condition Score: https://wsava.org/wp-content/uploads/2020/01/Muscle-Condition-Score-Chart-for-Cats.pdf).

Hypertension

Hypertension is a common problem in cats, mostly secondary to other diseases (ie, CKD, hyperthyroidism, hyperaldosteronism), but also occurs as a primary problem (essential hypertension). Because of the effects of untreated hypertension on highly vascular target organs (ie, eyes, brain, kidneys, and cardiovascular system), it is very important to detect elevations in blood pressure early to prevent permanent damage.[19]

As many as 65% of cats with CKD are hypertensive irrespective of the degree of severity of the renal disease.[20–22] Hypertension is less common in cats with hyperthyroidism (approximately 10%–23% at time of diagnosis), but approximately 25% of cats develop hypertension after initiation of therapy or even once euthyroidism has been achieved.[23–25] Diabetes mellitus is associated with hypertension in humans, but this does not appear to occur in cats. As many cats with diabetes have concurrent conditions that may be a risk factor for hypertension, it is difficult to unequivocally rule out any association.[26,27]

Nephrosclerosis (renal arteriosclerosis and glomerulosclerosis) is seen in hypertensive cats with CKD.[28] It is unclear, however, whether the hypertension contributes to progression of CKD (as it does in humans and in dogs). Hypertension can, however, contribute to proteinuria in CKD, and proteinuria is associated with shorter survival in cats.[29–31] Control of hypertension is important for its negative effects on cardiac function as well as progression of CKD.

The goal of treatment is to reduce the risk of TOD with an initial goal of 160 mm Hg and a long-term target of 140 mm Hg.[32] Amlodipine will reduce blood pressure by 30 to 70 mm Hg.[33,34] Starting dose is 0.625 mg/cat orally every 24 hours. Cats with blood pressure of $\geq$200 mm Hg may be started at 1.25 mg/cat orally every 24 hours, titrating cautiously up to 2.5 mg/cat orally every 24 hours.[35] In cats with proteinuric CKD, it may also reduce proteinuria. Telmisartan, an angiotensin receptor blocker, is licensed for treatment of CKD-associated proteinuria and has a beneficial effect on hypertension at 1.5 to 2 mg/kg orally every 24 hours.[36–38]

Hyperthyroidism

Renal disease is fairly common in untreated hyperthyroid cats. It may be masked due to increased cardiac output, renal blood flow, and glomerular filtration rate (GFR). The effects of muscle wasting exacerbate the lower creatinine concentrations. Monitoring renal parameters and muscle condition during therapy is advised. Similarly, hypertension may become evident only during the course of therapy or even after the patient is euthyroid. It is well recognized that amelioration of the hyperthyroid state by any method (ie, medical therapy, 131I treatment, or surgery) can result in decreased GFR, elevations in serum urea nitrogen and creatinine, and, in some cases, overt azotemia. The decline in GFR stabilizes by approximately 4 weeks.[39,40]

A practical approach to a patient with concurrent hyperthyroidism and CKD is to treat medically until the serum T4 is adequately controlled, at which time the effect of permanent therapy (radioiodine or surgery) may be predicted. If renal decline becomes apparent once euthyroidism has been achieved by an irreversible method, or if the cat becomes hypothyroid, exogenous thyroid hormone can be supplemented to support the kidneys. A balance must then be struck between creating iatrogenic hypothyroidism and maintaining renal function, as iatrogenic hypothyroidism appears to contribute to azotemia and decreased survival.[41–45] It is recommended to monitor serum thyroid-stimulating hormone (TSH) levels after radioiodine or during medical therapy to avoid iatrogenic hypothyroidism.[43,46] These cats should either receive a lower dose of medication or be supplemented with thyroxine before they develop overt disease or CKD.

From a nutritional perspective, hyperthyroidism is a hypermetabolic state that has profound effects not just on the kidneys, but also on body condition, muscle, the parathyroid, and endocrine pancreas. Peterson and Eirmann[47] recommend feeding "a diet containing a large amount of dietary protein (>40% of daily calories or metabolizable energy [ME] as protein; >12 g/100 kcal), a small amount of carbohydrate (<15% of total calories or ME; <4.5 g/100 kcal), and a moderate amount of phosphate (<250 mg of phosphate per 100 kcal)." For diabetes, a catabolic condition, they recommend feeding high protein (>40% ME; >12 g/100 kcal) to help maintain muscle mass.[47]

Diabetes

In addition to feeding a higher protein diet with restricted carbohydrate (cho) content, insulin is required to reverse glucose toxicity induced by the hyperglycemic state. Although evidence for benefit of feeding a high-protein low-carbohydrate diet is weak because of small sample size, variability in study design, and the impossibility to adjust a diet for just 1 nutrient, it suggests that feeding a diet with <3 g cho/100 g ME may be beneficial. Feeding canned food may be preferable to dry low-carbohydrate food, which may be preferable to feeding other dry food.[48]

Insulin choice is patient dependent, as there is no one best insulin. In fact, because diabetes is such a dynamic process, the insulin dose and even type may change for optimal therapy over the lifetime of a given individual. In general, it is advisable to start with an insulin licensed for cats or veterinary patients. Although not without challenges, blood glucose curves can be helpful in determining how a given patient is responding to a given insulin type. Alternately, monitoring interstitial glucose continuously (using a continuous glucose monitoring system or a flash device) is an option to replace curves in some patients.[49–53]

Diabetes in cats tends to be associated with chronic inflammatory conditions. Wherever possible, the source of inflammation should be identified and treated or controlled. Due to poor glycemic control, as well as low urine specific gravity, this patient also may be at risk for infectious problems, such as bacterial urinary tract infections. However, as bacteriuria may be subclinical and not require treatment in some individuals, a culture and sensitivity profile should be determined for appropriate and efficacious antimicrobial therapy. Should anesthesia be required to diagnose or modulate the underlying problem (eg, gastrointestinal inflammation and gingivitis, respectively), administer half of the insulin dose on the morning of anesthesia to a fed and hydrated cat. As with any preoperative cat, food should be withheld only for 3 to 4 hours.[54] Blood glucose should be monitored in diabetic patients during and after the procedure.

Degenerative Joint Disease

The cat with joint pain is often an older patient who may have concurrent problems including some that may affect drug metabolism (eg, CKD). Like painful patients of any age, they may be in a physiologic state that affects drug disposition, the most common ones being dehydration, inadequate tissue oxygenation (from anemia, hypotension, or hypovolemia), electrolyte or acid-base imbalances, and malnutrition. The greatest concern regarding potential adverse effects of NSAIDs should be in a patient with dehydration or anesthesia-related hypotension, as these could result in negative effects on gastric mucosal health or on renal function. Correction or prevention of these problems allows the NSAID to be used in most cases.

Opioids are safe for pain relief in any age group, and are excellent when used at the same time as other agents, especially NSAIDs. They are not, however, a first drug of choice for cats with arthritic pain, as they are not very effective for DJD. Metacam 0.5 mg/mL oral suspension has been granted a license in the European Union for the alleviation of inflammation and pain in chronic musculoskeletal disorders in cats. The registered dose is 0.1 mg/kg on the first day followed by 0.05 mg/kg orally once daily. Another brand of meloxicam (Loxicam) is also licensed for long-term use in cats in the European Union at the same dosage.

Three studies have evaluated long-term safety of meloxicam in older cats; one concluded that this agent is safe and efficacious for musculoskeletal pain administered at 0.01 to 0.03 mg/kg orally every 24 hours for a mean treatment duration of 5.8 months; no deleterious effect on renal function was detected. Gastrointestinal upset in 4% of cats was the only adverse effect noted.[55] The second and third studies reviewed the medical records of cats older than 7 years treated for a minimum of 6 months with a daily maintenance dose of 0.02 mg/kg meloxicam and concluded that this dose does not hasten progression of renal disease in aged cats or aged cats with preexistent stable IRIS stage 1 to 3 renal disease.[56,57]

In 2015, an article reported on the safety of robenacoxib (1–2.4 mg/kg) for daily, month-long treatment of DJD in cats, including 40 with CKD IRIS stages 2 to 4. There was no evidence of increased risk in the frequency of reported adverse events, or in deterioration in renal variables in the subgroup of cats with concurrent CKD.[58] Since 2018, the license for Onsior in Canada and the European Union allows for duration of treatment to be determined on an individual basis.

A suitable protocol for a cat with pain from musculoskeletal disease might be baseline NSAID with intermittent use of an opioid (such as buprenorphine) when "breakthrough" pain is evidenced by a decrease in appetite, mobility, or social interaction. Gabapentin may be added for ongoing care.

Environmental modifications: All resources should be easily accessible. Ramps and steps to favorite sleeping spots are helpful. Warm, soft, padded sleeping places for stiff, painful, possibly bony joints should be considered. Raising food and water bowls may help the cat with cervical vertebral changes. Adding a litter tray to reduce the distance between boxes may reduce accidents as well as encourage regular voiding and defecation. The rim of the tray must not be too high, nor the opening into the box too small. It should be scooped several times a day to encourage use. Regular nail trimming helps by maintaining proper joint relationships.

Feeding a diet that is supplemented with eicosapentaenoic acid, and docosahexaenoic acid ± green-lipped mussel extract and glucosamine/chondroitin sulfate may be beneficial. Disease-modifying agents such as polysulfated glycosaminoglycan, glucosamine, and chondroitin sulfate may improve mobility.[59] Additional modalities (therapeutic exercise, acupuncture, cold laser therapy), although no scientific studies have been done to support efficacy, may also play a role in providing comfort for a cat with musculoskeletal discomfort.

MANAGEMENT PLAN FOR A PATIENT WITH INTERNATIONAL RENAL INTEREST SOCIETY STAGE 2 TO 3 CHRONIC KIDNEY DISEASE, HYPERTENSION, HYPERTHYROIDISM, DIABETES MELLITUS, AND DEGENERATIVE JOINT DISEASE

Taking all of these factors into consideration, a reasonable plan would be as follows:

Hydration: Consider administering daily subcutaneous fluids once rehydrated starting at 2 to 3 mL/kg ideal weight per day based on the individual's needs.[60] Ensure availability of multiple, accessible fresh water stations. In addition, a "third bowl" containing a "nutrient-enriched" water supplement may be considered. Assess hydration based on completeness of fluid absorption and stool character.

Nutrition: Feed enough of an alkalinizing diet that provides the cat with adequate protein to optimize muscle condition based on reassessment. Should phosphorus restriction be indicated, consider feeding an early renal diet or using an intestinal phosphate binder.

Analgesia: Administer an NSAID daily, starting at label dose and titrating down to as low a dose that controls the discomfort. Consider multimodal additions of gabapentin and an opioid.

Meeting behavioral and environmental needs: Endure easy access to all key resources.[61]

Medical therapies: Amlodipine or telmisartan, methimazole, insulin, treatment for underlying inflammatory conditions.

DISCLOSURE

The author has nothing to disclose.

REFERENCES

1. Williams J, Phillips C, Byrd HM. Factors which influence owners when deciding to use chemotherapy in terminally ill pets. Animals 2017;7. https://doi.org/10.3390/ani7030018.
2. Zanghi BM, Gerheart L, Gardner CL. Effects of a nutrient-enriched water on water intake and indices of hydration in healthy domestic cats fed a dry kibble diet. Am J Vet Res 2018;79(7):733–44.
3. Zanghi BM, Wils-Plotz E, DeGeer S, et al. Effects of a nutrient-enriched water with and without poultry flavoring on water intake, urine specific gravity, and urine output in healthy domestic cats fed a dry kibble diet. Am J Vet Res 2018;79(11):1150–9.
4. Parkinson S, Tolbert K, Messenger K, et al. Evaluation of the effect of orally administered acid suppressants on intragastric pH in cats. J Vet Intern Med 2015;29:104–12.
5. Šutalo S, Ruetten M, Hartnack S, et al. The effect of orally administered ranitidine and once-daily or twice-daily orally administered omeprazole on intragastric pH in cats. J Vet Intern Med 2015;29:840–6.
6. Marks SL, Kook PH, Papich MG, et al. consensus statement: Support for rational administration of gastrointestinal protectants to dogs and cats. J Vet Intern Med 2018;32:1823–40.
7. Quimby JM, Lunn KF. Mirtazapine as an appetite stimulant and anti-emetic in cats with chronic kidney disease: a masked placebo-controlled crossover clinical trial. Vet J 2013;197:651–5.
8. Quimby JM, Brock WT, Moses K, et al. Chronic use of maropitant for the management of vomiting and inappetence in cats with chronic kidney disease: a blinded, placebo-controlled clinical trial. J Feline Med Surg 2015;17:692–7.
9. Freeman LM, Lachaud MP, Matthews S, et al. Evaluation of weight loss over time in cats with chronic kidney disease. J Vet Intern Med 2016;30:1661–6.
10. Scarlett JM, Donoghue S. Associations between body condition and disease in cats. J Am Vet Med Assoc 1998;212:1725–31.
11. Doria-Rose VP, Scarlett JM. Mortality rates and causes of death among emaciated cats. J Am Vet Med Assoc 2000;216:347–51.
12. Freeman LM. Cachexia and sarcopenia: emerging syndromes of importance in dogs and cats. J Vet Intern Med 2012;26:3–17.
13. Johnson LN, Freeman LM. Recognizing, describing, and managing reduced food intake in dogs and cats. J Am Vet Med Assoc 2017;251:1260–6.
14. Reynolds BS, Lefebvre HP, Feline CKD. Pathophysiology and risk factors—what do we know? J Feline Med Surg 2013;15(1_suppl):3–14.
15. Ross SJ, Osborne CA, Kirk CA, et al. Clinical evaluation of dietary modification for treatment of spontaneous chronic kidney disease in cats. J Am Vet Med Assoc 2006;229:949–57.
16. Polzin DJ, Churchill JA. Controversies in veterinary nephrology: renal diets are indicated for cats with International Renal Interest Society chronic kidney disease stages 2 to 4: the pro view. Vet Clin Small Anim 2016;46:1049–65.
17. Scherk MA, Laflamme DP. Controversies in veterinary nephrology: renal diets are indicated for cats with International Renal Interest Society chronic kidney disease stages 2 to 4: the con view. Vet Clin Small Anim 2016;46:1067–94.
18. Vanholder R, Glorieux G, Lameire N. The other side of the coin: impact of toxin generation and nutrition on the uremic syndrome. Semin Dial 2002;15:311–4.

19. Taylor SS, Sparkes AH, Briscoe K, et al. ISFM consensus guidelines on the diagnosis and management of hypertension in cats. J Feline Med Surg 2017;19(3): 288–303.

20. Kobayashi DL, Peterson ME, Graves TK, et al. Hypertension in cats with chronic renal failure or hyperthyroidism. J Vet Intern Med 1990;4:58–62.

21. Syme HM, Barber PJ, Markwell PJ, et al. Prevalence of systolic hypertension in cats with chronic renal failure at initial evaluation. J Am Vet Med Assoc 2002; 220:1799–804.

22. Bijsmans ES, Jepson RE, Chang YM, et al. Changes in systolic blood pressure over time in healthy cats and cats with chronic kidney disease. J Vet Intern Med 2015;29:855–61.

23. Morrow LD, Adams VJ, Elliott J, et al. Hypertension in hyperthyroid cats: prevalence, incidence and predictors of its development [abstract]. J Vet Intern Med 2009;23:699.

24. Syme HM, Elliott J. The prevalence of hypertension in hyperthyroid cats at diagnosis and following treatment [abstract]. J Vet Intern Med 2003;17:754.

25. Williams TL, Elliott J, Syme HM. Renin-angiotensin- aldosterone system activity in hyperthyroid cats with and without concurrent hypertension. J Vet Intern Med 2013;27:522–9.

26. Sennello KA, Schulman RL, Prosek R, et al. Systolic blood pressure in cats with diabetes mellitus. J Am Vet Med Assoc 2003;223:198–201.

27. Bloom CA, Rand JS. Diabetes and the kidney in human and veterinary medicine. Vet Clin North Am Small Anim Pract 2013;43:351–65.

28. Chakrabarti S, Syme HM, Elliott J. Clinicopathological variables predicting progression of azotemia in cats with chronic kidney disease. J Vet Intern Med 2012;26:275–81.

29. Syme HM, Markwell PJ, Pfeiffer D, et al. Survival of cats with naturally occurring chronic renal failure is related to severity of proteinuria. J Vet Intern Med 2006;20: 528–35.

30. Jepson RE, Elliott J, Brodbelt D, et al. Effect of control of systolic blood pressure on survival in cats with systemic hypertension. J Vet Intern Med 2007;21:402–9.

31. King JN, Tasker S, Gunn-Moore DA, et al. Prognostic factors in cats with chronic kidney disease. J Vet Intern Med 2007;21:906–16.

32. Acierno MJ, Brown S, Coleman AE, et al. ACVIM consensus statement: Guidelines for the identification, evaluation, and management of systemic hypertension in dogs and cats. J Vet Intern Med 2018;32(6):1803–22.

33. Elliott J, Barber PJ, Syme HM, et al. Feline hypertension: clinical findings and response to antihypertensive treatment in 30 cases. J Small Anim Pract 2001; 42:122–9.

34. Bijsmans ES, Doig M, Jepson RE, et al. Factors influencing the relationship between the dose of amlodipine required for blood pressure control and change in blood pressure in hypertensive cats. J Vet Intern Med 2016;30:1630–6.

35. Huhtinen M, Derre G, Renoldi HJ, et al. Randomized placebo-controlled clinical trial of a chewable formulation of amlodipine for the treatment of hypertension in client-owned cats. J Vet Intern Med 2015;29:786–93.

36. Glaus TM, Elliott J, Herberich E, et al. Efficacy of long-term oral telmisartan treatment in cats with hypertension: Results of a prospective European clinical trial. J Vet Intern Med 2019;33(2):413–22.

37. Coleman AE, Brown SA, Traas AM, et al. Safety and efficacy of orally administered telmisartan for the treatment of systemic hypertension in cats: results of a

double-blind, placebo-controlled, randomized clinical trial. J Vet Intern Med 2019;33(2):478–88.

38. Sent U, Gössl R, Elliott J, et al. Comparison of efficacy of long-term oral treatment with telmisartan and benazepril in cats with chronic kidney disease. J Vet Intern Med 2015;29:1479–87.

39. Becker TJ, Graves TK, Kruger JM, et al. Effects of methimazole on renal function in cats with hyperthyroidism. J Am Anim Hosp Assoc 2000;36:215.

40. Boag AK, Neiger R, Slater L, et al. Changes in the glomerular filtration rate of 27 cats with hyperthyroidism after treatment with radioactive iodine. Vet Rec 2007; 161:711.

41. Peterson ME. Feline focus: diagnostic testing for feline thyroid disease: hypothyroidism. Compendium 2013;35:E4.

42. Peterson ME. Diagnosis and management of iatrogenic hypothyroidism. In: Little SE, editor. August's consultations in feline internal medicine, vol. 7. St Louis (MO): Elsevier; 2016. p. 260–9.

43. Peterson ME. Advances in the treatment of feline hyperthyroidism: a strategy to slow the progression of CKD Proceedings ACVIM Forum Nashville, TN, June 4-7, 2014. p. 1083–5.

44. Williams TL, Elliott J, Syme HM. Effect on renal function of restoration of euthyroidism in hyperthyroid cats with iatrogenic hypothyroidism. J Vet Intern Med 2014; 28:1251–5.

45. Aldridge C, Behrend EN, Martin LG, et al. Evaluation of thyroid-stimulating hormone, total thyroxine, and free thyroxine concentrations in hyperthyroid cats receiving methimazole treatment. J Vet Intern Med 2015;29:862–8.

46. Peterson ME. Clinical study: information for veterinarians regarding enrolling cats into study - monitoring the effects of radioiodine treatment with a complete thyroid panel (T4, T3, Free T4, TSH). Available at: https://www.animalendocrine.com/wp-content/uploads/2012/09/Vets-Complete-Thyroid-Panel-T4-T3-Free-T4-TSH-to-Diagnose-Iatrogenic-Hypothyroidism-in-Cats.pdf. Accessed March 15, 2020.

47. Peterson ME, Eirmann L. Dietary management of feline endocrine disease. Vet Clin Small Anim 2014;44:775–88.

48. Sparkes A, Cannon M, Church D, et al. ISFM consensus guidelines on the practical management of diabetes mellitus in cats. J Feline Med Surg 2015;17(3): 235–50.

49. Reusch CE, Kley S, Casella M. Home monitoring of the diabetic cat. J Feline Med Surg 2006;8:119–27.

50. Moretti S, Tschuor F, Osto M, et al. Evaluation of a novel real-time continuous glucose-monitoring system for use in cats. J Vet Intern Med 2010;24:120–6.

51. Salesov E, Zini E, Riederer A, et al. Comparison of the pharmacodynamics of protamine zinc insulin and insulin degludec and validation of the continuous glucose monitoring system iPro2 in healthy cats. Res Vet Sci 2018;118:79–85.

52. Corradini S, Pilosio B, Dondi F, et al. Accuracy of a flash glucose monitoring system in diabetic dogs. J Vet Intern Med 2016;30(4):983–8.

53. Gottlieb S, Rand J. Managing feline diabetes: current perspectives (Review). Vet Med Res Rep 2018;9:33.

54. Robertson SA, Gogolski SM, Pascoe P, et al. AAFP feline anesthesia guidelines. J Feline Med Surg 2018;20(7):602–34.

55. Gunew MN, Menrath VH, Marshall RD. Long-term safety, efficacy and palatability of oral meloxicam at 0.01-0.03 mg/kg for treatment of osteoarthritic pain in cats. J Feline Med Surg 2008;10:235–41.

56. Gowan R, Lingard A, Johnston L, et al. Retrospective case control study of the effects of long-term dosing with meloxicam on renal function in aged cats with degenerative joint disease. J Feline Med Surg 2011;13:752–61.

57. Gowan RA, Baral RM, Lingard AE, et al. A retrospective analysis of the effects of meloxicam on the longevity of aged cats with and without overt chronic kidney disease. J Feline Med Surg 2012;14(12):876–81.

58. King JN, King S, Budsberg SC, et al. Clinical safety of robenacoxib in feline osteoarthritis: results of a randomized, blinded, placebo-controlled clinical trial. J Feline Med Surg 2016;18(8):632–42.

59. Lascelles BDX, Depuy V, Thomson A, et al. Evaluation of a therapeutic diet for feline degenerative joint disease. J Vet Intern Med 2010;24:487–95.

60. Davis H, Jensen T, Johnson A, et al. 2013 AAHA/AAFP fluid therapy guidelines for dogs and cats. J Am Anim Hosp Assoc 2013;49(3):149–59.

61. Ellis SL, Rodan I, Carney HC, et al. AAFP and ISFM feline environmental needs guidelines. J Feline Med Surg 2013;15(3):219–30.

Distinguishing Between Dermatologic Disorders of the Face, Nasal Planum, and Ears

Great Lookalikes in Feline Dermatology

Kimberly Coyner, DVM

KEYWORDS

- Feline facial dermatitis • Dermatophytosis • Herpesvirus • Atopy • Food allergy
- Mosquito bite hypersensitivity • Squamous cell carcinoma • Bowen's disease

KEY POINTS

- Facial dermatitis in cats can be caused by a broad range of infectious, allergic, immune-mediated and neoplastic disorders with very different treatments and prognoses.
- Baseline dermatologic diagnostics (skin scrapings for mites, cytology for infection and to characterize inflammatory infiltrate, and dermatophyte culture) are indicated in all cases; aerobic bacterial skin culture is indicated if bacteria are found on cytology despite empiric antibiotics.
- Biopsies for dermatohistopathology ± tissue cultures are indicated in cases that are not diagnosed on screening tests and that do not respond to empiric therapy.

INTRODUCTION

Facial dermatitis in cats can be a frustrating clinical entity to diagnose, because many disorders look similar. This article presents facial disorders as they present clinically: pruritic, alopecic, crusting, ulcerative, or nodular diseases on the face, nonhaired nasal planum, haired skin of the muzzle/face, pinna, and ear canal. Case approach, differential diagnoses, and diagnostic testing are discussed. General treatments for the most common presenting complaint of facial pruritus are presented; however specific treatments for every cause of facial dermatitis are beyond the scope of this article, and appropriate references are provided.

Dermatology Clinic for Animals, 8300 Quinault Drive NE, Suite A, Lacey, WA 98516, USA
E-mail address: dermvetwa@gmail.com

Vet Clin Small Anim 50 (2020) 823–882
https://doi.org/10.1016/j.cvsm.2020.03.008
0195-5616/20/© 2020 Elsevier Inc. All rights reserved.

vetsmall.theclinics.com

Table 1
Causes by clinical sign and location

	Nonhaired Nasal Planum	Haired Dorsal Nose/Chin/Lips/Eyelids/Face	Pinna	Ear Canal
Pruritic	Allergy, ± herpes, pemphigus foliaceus (which cause crusting ± erosions but are not necessarily pruritic)	Allergy, parasites, bacterial or yeast infection (2° to underlying 1° disease); ± herpes, dermatophytosis, pemphigus foliaceus (which cause hair loss/crusting but are not necessarily pruritic)	Allergy, parasites, bacterial or yeast infection (2° to underlying 1° disease); ± dermatophytosis, pemphigus foliaceus (which cause hair loss/crusting but are not necessarily pruritic)	Allergy, parasites, bacterial or yeast infection (2° to underlying 1° disease); ± pemphigus foliaceus
Alopecic	NA	Dermatophyte, Demodex, rubbing caused by allergy, rarely immune-mediated follicular or paraneoplastic disorders	Dermatophyte, Demodex, self-trauma caused by allergy, idiopathic pinnal alopecia, solar dermatosis, overuse of topical steroids	NA
Ulcerative	Herpes, deep fungal or mycobacterial infection, mosquito bite hypersensitivity, trauma caused by allergy, Bengal nasal ulcerative dermatitis, neoplasia, immune mediated (vasculitis, pemphigus vulgaris; very rare)	Herpes, eroded eosinophilic granuloma, deep fungal or mycobacterial infection, mosquito bite hypersensitivity, trauma caused by allergy, neoplasia, immune mediated (vasculitis, pemphigus vulgaris; very rare)	Deep bacterial or fungal infection, mycobacterial, self-trauma caused by allergy/parasites, immune-mediated disease, neoplasia	Severe infection, self-trauma secondary to allergy/parasites, immune-mediated disease, neoplasia
Nodular	Deep fungal or mycobacterial infection, neoplasia	Deep fungal or mycobacterial infection, eosinophilic granuloma (lips/chin), neoplasia, severe feline acne (chin), apocrine cystomatosis (lips/eyelids), nasal plasma cell dermatitis	Deep fungal or mycobacterial infection, neoplasia	Inflammatory polyp, neoplasia, apocrine cystomatosis

| Crusting | Pemphigus foliaceus, herpes, deep fungal, mosquito bite hypersensitivity, trauma caused by allergy, Bengal nasal ulcerative dermatitis, neoplasia | Dermatophyte, Demodex, pemphigus foliaceus, allergy, Notoedres, severe feline acne (chin), neoplasia. Rare: sebaceous adenitis, erythema multiforme, paraneoplastic, thymoma-induced exfoliative dermatitis, idiopathic facial dermatosis/dirty face syndrome | Dermatophyte, Notoedres, pemphigus foliaceus, self-trauma ± bacterial infection secondary to underlying allergy. neoplasia. Rare: sebaceous adenitis, erythema multiforme, paraneoplastic, thymoma-induced exfoliative dermatitis | Otodectes, bacterial infection secondary to underlying disease, self-trauma secondary to allergy/ parasites, pemphigus foliaceus, neoplasia, proliferative necrotizing otitis externa |

Abbreviation: NA, not applicable.

FACIAL DERMATOSES
Facial Pruritus

Key points
Facial pruritus is a common clinical presentation in cats and has 3 main causes (**Table 1**)[1]: (1) allergy (eg, food allergy, atopy [**Fig. 1**], flea bite hypersensitivity, mosquito bite hypersensitivity)[1]; (2) parasites, including *Notoedres* (**Fig. 2**), *Demodex*, *Otodectes*,[2,3] and fleas; and (3) bacterial and/or yeast infections commonly occurring secondarily to an underlying primary disease, such as allergy (**Fig. 3**) or parasites. These infections can also complicate rare dermatoses such as paraneoplastic alopecia or thymoma-induced exfoliative dermatitis. Less common causes for facial pruritus in cats include dermatophytosis, herpesvirus dermatitis, and pemphigus foliaceus[4–6]; these disorders tend to cause hair loss and crusting but are not necessarily pruritic.

Diagnosis/clinical management
As with all dermatoses, baseline dermatologic diagnostics (skin scrapings for mites, cytology for infection and to characterize inflammatory infiltrate, and dermatophyte culture) are indicated in all cases (see **Table 1**). Should secondary bacterial or yeast infection be present (based on cytology), treat with a 3-week course of appropriate antimicrobial therapy and perform aerobic bacterial culture if bacteria persist cytologically despite empiric antibiotics. To ensure hard-to-find parasites (eg, feline *Demodex*) are not present, a therapeutic trial with an isoxazoline or imidacloprid plus moxidectin is indicated (these products also kill *Otodectes* and *Notoedres*).[7,8] If pruritus persists despite these treatments, a prescription hypoallergenic diet trial for 8 to 12 weeks is warranted (**Box 1**). If pruritus is moderate to severe, oral corticosteroids may be helpful to reduce self-trauma during the first 3 to 4 weeks on the hypoallergenic diet.

Corticosteroid options include prednisolone 1 mg/kg by mouth twice a day for 5 days then taper, dexamethasone 0.1 to 0.2 mg/kg by mouth once daily for 3 days then taper, or triamcinolone 0.1 to 0.2 mg/kg by mouth once daily for 3 to 5 days then taper. Long-acting repositol corticosteroid injections should only be used if the cat cannot be orally medicated; most cats tolerate dexamethasone sodium phosphate given orally, because of the small volume (0.15–0.25 mL per dose for most cats).

Atopic dermatitis is likely if facial pruritus improves markedly on corticosteroids but recurs despite treatment of parasites/infection and being fed solely a prescription hypoallergenic diet. Treatment options for atopy include continued medical management with corticosteroids at the lowest possible dose/frequency, oral cyclosporine, and allergy testing/desensitization therapy to identify and treat the underlying cause and reduce the need for symptomatic drugs.[1] Biopsy for dermatohistopathology is indicated in cases that do not respond to empiric therapy and in which no infection is present, or in which crusting without pruritus is present.

Pemphigus foliaceus and herpesvirus dermatitis lesions may partially improve on corticosteroids then relapse quickly in the same locations ± new locations often without significant pruritus. Rarely, idiopathic head (± neck) ulcerative dermatitis is a disorder with a poor response to parasite treatments, antibiotics, hypoallergenic diets, corticosteroids, and cyclosporine.[9,10] In these cases, neuropathic itch or behavioral issues may play a role, and treatment with gabapentin, fluoxetine, amitriptyline, oclacitinib (extralabel), or topiramate may be attempted.[11–13] Dermatology referral is ideal in these cases.

Diseases of the Nonhaired Nasal Planum

Ulcerative dermatoses

Causes Nasal planum ulcerations can be caused by infectious agents, including herpesvirus (**Fig. 4**),[5,16] deep fungi (eg, *Cryptococcus, Blastomyces, Histoplasma, Sporothrix*, saprophytes; **Figs. 5** and **6**),[17,18] and mycobacteria (see **Table 1**).[19,20] Other causes include mosquito bite hypersensitivity (**Fig. 7**),[21] trauma caused by rubbing (eg, atopy (**Fig. 8**), food allergy), and neoplasia (eg, squamous cell carcinoma [SCC]; **Figs. 9** and **10**).[22] Nasal ulcerative dermatitis is a breed-related disorder reported rarely in young Bengal cats.[23] Rarely, immune-mediated diseases (eg, vasculitis, systemic lupus, pemphigus vulgaris) can cause ulceration on the nasal planum.

Diagnostics Cytology is used to screen for infectious organisms and to characterize the inflammatory cell population. In most cases, biopsy/dermatohistopathology is necessary; if eosinophilic inflammation is noted, then careful evaluation for herpesvirus is needed,[5] and, if pyogranulomatous inflammation is found, then special stains for infectious organisms are indicated.

Crusting dermatoses

Causes Crusting of the nonhaired nasal planum can be caused by the same diseases as noted for ulceration (see **Fig. 10**; **Figs. 11** and **12**), as well as pemphigus foliaceus (**Fig. 13**).

Diagnostics Cytology is used to screen for infection and to characterize the inflammatory cell population. Acantholysis suggests pemphigus foliaceus. In most cases biopsy/dermatohistopathology is necessary.

Nodular dermatoses

Causes Masses/nodules affecting the nonhaired nasal planum can be caused by infectious agents, including deep fungi (see **Fig. 5**), mycobacteria (**Fig. 14**), bovine papillomaviral-induced feline sarcoid (**Fig. 15**),[24] as well as neoplasia (**Figs. 16** and **17**).

Diagnostics Aspirate/cytology, biopsy/dermatohistopathology are used.

Pigmentary disorders

Causes Lentigo is a unique but normal finding in orange cats in which flat pigmented macules develop on facial mucosal surfaces, including the planum, lips, and eyelids (**Fig. 18**). This condition is a cosmetic issue with no clinical relevance.

Diseases of the Haired Dorsal Nose/Muzzle, Chin, Lips, Eyelids, and Lateral Face

Alopecia

Causes Hair loss on the dorsal nose/muzzle, chin, and other areas on the face is commonly caused by infectious diseases, such as dermatophytosis (**Figs. 19** and **20**) and less commonly demodicosis (**Fig. 21**), by self-trauma caused by hypersensitivity disorders (atopy [see **Figs. 1** and **8**], food allergy, mosquito bite hypersensitivity), and rarely by immune-mediated follicular disorders such as mural folliculitis (**Fig. 22**, see **Table 1**).[25,26] In addition, feline acne can cause chin alopecia with dark debris in mild cases, as well as comedones, crusts, furuncles, and swelling in severe cases (**Fig. 23**).[27] Dermatophytosis may mimic acne (**Fig. 24**). Paraneoplastic alopecia is a rare cause of alopecia that can involve the face as well as the medial limbs and ventrum, and is associated with pancreatic or liver neoplasia (**Fig. 25**).[28]

Diagnostics Dermatophyte culture and skin scrapings/hair plucks for *Demodex* mites are first-line diagnostics. If screening tests are negative and if pruritus is not present, then biopsy/dermatohistopathology are indicated.

Ulcerative dermatoses

Causes Causes include infectious diseases, such as herpesvirus dermatitis (most commonly on the dorsal nose and eyelids; **Figs. 26–29**), deep fungal infection (**Figs. 30–32**), and mycobacterial infection; hypersensitivity disorders, such as mosquito bite hypersensitivity (on the dorsal nose; see **Fig. 7**), atopy, or food allergy causing excoriations or eroded eosinophilic granulomas, which are commonly secondarily infected with bacteria (see **Fig. 3**; **Figs. 33–37**)[29]; and neoplasia, most commonly SCC (**Fig. 38**). Idiopathic head/neck dermatitis is a rare cause for facial ulcerations,[9] as are immune-mediated diseases such as vasculitis, systemic lupus, and pemphigus vulgaris.

Diagnostics Cytology is indicated to screen for infectious organisms and to characterize inflammatory cell population. In most cases, biopsy/dermatohistopathology is necessary.

Crusting dermatoses

Causes In addition to the aforementioned infectious agents (see **Fig. 30**; **Figs. 39–44**), crusting of the haired skin on the face can be caused by dermatophytosis (see **Figs. 19, 20** and **24**); *Demodex*; pemphigus foliaceus (**Figs. 45** and **46**); hypersensitivity disorders (see **Fig. 1**; **Figs. 47–49**); *Notoedres* (**Fig. 50**); neoplasia (eg, SCC; see **Fig. 10**; **Fig. 51**); or Bowen's disease/SCC in situ, which is triggered by feline papillomavirus (**Figs. 52** and **53**).[30] Rare disorders that can cause adherent symmetric facial crusting in older cats are sebaceous adenitis, erythema multiforme, paraneoplastic disease, and exfoliative dermatitis (which may or may not be associated with thymoma) (**Fig. 54**).[31–33] In addition, feline acne can cause crusts as well as furuncles and swelling of the chin in severe cases (**Fig. 55**).[27] Rarely, feline idiopathic facial dermatosis/dirty face syndrome causes periocular, facial, and chin dermatitis and dark crusting/exudate in young Persian and Himalayan cats (**Fig. 56**).[34]

Diagnostics Skin scrapings for mites, cytology, and dermatophyte culture are first-line diagnostics ± biopsy/dermatohistopathology.

Nodular dermatoses

Causes Masses/nodules affecting the haired facial skin can be caused by infectious agents already mentioned (see **Figs. 5, 11** and **14**; **Figs. 57–61**, see **Table 1**) and neoplasia (see **Fig. 16**; **Figs. 62–66**).[22,35] In addition, keratinization disorders such as cystic feline acne can cause inflamed cystic chin masses (see **Fig. 55**), and chin swelling can also occur because of eosinophilic granuloma complex (fat chin syndrome) triggered by underlying allergies (**Fig. 67**).[29] Apocrine cystomatosis can affect the lip and eyelid margins to cause cystic masses (**Figs. 68** and **69**).[36] Rarely, immune-mediated plasma cell infiltration can occur on the haired dorsal nose alone or concurrently with plasma cell pododermatitis (**Fig. 70**).[37]

Diagnostics Diagnostics include aspirate/cytology and biopsy/dermatohistopathology.

Diseases of the Pinnae

Alopecia

Causes Causes include infectious diseases, such as dermatophytosis (**Fig. 71**) and less commonly demodicosis (**Fig. 72**), as well as self-trauma caused by hypersensitivity disorders (see **Table 1**). Idiopathic pinnal alopecia is a rare and poorly understood disorder of nonpruritic pinnal hair loss that occurs symmetrically, is more common in Siamese cats, and spontaneously resolves within a few months (**Fig. 73**).[38] In older cats with white pinnae, chronic sun damage/solar dermatosis can cause alopecia and thickening of the pinnal margins (**Fig. 74**).[39] In addition, pinnal hair loss ± curling can be seen in some cats chronically treated with topical or systemic corticosteroid-containing medications (**Fig. 75**).

Diagnostics Dermatophyte culture and skin scrapings/hair plucks for *Demodex* mites are first-line diagnostics. Consider breed and symmetry, and obtain a history of prior topical medications. If screening tests are negative, if pruritus is not present, and if history is not informative, then biopsy/dermatohistopathology may be indicated.

Ulcerative dermatoses

Causes Ulcerations of the pinna can be caused by infectious diseases detailed earlier; trauma caused by scratching caused by hypersensitivity disorders; immune-mediated disease (rare); or neoplasia, most commonly SCC (**Fig. 76**).

Diagnostics Cytology is indicated to screen for infectious organisms and to characterize the inflammatory cell population. In most cases, biopsy/dermatohistopathology is necessary.

Crusting dermatoses

Causes Causes include infectious diseases such as dermatophytosis, bacterial infection (usually secondary to allergies), parasites such as *Notoedres* (**Fig. 77**), immune-mediated diseases such as pemphigus foliaceus (**Figs. 78** and **79**), hypersensitivity disorders/trauma caused by scratching (**Figs. 80** and **81**), or Bowen's disease/SCC in situ (**Fig. 82**). Rare disorders that can cause pinnal crusting in older cats include sebaceous adenitis, erythema multiforme, and thymoma-induced exfoliative dermatitis (**Fig. 83**).

Diagnostics Skin scrapings for mites, dermatophyte culture, and cytology are first-line diagnostics, ± biopsy/dermatohistopathology.

Nodular dermatoses

Causes Infectious granulomas (fungal or mycobacterial) and neoplasia (**Fig. 84**) are most common. A rare immune-mediated disorder called auricular chondritis causes irregular swelling of the pinnal cartilage (**Fig. 85**).[40]

Diagnostics Diagnostics include aspirate/cytology and biopsy/dermatohistopathology.

Miscellaneous pinnal disorders

Drooping of the distal pinnae can occur because of chronic corticosteroid use (**Fig. 86**). Frostbite of the pinnae can cause acute erythema or purplish pinnal skin discoloration followed by necrosis and ulceration (**Fig. 87**).

Diseases of the Ear Canals

Ulcerative dermatoses

Causes Causes include severe bacterial infection (usually secondary to otic parasites, allergy, or ear canal polyp or neoplasia); trauma of external canals caused by scratching caused by hypersensitivity disorders (including contact allergy to topical medications); immune-mediated disease (**Fig. 88**); and neoplasia, most commonly SCC (see **Table 1**).

Diagnostics Otic swabs for mites and cytology are indicated to screen for infectious organisms and to characterize the inflammatory cell population ± culture if bacteria are present; if pruritus/self-trauma are present, then allergy work-up may be indicated ± biopsy/dermatohistopathology.

Crusting dermatoses

Causes In addition to the diseases described earlier, ear canal crusting/dark granular otic debris can be caused by *Otodectes*. In addition, proliferative necrotizing otitis externa is a unique, uncommon immune-mediated disorder in young cats that causes adherent brown crusting and inflammation in the distal ear canal (**Fig. 89**).[41]

Diagnostics Otic swabs for mites and cytology are indicated to screen for infectious organisms and to characterize the inflammatory cell population ± culture if bacteria are present despite empiric antibiotics. In cases in which parasites are ruled out and ear infections are recurrent, and/or crusting is caused by pruritus/self-trauma, then allergy work-up may be indicated (hypoallergenic diet trial ± environmental allergy testing if pruritus/infections persist despite diet trial). Biopsy/dermatohistopathology may be needed in cases in which no parasites/infection are found on screening tests, in nonpruritic cats, or cats with persistent crusting despite prevention of self-trauma using an Elizabethan collar.

Nodular ear canal dermatoses

Causes Causes include inflammatory polyps and, in older cats, neoplasia (SCC, ceruminous adenocarcinoma).[42] Apocrine cystomatosis causes blue to black firm cystic masses in the ear canals and outer ears, which can eventually obstruct the ear canal resulting in secondary infections. Although documented most commonly in Persian/Himalayan cats, it can occur in any breed (**Fig. 90**).[43]

Diagnostics Diagnostics include biopsy/dermatohistopathology.

The Importance of Signalment/History

As with all conditions, the list of possible differential diagnoses for a cat with facial dermatitis can often be narrowed by considering the signalment and history.

- Pruritus with secondary excoriations can increase the suspicion of atopy, food allergy, or parasites; conversely, lack of pruritus means atopy and food allergy are unlikely.

- A history of seasonality can lead to a clinical suspicion of atopy or mosquito bite hypersensitivity.
- Infectious diseases such as parasites and dermatophytosis are more likely to occur in kittens, multicat households, and in cats allowed to roam outside, as well as in immunosuppressed cats (retrovirus positive, on immunomodulatory medications), and careful questioning about involvement of other pets and humans is important.
- Some unique disorders, such as proliferative necrotizing otitis externa, tend to occur in kittens and young cats.[41]
- Consideration of breed can be important, such as nasal dermatosis in Bengal cats.[23] Apocrine cystomatosis and idiopathic facial dermatitis (feline dirty face syndrome) occur more commonly in Persian or Himalayan cats.[34,43]
- Concurrent clinical signs should be considered; a cat with crusting nasal dermatitis that is also sneezing or having oculonasal discharge can increase the suspicion for herpesvirus dermatitis (although herpesvirus dermatitis can also occur without respiratory signs).
- A cat receiving chronic systemic, topical, or inhaled corticosteroid treatment (including exposure to human steroid creams) is at risk for pinnal drooping, pinnal alopecia, and facial *Demodex*.[44]
- Neoplastic disorders are more common in older animals.
  ○ SCC is more common in middle-aged to older cats with nonpigmented noses, eyelids, and ears.
  ○ Facial dermatitis/alopecia as well as hair loss and thin, shiny skin on the limbs/ventrum and weight loss in an elderly cat are concerning for paraneoplastic alopecia.
  ○ Adherent scaling/crusting on the dorsal head of an older cat is concerning for erythema multiforme or thymoma-associated exfoliative dermatosis.
  ○ Dark, slightly raised ± crusted multifocal lesions on the temporal areas ± outer ears are suspicious for Bowen's disease (SCC in situ triggered by papillomavirus).

Dermatology Diagnostics

Baseline dermatology diagnostics include skin scrapings for mites, surface skin (touch impression) or mass aspirate cytology to evaluate inflammatory infiltrate and screen for infectious organisms, Wood lamp examination, and dermatophyte culture ± dermatophyte polymerase chain reaction (PCR); surface or tissue cultures for bacterial or deep fungal organisms and biopsies may be indicated in cases of ulcerative or nodular lesions, or cases in which screening tests are not informative and/or when the cat does not respond to initial treatments (**Table 2**).

SUMMARY

It is clear that there are many possible causes for feline nasal and facial dermatitis, but, with careful consideration of signalment, history, concurrent clinical signs, and results of baseline dermatology diagnostics informing possible further diagnostics, such as cultures and biopsies, each feline facial dermatologic disease is a unique puzzle that can be solved.

DISCLOSURE

The author has nothing to disclose.

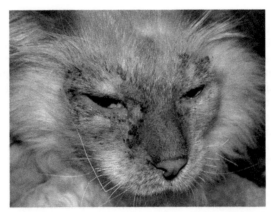

Fig. 1. Facial barbering/excoriations caused by atopy. (*From* Coyner K. Clinical Atlas of Canine and Feline Dermatology. Hoboken, NJ: Wiley; 2020; with permission.)

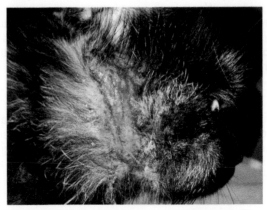

Fig. 2. Facial and pinnal crusting and pruritus caused by *Notoedres* infestation. (*From* Coyner K. Clinical Atlas of Canine and Feline Dermatology. Hoboken, NJ: Wiley; 2020; with permission.)

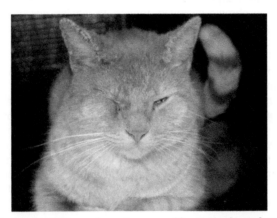

Fig. 3. Facial excoriations and bacterial pyoderma caused by atopy. (*From* Coyner K. Clinical Atlas of Canine and Feline Dermatology. Hoboken, NJ: Wiley; 2020; with permission.)

Box 1
Tips for performing a hypoallergenic diet trial

- Food allergy can occur at any time in life, even after eating the same food for years.
- Food allergy can cause facial and/or generalized pruritus and/or recurrent otitis.
- Food allergy is diagnosed and treated with a strict prescription hypoallergenic diet trial for 8 to 12 weeks.
- Options include novel protein or hydrolyzed diets; a careful dietary history is necessary to select an appropriate food.
- Over-the-counter novel protein diets are not ideal because they can be microscopically contaminated with other ingredients.[14]
- Serology for food allergy is inaccurate and should not be used.[15]
- Perform a slow diet transition over 10 to 14 days to increase the chance of acceptance of the new food.
- If the cat refuses the new diet, try a different brand/flavor; it can take several tries to find the right food for each cat.
- Eliminate all other foods/treats/supplements.
- Feed all cats in the home the same food if possible.

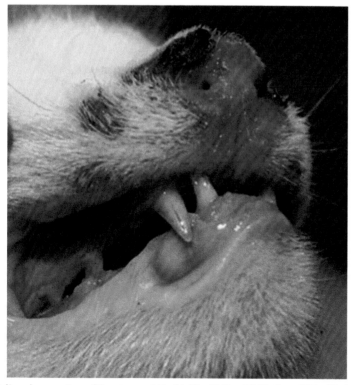

Fig. 4. Feline herpesvirus. (*Courtesy of* R. Malik, DVSc, DipVetAn, MVetClinStud, PhD, FACVSc, FASM, MASID, Sydney, Australia.)

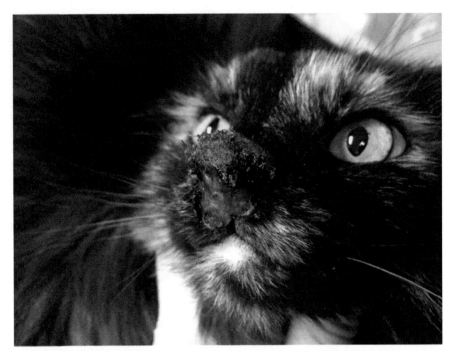

Fig. 5. Cryptococcosis. (*From* Coyner K. Clinical Atlas of Canine and Feline Dermatology. Hoboken, NJ: Wiley; 2020; with permission.)

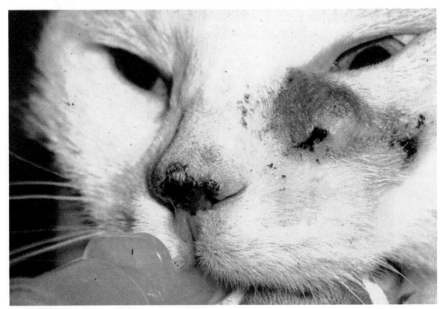

Fig. 6. Phaeohyphomycosis. (*Courtesy of* R. Malik, DVSc, DipVetAn, MVetClinStud, PhD, FACVSc, FASM, MASID, Sydney, Australia.)

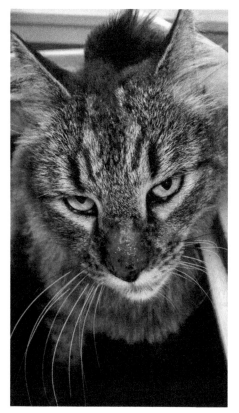

Fig. 7. Mosquito bite hypersensitivity. (*From* Coyner K. Clinical Atlas of Canine and Feline Dermatology. Hoboken, NJ: Wiley; 2020; with permission.)

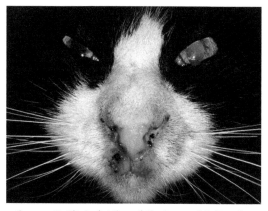

Fig. 8. Atopy. (*From* Coyner K. Clinical Atlas of Canine and Feline Dermatology. Hoboken, NJ: Wiley; 2020; with permission.)

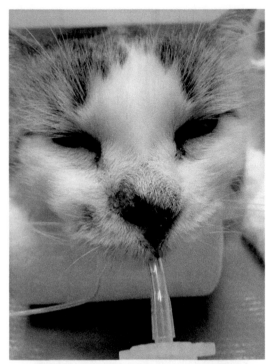

Fig. 9. Squamous cell carcinoma. (*Courtesy of* C. Souza DVM, MSC, PhD, Urbana, IL.)

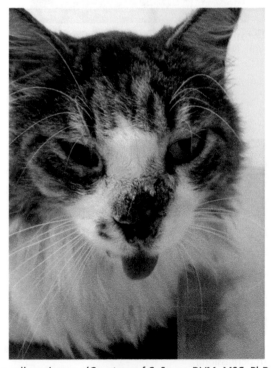

Fig. 10. Squamous cell carcinoma. (*Courtesy of* C. Souza DVM, MSC, PhD, Urbana, IL.)

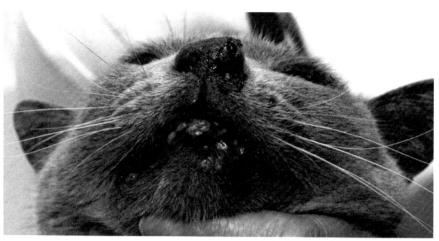

Fig. 11. Cryptococcosis. (*Courtesy of* R. Malik, DVSc, DipVetAn, MVetClinStud, PhD, FACVSc, FASM, MASID, Sydney, Australia.)

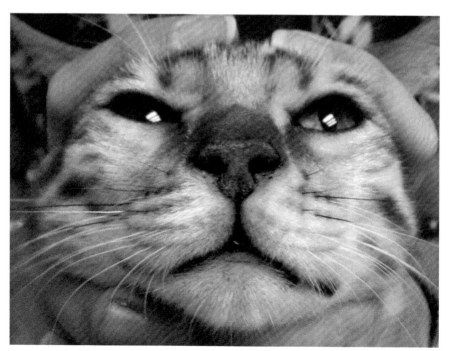

Fig. 12. Adherent crusting on the nasal planum margins in a Bengal cat. (© Veterinary Information Network®, Inc.; Image by Cherry Douglas, DVM.)

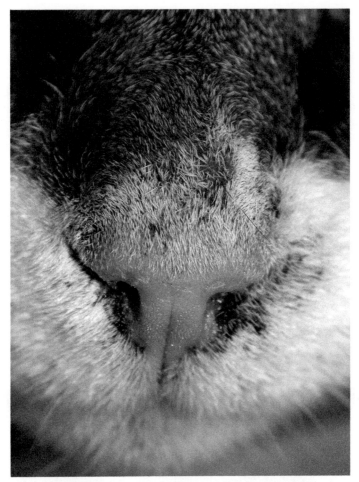

Fig. 13. Pemphigus foliaceus. Note the similarity to herpesvirus dermatitis.

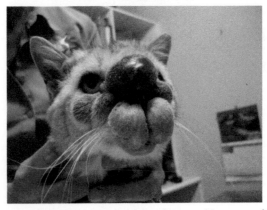

Fig. 14. *Mycobacteria tarwinense*, a type of feline leprosy. (*Courtesy of* Dr. Richard Malik, DVSc, DipVetAn, MVetClinStud, PhD, FACVSc, FASM, MASID, Sydney, Australia.)

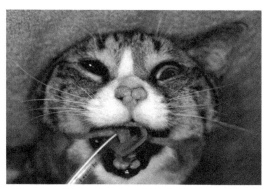

Fig. 15. Feline sarcoid. (*From* Coyner K. Clinical Atlas of Canine and Feline Dermatology. Hoboken, NJ: Wiley; 2020; with permission.)

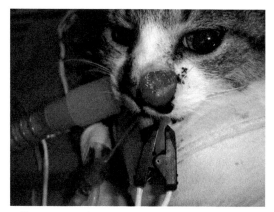

Fig. 16. Squamous cell carcinoma. (*Courtesy of* C. Souza DVM, MSC, PhD, Urbana, IL.)

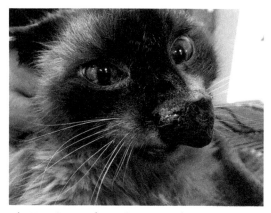

Fig. 17. Melanoma. (© Veterinary Information Network®, Inc.; Image by Adam Boardman DVM.)

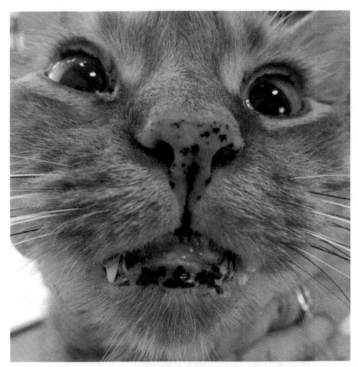

Fig. 18. Lentigo. (*From* Coyner K. Clinical Atlas of Canine and Feline Dermatology. Hoboken, NJ: Wiley; 2020; with permission.)

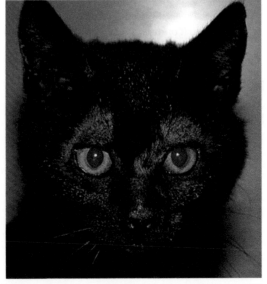

Fig. 19. Dermatophytosis. (*From* Coyner K. Clinical Atlas of Canine and Feline Dermatology. Hoboken, NJ: Wiley; 2020; with permission.)

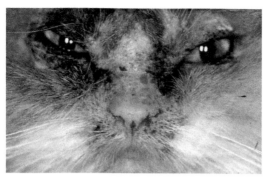

Fig. 20. Dermatophytosis as seen in this cat can be clinically similar to immune-mediated disease. (*From* Coyner K. Clinical Atlas of Canine and Feline Dermatology. Hoboken, NJ: Wiley; 2020; with permission.)

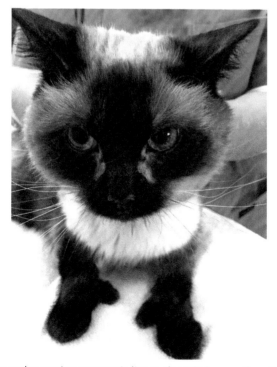

Fig. 21. Feline *Demodex* causing symmetric linear alopecia in an asthmatic cat corresponding with contact areas of a mask designed to deliver inhaled corticosteroids. (*From* Coyner K. Clinical Atlas of Canine and Feline Dermatology. Hoboken, NJ: Wiley; 2020; with permission.)

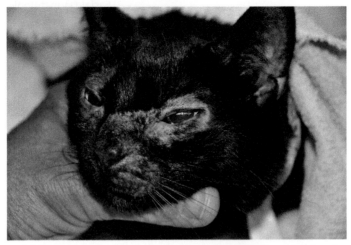

Fig. 22. Mural folliculitis. (*From* Coyner K. Clinical Atlas of Canine and Feline Dermatology. Hoboken, NJ: Wiley; 2020; with permission.)

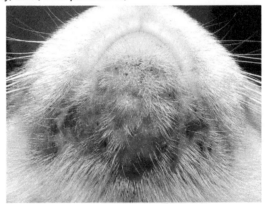

Fig. 23. Severe feline acne. (*From* Coyner K. Clinical Atlas of Canine and Feline Dermatology. Hoboken, NJ: Wiley; 2020; with permission.)

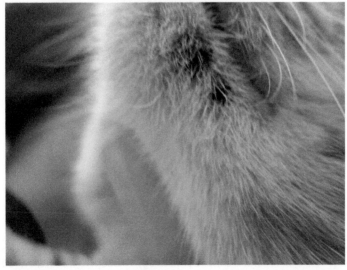

Fig. 24. Dark chin debris mimicking feline acne in a cat with dermatophytosis. (*From* Coyner K. Clinical Atlas of Canine and Feline Dermatology. Hoboken, NJ: Wiley; 2020; with permission.)

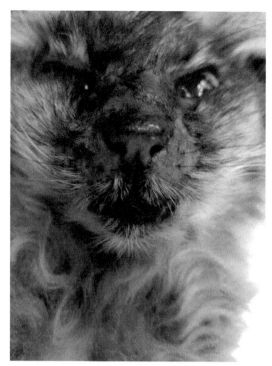

Fig. 25. Paraneoplastic disease. (© Veterinary Information Network®, Inc.; Image by Eric Clough DVM.)

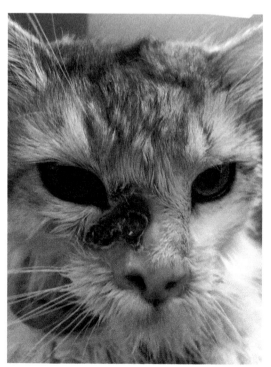

Fig. 26. Herpesvirus dermatitis. (*From* Coyner K. Clinical Atlas of Canine and Feline Dermatology. Hoboken, NJ: Wiley; 2020; with permission.)

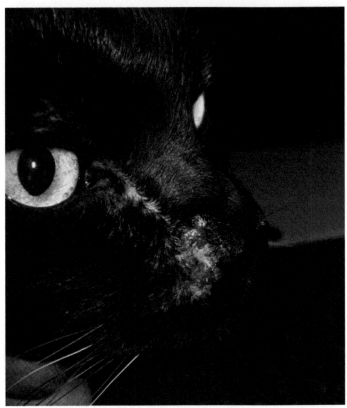

Fig. 27. Herpesvirus dermatitis. (*Courtesy of* R. Malik, DVSc, DipVetAn, MVetClinStud, PhD, FACVSc, FASM, MASID, Sydney, Australia.)

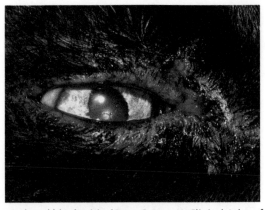

Fig. 28. Herpesvirus-induced blepharitis. (*From* Coyner K. Clinical Atlas of Canine and Feline Dermatology. Hoboken, NJ: Wiley; 2020; with permission.)

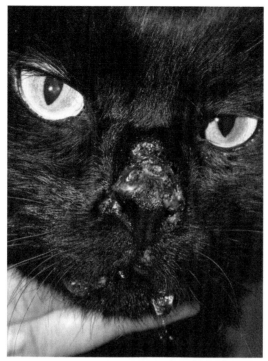

Fig. 29. Herpesvirus dermatitis. (*From* Coyner K. Clinical Atlas of Canine and Feline Dermatology. Hoboken, NJ: Wiley; 2020; with permission.)

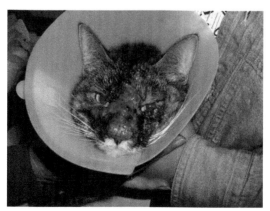

Fig. 30. Cryptococcosis. (*Courtesy of* R. Malik, DVSc, DipVetAn, MVetClinStud, PhD, FACVSc, FASM, MASID, Sydney, Australia.)

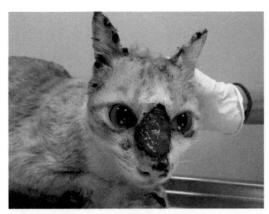

Fig. 31. Sporotrichosis. (*From* Coyner K. Clinical Atlas of Canine and Feline Dermatology. Hoboken, NJ: Wiley; 2020; with permission.)

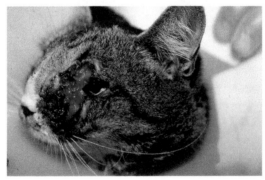

Fig. 32. Histoplasmosis. (*From* Coyner K. Clinical Atlas of Canine and Feline Dermatology. Hoboken, NJ: Wiley; 2020; with permission.)

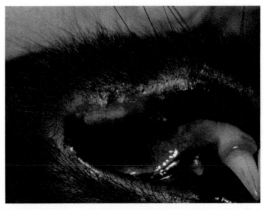

Fig. 33. Eosinophilic granuloma caused by atopy. (*From* Coyner K. Clinical Atlas of Canine and Feline Dermatology. Hoboken, NJ: Wiley; 2020; with permission.)

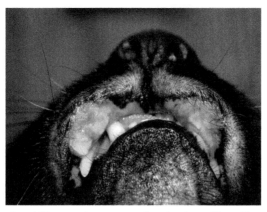

Fig. 34. Infected eosinophilic granulomas secondary to atopy. (*From* Coyner K. Clinical Atlas of Canine and Feline Dermatology. Hoboken, NJ: Wiley; 2020; with permission.)

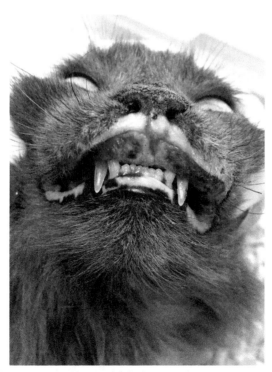

Fig. 35. Severe chronic untreated eosinophilic lip granulomas causing severe scarring in an allergic cat. (*From* Coyner K. Clinical Atlas of Canine and Feline Dermatology. Hoboken, NJ: Wiley; 2020; with permission.)

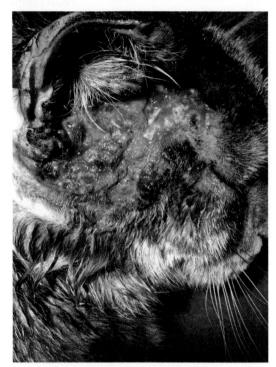

Fig. 36. Deep pyoderma caused by food allergy. (*From* Coyner K. Clinical Atlas of Canine and Feline Dermatology. Hoboken, NJ: Wiley; 2020; with permission.)

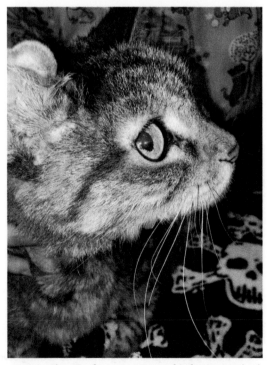

Fig. 37. The same cat as in **Fig. 46** after treatment of infection and a hypoallergenic diet. (*From* Coyner K. Clinical Atlas of Canine and Feline Dermatology. Hoboken, NJ: Wiley; 2020; with permission.)

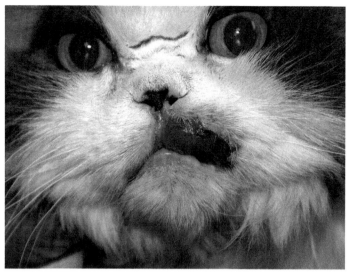

Fig. 38. Squamous cell carcinoma. (*From* Coyner K. Clinical Atlas of Canine and Feline Dermatology. Hoboken, NJ: Wiley; 2020; with permission.)

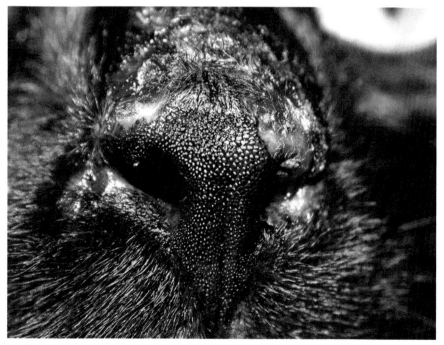

Fig. 39. Herpesvirus dermatitis. (*From* Coyner K. Clinical Atlas of Canine and Feline Dermatology. Hoboken, NJ: Wiley; 2020; with permission.)

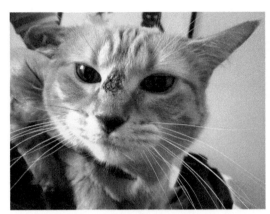

Fig. 40. Herpesvirus dermatitis. (*From* Coyner K. Clinical Atlas of Canine and Feline Dermatology. Hoboken, NJ: Wiley; 2020; with permission.)

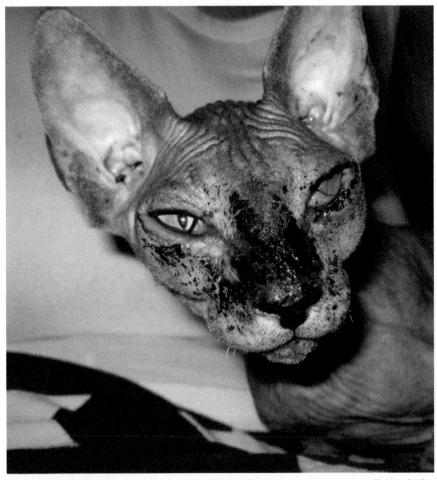

Fig. 41. Herpesvirus dermatitis. (*Courtesy of* R. Malik, DVSc, DipVetAn, MVetClinStud, PhD, FACVSc, FASM, MASID, Sydney, Australia.)

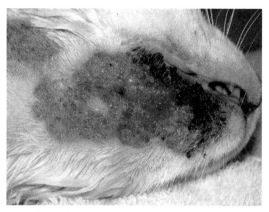

Fig. 42. Chronic bacterial pyoderma. (*From* Coyner K. Clinical Atlas of Canine and Feline Dermatology. Hoboken, NJ: Wiley; 2020; with permission.)

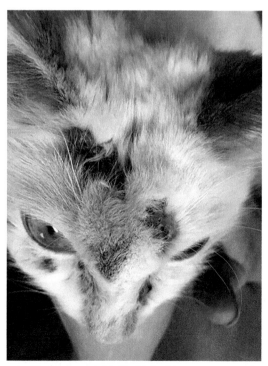

Fig. 43. Cryptococcosis. (*Courtesy of* R. Malik, DVSc, DipVetAn, MVetClinStud, PhD, FACVSc, FASM, MASID, Sydney, Australia.)

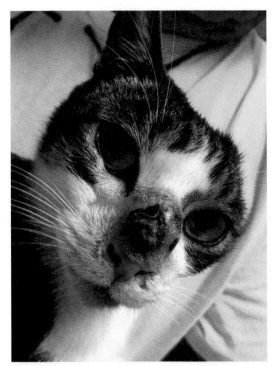

Fig. 44. Phaeohyphomycosis. (© Veterinary Information Network®, Inc.; Image by Tammy Brown DVM.)

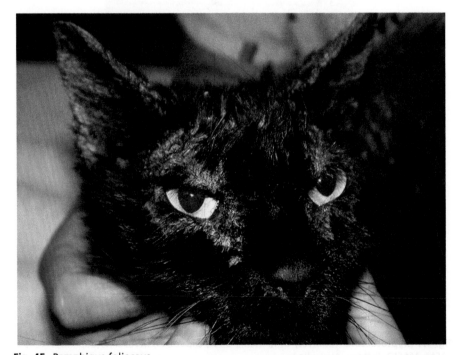

Fig. 45. Pemphigus foliaceus.

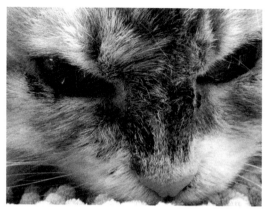

Fig. 46. Pemphigus foliaceus.

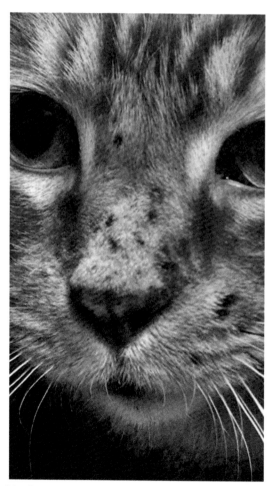

Fig. 47. Mosquito bite hypersensitivity. (*From* Coyner K. Clinical Atlas of Canine and Feline Dermatology. Hoboken, NJ: Wiley; 2020; with permission.)

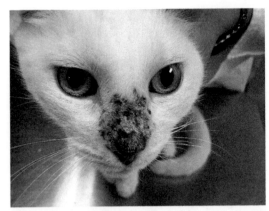

Fig. 48. Mosquito bite hypersensitivity. (*From* Coyner K. Clinical Atlas of Canine and Feline Dermatology. Hoboken, NJ: Wiley; 2020; with permission.)

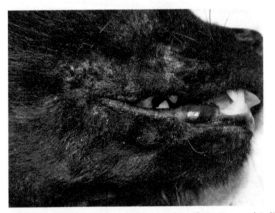

Fig. 49. Atopic dermatitis. (*From* Coyner K. Clinical Atlas of Canine and Feline Dermatology. Hoboken, NJ: Wiley; 2020; with permission.)

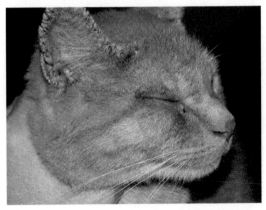

Fig. 50. *Notoedres* infestation. (*From* Coyner K. Clinical Atlas of Canine and Feline Dermatology. Hoboken, NJ: Wiley; 2020; with permission.)

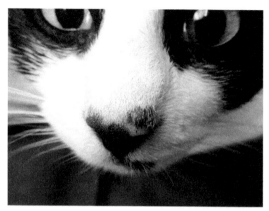

Fig. 51. SCC in situ at the nasal mucocutaneous junction. (*From* Coyner K. Clinical Atlas of Canine and Feline Dermatology. Hoboken, NJ: Wiley; 2020; with permission.)

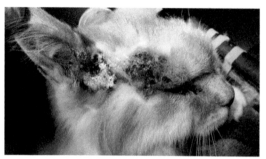

Fig. 52. Bowen's disease. (*Courtesy of* R. Malik, DVSc, DipVetAn, MVetClinStud, PhD, FACVSc, FASM, MASID, Sydney, Australia.)

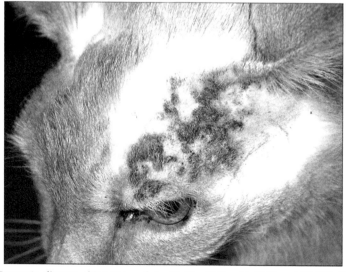

Fig. 53. Bowen's disease. (*Courtesy of* R. Malik, DVSc, DipVetAn, MVetClinStud, PhD, FACVSc, FASM, MASID, Sydney, Australia.)

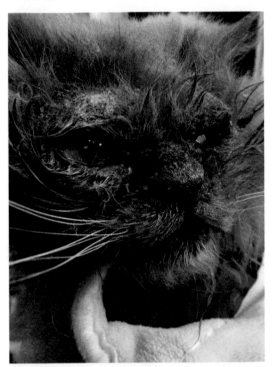

Fig. 54. Thymoma-induced exfoliative dermatitis; secondary bacterial and malassezia infections contributed to inflammation and pruritus. (*From* Coyner K. Clinical Atlas of Canine and Feline Dermatology. Hoboken, NJ: Wiley; 2020; with permission.)

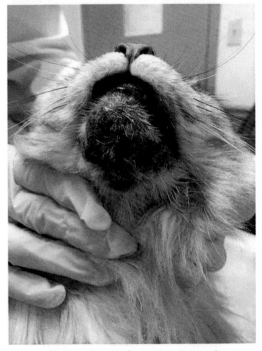

Fig. 55. Severe feline acne. (© Veterinary Information Network®, Inc.; Image by Elizabeth Noyes DVM.)

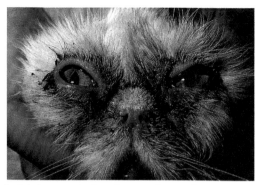

Fig. 56. Idiopathic facial dermatosis/dirty face syndrome. (*From* Coyner K. Clinical Atlas of Canine and Feline Dermatology. Hoboken, NJ: Wiley; 2020; with permission.)

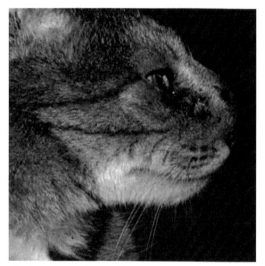

Fig. 57. Cryptococcosis. (*Courtesy of* R. Malik, DVSc, DipVetAn, MVetClinStud, PhD, FACVSc, FASM, MASID, Sydney, Australia.)

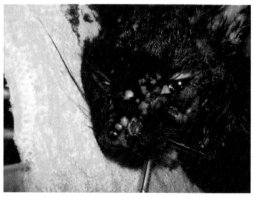

Fig. 58. Cryptococcosis. (*Courtesy of* R. Malik, DVSc, DipVetAn, MVetClinStud, PhD, FACVSc, FASM, MASID, Sydney, Australia.)

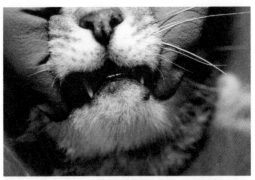

Fig. 59. Sporotrichosis. (*From* Coyner K. Clinical Atlas of Canine and Feline Dermatology. Hoboken, NJ: Wiley; 2020; with permission.)

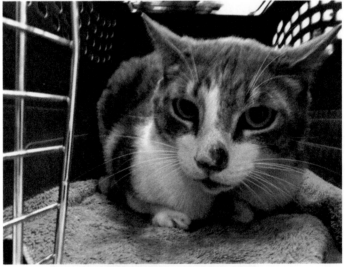

Fig. 60. Sporotrichosis. (*From* Coyner K. Clinical Atlas of Canine and Feline Dermatology. Hoboken, NJ: Wiley; 2020; with permission.)

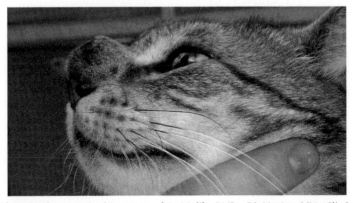

Fig. 61. Phaeohyphomycosis. (*Courtesy of* R. Malik, DVSc, DipVetAn, MVetClinStud, PhD, FACVSc, FASM, MASID, Sydney, Australia.)

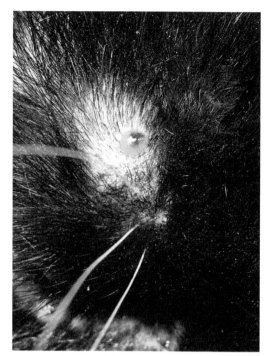

Fig. 62. Mast cell tumor. (*From* Coyner K. Clinical Atlas of Canine and Feline Dermatology. Hoboken, NJ: Wiley; 2020; with permission.)

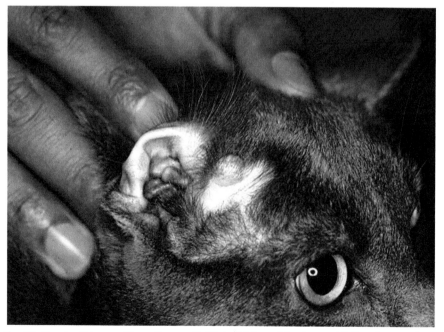

Fig. 63. Basal cell tumor. (*From* Coyner K. Clinical Atlas of Canine and Feline Dermatology. Hoboken, NJ: Wiley; 2020; with permission.)

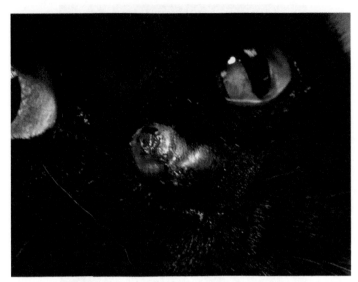

Fig. 64. Melanoma. (© Veterinary Information Network®, Inc.; Image by Karen Fischer DVM.)

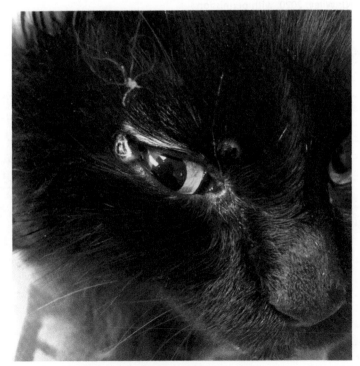

Fig. 65. Progressive dendritic cell histiocytosis. (*From* Coyner K. Clinical Atlas of Canine and Feline Dermatology. Hoboken, NJ: Wiley; 2020; with permission.)

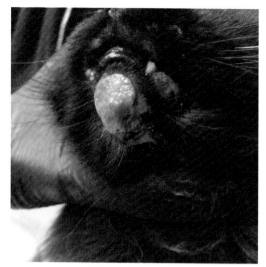

Fig. 66. The same cat as in **Fig. 85**: larger ulcerated masses were present on the lips and chin. (*From* Coyner K. Clinical Atlas of Canine and Feline Dermatology. Hoboken, NJ: Wiley; 2020; with permission.)

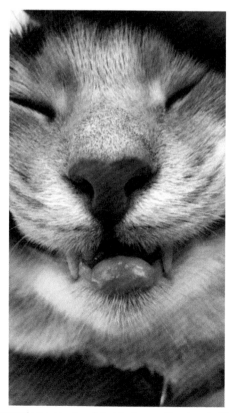

Fig. 67. Eosinophilic granuloma causing fat chin in an allergic cat. (*Courtesy of* A. Simpson, DVM, MS, DACVD, Aurora, IL.)

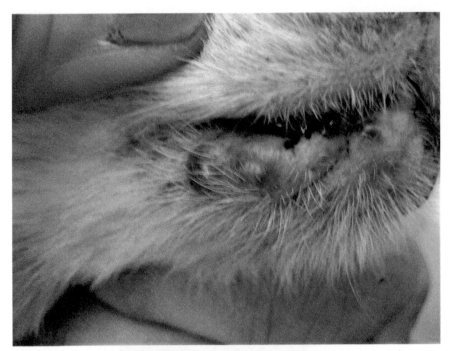

Fig. 68. Blue cystic lip masses caused by apocrine cystomatosis. (© Veterinary Information Network®, Inc.; Image by Daniel Hall DVM.)

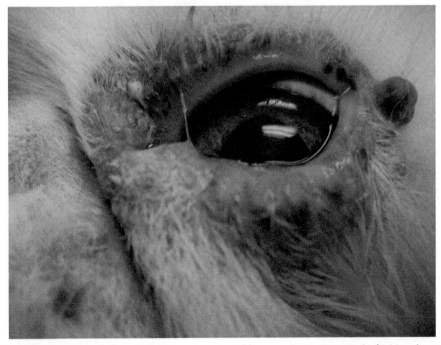

Fig. 69. Numerous dark eyelid masses also caused by apocrine cystomatosis. (© Veterinary Information Network®, Inc.; Image by Mike Bloomer DVM.)

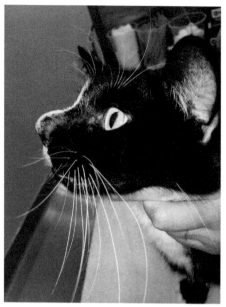

Fig. 70. Nasal swelling caused by plasmacytic inflammation; the cat also had plasma cell pododermatitis. (*From* Coyner K. Clinical Atlas of Canine and Feline Dermatology. Hoboken, NJ: Wiley; 2020; with permission.)

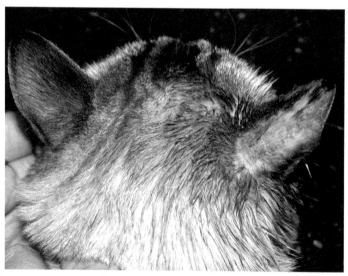

Fig. 71. Asymmetrical pinnal alopecia caused by dermatophytosis. (*From* Coyner K. Clinical Atlas of Canine and Feline Dermatology. Hoboken, NJ: Wiley; 2020; with permission.)

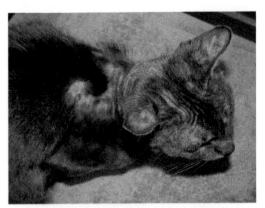

Fig. 72. Patchy pinnal alopecia in a cat with demodicosis. (*From* Coyner K. Clinical Atlas of Canine and Feline Dermatology. Hoboken, NJ: Wiley; 2020; with permission.)

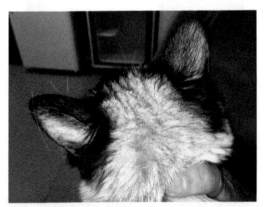

Fig. 73. Idiopathic pinnal alopecia in a Siamese cat. (*From* Coyner K. Clinical Atlas of Canine and Feline Dermatology. Hoboken, NJ: Wiley; 2020; with permission.)

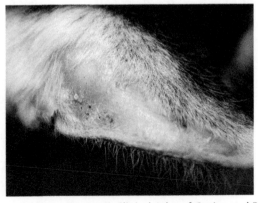

Fig. 74. Solar dermatosis. (*From* Coyner K. Clinical Atlas of Canine and Feline Dermatology. Hoboken, NJ: Wiley; 2020; with permission.)

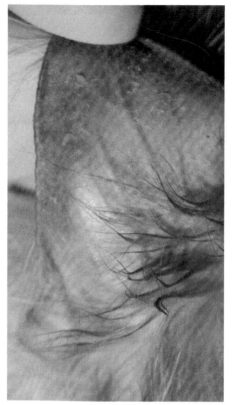

Fig. 75. Pinnal alopecia with cutaneous atrophy in an atopic cat treated with prolonged topical corticosteroids. (*From* Coyner K. Clinical Atlas of Canine and Feline Dermatology. Hoboken, NJ: Wiley; 2020; with permission.)

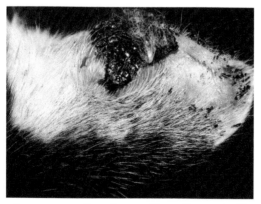

Fig. 76. Solar-induced squamous cell carcinoma. (*From* Coyner K. Clinical Atlas of Canine and Feline Dermatology. Hoboken, NJ: Wiley; 2020; with permission.)

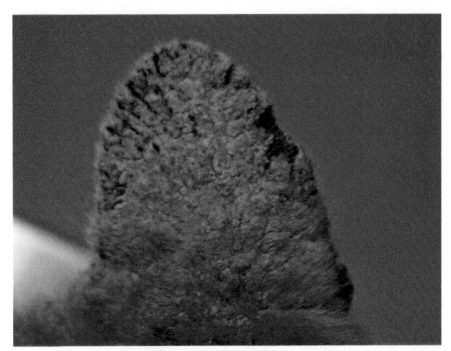

Fig. 77. *Notoedres* infestation. (*From* Coyner K. Clinical Atlas of Canine and Feline Dermatology. Hoboken, NJ: Wiley; 2020; with permission.)

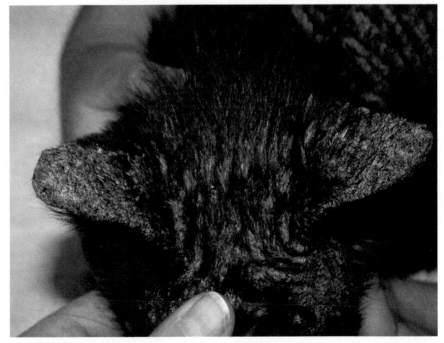

Fig. 78. Pemphigus foliaceus. (*From* Coyner K. Clinical Atlas of Canine and Feline Dermatology. Hoboken, NJ: Wiley; 2020; with permission.)

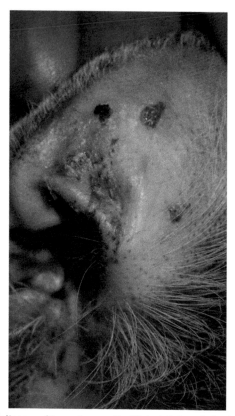

Fig. 79. Pemphigus foliaceus. (*From* Coyner K. Clinical Atlas of Canine and Feline Dermatology. Hoboken, NJ: Wiley; 2020; with permission.)

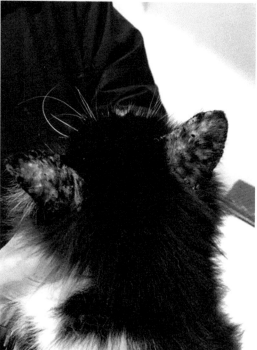

Fig. 80. Mosquito bite hypersensitivity. (*Courtesy of* R. Malik, DVSc, DipVetAn, MVetClinStud, PhD, FACVSc, FASM, MASID, Sydney, Australia.)

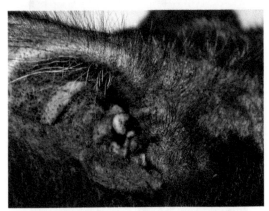

Fig. 81. Pinnal and preauricular crusted excoriations caused by atopy. (*From* Coyner K. Clinical Atlas of Canine and Feline Dermatology. Hoboken, NJ: Wiley; 2020; with permission.)

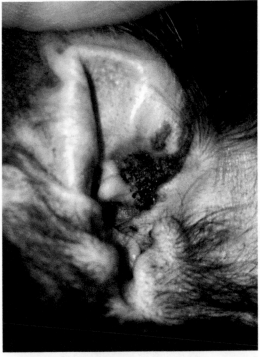

Fig. 82. Bowen's disease. (*From* Coyner K. Clinical Atlas of Canine and Feline Dermatology. Hoboken, NJ: Wiley; 2020; with permission.)

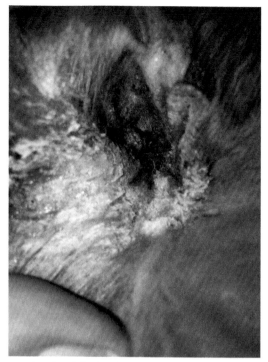

Fig. 83. Thymoma-associated exfoliative dermatitis.

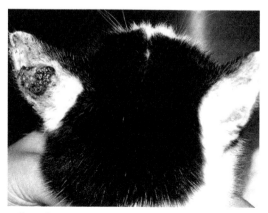

Fig. 84. Squamous cell carcinoma.

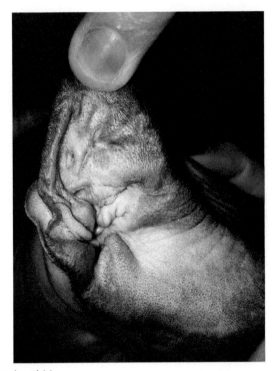

Fig. 85. Auricular chondritis.

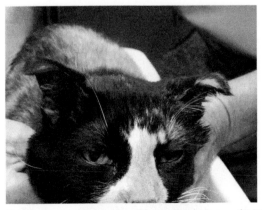

Fig. 86. Iatrogenic Cushing caused drooping of both distal pinnae. (© Veterinary Information Network®, Inc.; Image by Sue Fluhr DVM.)

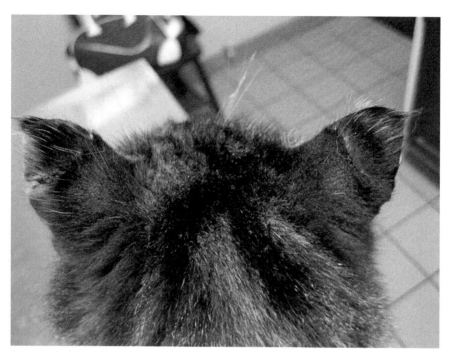

Fig. 87. Frostbite-induced distal pinnal necrosis. (© Veterinary Information Network®, Inc.; Image by Tamara Goff DVM.)

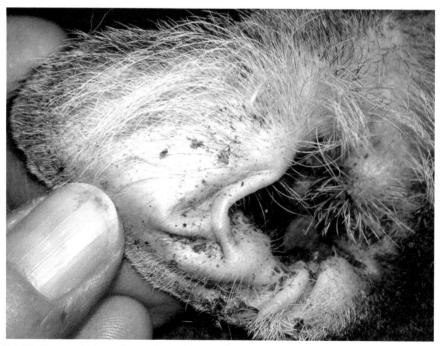

Fig. 88. Ear canal ulceration and purulent exudate caused by pemphigus foliaceus and secondary bacterial otitis. (*From* Coyner K. Clinical Atlas of Canine and Feline Dermatology. Hoboken, NJ: Wiley; 2020; with permission.)

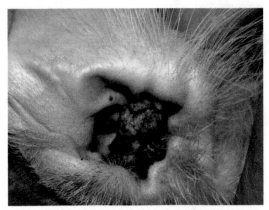

Fig. 89. Proliferative necrotizing otitis externa. (*From* Coyner K. Clinical Atlas of Canine and Feline Dermatology. Hoboken, NJ: Wiley; 2020; with permission.)

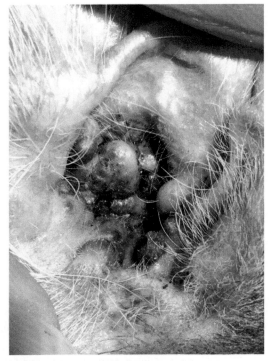

Fig. 90. Ceruminous (apocrine) cystomatosis.

Table 2
Dermatology diagnostics

Diagnostic Test and Technique	Uses/Indications	Limitations/Disadvantages	Caveats/Comments
Skin scrapings A dulled #10 scalpel blade or medical curette/spatula and mineral oil are used to collect skin debris, which is then mixed with more mineral oil on a microscope slide and observed under 4–10× power	To screen for mites such as *Notoedres*, *Otodectes*, and *Demodex* Can also be used to examine hair shafts (trichogram) for possible fungal organisms	False-negative scrapings can occur	Some parasites, especially feline *Demodex* or ectopic *Otodectes*, can be difficult to find on scrapings, and trial treatment with an isoxazoline insecticide is often indicated in cats with facial hair loss and/or pruritus Selamectin does not treat *Demodex Demodex* mites can also be obtained using hair plucks placed into mineral oil, a technique especially helpful for hard-to-scrape areas such as eyelids and lips
Surface skin cytology Samples are applied to a microscope slide and stained with Diff-Quik or similar stain, scanned under 10× to identify an area with well stained cells, then observed under 40–100×	To screen for infectious organisms and to characterize inflammatory cell population Infectious agents that can be found on skin cytology include bacteria, *Malassezia*, and other fungi, including dermatophyte arthroconidia and deep fungal organisms	Requires practice and a good microscope for accurate interpretation Cannot speciate bacteria, can only give bacterial morphology	Cytology must be performed when performing skin or ear culture in order to be able to interpret culture results Neutrophilic or pyogranulomatous inflammation is consistent with an infectious or inflammatory process Eosinophilic inflammation is suggestive of a hypersensitivity dermatitis (atopy, food allergy, mosquito bite hypersensitivity), parasitic infestation, or feline herpesvirus dermatitis Acantholytic cells can suggest pemphigus complex but can also be seen with chronic infection and support the need for biopsy and dermatophyte culture

(continued on next page)

Table 2
(continued)

Diagnostic Test and Technique	Uses/Indications	Limitations/Disadvantages	Caveats/Comments
Mass aspirate cytology Use 25–22-G needle core lesion, redirect and repeat, then attach a 3–6 mL syringe, expel needle contents onto slide, make gentle squash prep to obtain a monolayer, stain, and observe under 10–100×	Performed to determine whether: 1. A mass is inflammatory vs cyst vs potential neoplasia 2. The potential need for biopsy or tissue cultures (if neoplastic cells or inflammatory cells are seen) 3. Send-out cytology for evaluation by a pathologist will be needed or diagnostic (eg, if suspected neoplastic cells are found)	Can be difficult to perform in sensitive areas and may require sedation Cannot be used as an alternative to biopsy for definitive diagnosis of a mass, because some tumors do not exfoliate well and cannot grade a tumor on cytology	If aspiration for cytology does not harvest diagnostic cells on in-house cytology, then biopsy is indicated If aspiration cytology reveals pyogranulomatous inflammation, then perform biopsies for both histopathology/special stains for organisms as well as tissue cultures
Bacterial culture Use a sterile culturette to swab a freshly ruptured pustule or lift a crust and use the swab to sample the exudate under crust. In dry lesions, use a saline-moistened swab to vigorously rub several scaly areas Alternatively, bacterial skin cultures can be performed by obtaining a 4-mm to 6-mm punch biopsy of papule, pustule, or crusted lesion, which is then placed in sterile red-top tube (± with 0.25–0.5 mL sterile, not bacteriostatic, saline to keep it moist), then submit for macerated tissue culture	Culture is indicated if bacteria are found on skin cytology despite empiric antibiotics, or in cases of deep pyoderma (draining or ulcerated areas) In superficial infections, aerobic bacterial culture is the only culture needed In animals with draining tracts or nodules, samples may also be needed for anaerobic culture, fungal culture, or mycobacterial culture In these cases, a deep tissue biopsy rather than a swab is the best sample; submit part for cultures and part in formalin for histopathology, including special stains for organisms	Costly test Some laboratories speciate and perform sensitivities on all organisms obtained, even if they are not significant, leading to risk of overtreatment	Before culture, stop topical and systemic antimicrobials for 48 h if possible (however, if numerous bacteria are found on cytology despite antibiotic treatment, delaying culture is not necessary) Cytology must be performed when performing skin or ear culture in order to be able to interpret culture results If biopsying a mass or draining area for culture, save a tissue sample in aluminum foil in the freezer in case further diagnostics, such as PCR, are indicated

Wood lamp examination Look for apple green fluorescence incorporated into hair shafts Pluck fluorescing hairs for dermatophyte culture and direct microscopic examination	To screen for dermatophytosis caused by *Microsporum canis*	*Microsporum gypseum* and *Trichophyton* do not fluoresce False-negative Wood lamp results can occur in 20%–50% of *M canis* cases, in all *M gypseum* and *Trichophyton mentagrophytes* cases, and after use of topical iodine False-positive Wood lamp reactions can occur because of misinterpretation of nonspecific fluorescence of keratin debris generated by other infections, topical medications, and carpet fibers	A Wood lamp with electric plug and magnification is more accurate than battery operated units Warm up for 5–10 min before use, examine in a dark room/allow eyes to adapt, holding lamp a few inches away from skin/fur

(continued on next page)

Table 2
(continued)

Diagnostic Test and Technique	Uses/Indications	Limitations/Disadvantages	Caveats/Comments
Dermatophyte culture Obtain samples with both hair plucks and sterile toothbrush Ideal hairs to select are those in areas of active crusting, and hairs that appear damaged or misshapen and/or fluoresce under a Wood lamp Use a round or rectangular flat dermatophyte culture plate, avoid screw-top vials Incubate at room temperature with 30% humidity/place in plastic bags to prevent dehydration of the media	To screen for dermatophytes	Because some nondermatophyte fungal organisms can cause positive media color change concurrent with colony growth and mimic dermatophytes, microscopic examination of all suspect colonies is essential to avoid misidentification	Dermatophyte growth usually appears within 7–10 d, but plates should be kept for 14–21 d, especially if the sample has been obtained from a cat currently under therapy with antifungal medications Dermatophytes appear as white, light yellow, tan, or buff-colored, cottony to powdery colonies with concurrent media color change Dermatophytes are never black, green, or gray Daily observation and logging of fungal growth correlated with media color change is critical in correctly interpreting dermatophyte culture results Follow-up dermatophyte cultures are obtained by toothbrush technique every 1–2 wk to determine when treatment may be discontinued (after 2 negative cultures)[4]

Dermatophyte identification

To obtain sample for cytology of dermatophyte culture, clear acetate tape is gently touched to the surface of the fungal colony and then the tape is applied to a glass slide over a drop of blue stain (such as methylene blue, or the blue Diff-Quik solution [basophilic thiazine dye])

The slide is examined under 10–40× looking for characteristic dermatophyte macroconidia

Microscopic evaluation of suspect fungal growth is essential, because some nonpathogenic environmental fungi can mimic dermatophytes in gross colony morphology and ability to turn the media red

False-negative results are possible if dermatophyte culture is overgrown by contaminant or not incubated in ideal conditions

False-positive results possible if similar environmental fungal spores such as *Alternaria* are misinterpreted as dermatophytes

M canis, the most common dermatophyte species infecting cats, has numerous large, spindle-shaped, thick-walled spores with 6 or more internal cells

M gypseum is very rarely identified in cats, lives on decaying keratin in the soil, and produces numerous large, spindle-shaped spores with thin walls and 6 or fewer internal cells

Trichophyton mentagrophytes is usually a rodent pathogen that occasionally causes infection in cats and produces long, cigar-shaped macroconidia with thin walls; spores may be few; spiral-shaped hyphae are also common

In early cultures, only fungal hyphae with immature or no macroconidia may be seen (especially in cases of *Trichophyton*), and these cultures should be incubated longer to allow for spore development

(continued on next page)

Table 2
(continued)

Diagnostic Test and Technique	Uses/Indications	Limitations/Disadvantages	Caveats/Comments
Dermatophyte PCR Samples for PCR should be obtained from lesions using a toothbrush and by collecting scales and crusts. If toothbrushes are submitted, wrap the head of the sample in a plastic bag (do not tape shut) and then place this into a second bag. If crusts or scales are submitted, use a sterile dry blood collection tube	To screen for dermatophytes[45]	False-negative results are rare but can occur if not enough material including intact hair roots is submitted for analysis PCR testing does not discriminate between live and dead fungal DNA Positive PCR may be misinterpreted as clinical infection when dead dermatophyte organisms are picked up on a successfully treated animal or a single environmental dermatophyte spore such as *M gypseum* or *Trichophyton* is coincidentally picked up	Ideally, both dermatophyte PCR and dermatophyte culture should be used concurrently for optimal diagnosis of dermatophytosis

Biopsy			
Nasal planum or pinnal lesions can be biopsied with a 4-mm punch or a small wedge biopsy and closed with a single simple interrupted absorbable suture	Performed in cases of suspected neoplasia, vesicular or ulcerative diseases, unusual or atypical cases, and in cases that have not responded to conventional therapy	Secondary infection can alter histopathologic findings; check cytology of superficial or crusty lesions before biopsy because pretreatment with antibiotics for 2-3 wk may be needed	If eosinophilic inflammation is noted on facial lesion biopsy, then careful evaluation for herpesvirus is needed, which may include immunohistochemistry or PCR. If pyogranulomatous inflammation is found, then special stains for infectious organisms are indicated
Pinnal marginal lesions can be sampled using a scalpel blade using a shave technique and then left open to heal by second intention		Corticosteroid therapy can also change biopsy results, and ideally patients should not receive oral or topical corticosteroids within 2-3 wk or injectable long-acting corticosteroids within 6-8 wk of performing the biopsy procedure (severe, life-threatening cases are an exception to this rule)	Do not prep or shave area to be biopsied to avoid removing diagnostic material. Crusts should be carefully preserved with the skin biopsies
Place the area of interest in the center of the biopsy punch and do not include a significant amount of normal skin with the biopsy. The only time a lesion should be biopsied on the margin is in the case of an ulcerative skin disease			If possible, choose primary lesions such as papules, pustules, vesicles, macules, or nodules. Lesions that are less likely to be diagnostic include excoriated, ulcerated, or chronically scarred areas
			More information is gained by performing multiple (3-5) 4-mm to 6-mm samples, obtained from a variety of lesions
			Biopsy samples from different lesions or nodules should be tagged with a suture or placed in individually labeled containers for differentiation
			Send to dermatopathologist with full signalment, history, and pictures of lesions for best interpretation

REFERENCES

1. Diesel A. Cutaneous hypersensitivity dermatoses in the feline patient: a review of allergic skin disease in cats. Vet Sci 2017;4(2):25.
2. Beale K. Feline demodicosis: a consideration in the itchy or overgrooming cat. J Feline Med Surg 2012;14(3):209–13.
3. Sotiraki ST, Koutinas AF, Leontides LS, et al. Factors affecting the frequency of ear canal and face infestation by *Otodectes cynotis* in the cat. Vet Parasitol 2001;96(4):309–15.
4. Moriello K, Coyner K, Paterson S, et al. Diagnosis and treatment of dermatophytosis in dogs and cats: Clinical Consensus Guidelines of the World Association for Veterinary Dermatology. Vet Dermatol 2017;28(3):266.e68.
5. Hargis AM, Ginn PE. Feline herpesvirus 1-associated facial and nasal dermatitis and stomatitis in domestic cats. Vet Clin North Am Small Anim Pract 1999;29(6): 1281–90.
6. Preziosi DE. Feline pemphigus foliaceus. Vet Clin North Am Small Anim Pract 2019;49(1):95–104.
7. Beccati MB, Pandolfi PP, Di Palma AD. Efficacy of fluralaner spot-on in cats affected by generalized demodicosis: seven cases. Vet Dermatol 2019;30:454.
8. Short J, Gram D. Successful treatment of *Demodex gatoi* with 10% Imidacloprid/ 1% Moxidectin. J Am Anim Hosp Assoc 2016;52(1):68–72.
9. Spaterna A, Mechelli L, Rueca F, et al. Feline idiopathic ulcerative dermatosis: three cases. Vet Res Commun 2003;27:795–8.
10. Titeux E, Gilbert C, Briand A, et al. From feline idiopathic ulcerative dermatitis to feline behavioral ulcerative dermatitis: Grooming repetitive behaviors indicators of poor welfare in cats. Front Vet Sci 2018;5:81.
11. Grant D, Rusbridge C. Topiramate in the management of feline idiopathic ulcerative dermatitis in a two-year-old cat. Vet Dermatol 2014;25:226–8.
12. Loft KE. Feline idiopathic ulcerative dermatosis treated successfully with oclacitinib. Vet Dermatol 2015;26:134–5.
13. Bowen J, Heath S, editors. Feline compulsive disorders. In: Behaviour problems in small animals: practical advice for the veterinarian team. Philadelphia: Elsevier Saunders; 2005. p. 177–81.
14. Olivry T, Mueller RS. Critically appraised topic on adverse food reactions of companion animals (5): discrepancies between ingredients and labeling in commercial pet foods. BMC Vet Res 2018;14(1):24.
15. Mueller RS, Olivry T. Critically appraised topic on adverse food reactions of companion animals (4): can we diagnose adverse food reactions in dogs and cats with in vivo or in vitro tests? BMC Vet Res 2017;13(1):275.
16. Thomasy SM, Shull O, Outerbridge CA, et al. Oral administration of famciclovir for treatment of spontaneous ocular, respiratory, or dermatologic disease attributed to feline herpesvirus type 1: 59 cases (2006-2013). J Am Vet Med Assoc 2016; 249(5):526–38.
17. Pennisi MG, Hartmann K, Lloret A, et al. Cryptococcosis in cats: ABCD guidelines on prevention and management. J Feline Med Surg 2013;15(7):611–8.
18. De Souza EW, Borba CM, Pereira SA, et al. Clinical features, fungal load, coinfections, histological skin changes, and itraconazole treatment response of cats with sporotrichosis caused by *Sporothrix brasiliensis*. Sci Rep 2018;8(1):9074.
19. Gunn-Moore DA. Feline mycobacterial infections. Vet J 2014;201(2):230–8.
20. Lloret A, Hartmann K, Pennisi MG, et al. Mycobacteriosis in cats. ABCD guidelines on prevention and management. J Feline Med Surg 2013;15:591–7.

21. Mason KV, Evans AG. Mosquito bite-caused eosinophilic dermatitis in cats. J Am Vet Med Assoc 1991;198(12):2086–8.
22. Murphy S. Cutaneous squamous cell carcinoma in the cat: current understanding and treatment approaches. J Feline Med Surg 2013;15(5):401–7.
23. Auxilia ST, Abramo F, Ficker C, et al. Juvenile idiopathic nasal scaling in three Bengal cats. Vet Dermatol 2004;15(1):52.
24. Munday JS, Thomson N, Dunowska M, et al. Genomic characterisation of the feline sarcoid-associated papillomavirus and proposed classification as *Bos taurus* papillomavirus type 14. Vet Microbiol 2015;177(3–4):289–95.
25. Gross TL, Olivry T, Vitale CB, et al. Degenerative mucinotic mural folliculitis in cats. Vet Dermatol 2001;12(5):279–83.
26. Rosenberg AS, Scott DW, Erb HN, et al. Infiltrative lymphocytic mural folliculitis: a histopathological reaction pattern in skin-biopsy specimens from cats with allergic skin disease. J Feline Med Surg 2010;12(2):80–5.
27. Jazic E, Coyner KS, Loeffler DG, et al. An evaluation of the clinical, cytological, infectious and histopathological features of feline acne. Vet Dermatol 2006; 17(2):134–40.
28. Marconato L, Albanese F, Viacava P, et al. Paraneoplastic alopecia associated with hepatocellular carcinoma in a cat. Vet Dermatol 2007;18(4):267–71.
29. Buckley L, Nuttall T. Feline eosinophilic granuloma complex(ities): some clinical clarification. J Feline Med Surg 2012;14(7):471–81.
30. Favrot C, Welle M, Heimann M, et al. Clinical, histologic, and immunohistochemical analyses of feline squamous cell carcinoma in situ. Vet Pathol 2009;46(1): 25–33.
31. Glos K, von Bomhard W, Bettenay S, et al. Sebaceous adenitis and mural folliculitis in a cat responsive to topical fatty acid supplementation. Vet Dermatol 2016; 27(1):57.e18.
32. Cavalcanti JV, Moura MP, Monteiro FO. Thymoma associated with exfoliative dermatitis in a cat. J Feline Med Surg 2014;16(12):1020–3.
33. Linek M, Rüfenacht S, Brachelente C, et al. Nonthymoma-associated exfoliative dermatitis in 18 cats. Vet Dermatol 2015;26(1):40–5, e12-3.
34. Fontaine J, Heimann M. Idiopathic facial dermatitis of the Persian cat: three cases controlled with cyclosporine. Vet Dermatol 2004;15(1):64.
35. Moore PF. A review of histiocytic diseases of dogs and cats. Vet Pathol 2014; 51(1):167–84.
36. Berger D. Feline ceruminous cystomatosis. Clinician's Brief 2015;13(6):25.
37. Bensignor E, Merven F. Nasal plasma cell dermatitis in cats. Vet Dermatol 2011; 22(3):286.
38. Miller W, Griffin C, Campbell K. Muller and Kirk's small animal dermatology. 7th edition. St Louis (MO): Saunders; 2012.
39. Scarff D. Solar dermatoses in companion animals Part 2: feline solar dermatoses. Companion Anim 2007;12(4):69–73.
40. Gerber B, Crottaz M, von Tscharner C, et al. Feline relapsing polychondritis: two cases and a review of the literature. J Feline Med Surg 2002;4(4):189–94.
41. Mauldin EA, Ness TA, Goldschmidt MH. Proliferative and necrotizing otitis externa in four cats. Vet Dermatol 2007;18(5):370–7.
42. Greci V, Mortellaro CM. Management of otic and nasopharyngeal, and nasal polyps in cats and dogs. Vet Clin North Am Small Anim Pract 2016;46(4): 643–61.

43. Soohoo J, Earl Loft K, Lange CE. Feline ceruminous cystomatosis in the ears of 25 cats (2014-2016). In: Proceedings of the North American Veterinary Dermatology Forum. Orlando, FL, USA, April 26-29, 2017. 107.
44. Bizikova P. Localized demodicosis due to *Demodex cati* on the muzzle of two cats treated with inhalant glucocorticoids. Vet Dermatol 2014;25(3):222.e58.
45. Jacobson LS, McIntyre L, Mykusz J. Comparison of real-time PCR with fungal culture for the diagnosis of *Microsporum canis* dermatophytosis in shelter cats: a field study. J Feline Med Surg 2018;20(2):103–7.

New Tests in Feline Veterinary Medicine
When to Use Them and When to Stick with Tried-and-True Tests

Sally Lester, DVM, MVSc[a,b,*]

KEYWORDS

- Reference intervals • Reference change intervals • Hematology • Biochemistries
- Endocrine disease • New tests

KEY POINTS

- Interpretation of test results should take into consideration analysis of trends, reference change intervals, and population-based reference intervals specific to the machine and practice.
- Despite improvements in hematology machines, a microscopic review of a blood smear remains necessary.
- Newer tests, which complement existing tests, include hepcidin, symmetric dimethylarginine, fibroblast growth factor 23, cardiac troponin I, N-terminal proB-type natriuretic peptide, serum amyloid A, β-hydroxybutyrate, and canine thyroid-stimulating hormone (cTSH).

INTRODUCTION

Recent developments in clinical pathology have more to do with the accessibility of in-clinic machines and new applications of reference intervals (RIs) than actual new tests. The focus of this article is on optimizing existing procedures while incorporating new tests and the tools needed to interpret the results.

Diagnostic tests do not stand alone! Interpreting test results requires consideration of factors that reflect

1. The patient, including clinical signs, history, and physical examination
2. Preanalytical procedures, including patient handling (restraint, occlusion of vessels, which veins, and sedation) and sample handling (tubes used, clotting of the sample, spinning of the sample, and so forth)

---
[a] True North Veterinary Diagnostics, Langley, British Columbia, Canada; [b] Pilchuck Veterinary Hospital, Snohomish, WA, USA
* 2106 Cedar Road, Lake Stevens, WA 98258.
E-mail address: slpathd@aol.com

Vet Clin Small Anim 50 (2020) 883–898
https://doi.org/10.1016/j.cvsm.2020.03.007
0195-5616/20/© 2020 Elsevier Inc. All rights reserved.
vetsmall.theclinics.com

3. Analytical procedures, including knowledge of the accuracy/precision of the test (www.asvcp.org/page/QALS_Guidelines)
4. Postanalytical considerations, including the appropriate use of RIs defined for the population or the individual and verification of abnormal results

It is the responsibility of veterinarians to

- Understand how their in-clinic equipment works
- Ensure that quality control procedures are in place, including documentation and training for personnel using the machines
- Ensure that the methodology provides the information that is required[1]

Similarly, when using external laboratories, it is important to be familiar with their quality assurance procedures and methodology.

POSTANALYTICAL INTERPRETATION

Determining whether a patient's status is healthy or sick requires more than comparing a result to an RI. Interpretation of results entails thoughtfulness and an understanding of what a "number" means.

Reference Intervals Are Not Universal

The population of cats within a region can vary and there are reports documenting differences in the RIs between cat breeds,[2–5] and age (**Box 1**). Breed variation appears significant with symmetric dimethylarginine (SDMA), creatinine, glucose, and total protein (TP). Elevations in alkaline phosphatase (ALP) along with calcium and phosphorus may be different in larger breed cat populations as well as kittens. For example, creatinine levels are related to body mass. Healthy Maine coons may have a higher upper limit for creatinine, above 1.6 mg/dL (141 μ/mol), the value used in International Renal Interest Society staging[5] (www.iris-kidney.com/pdf/IRIS_Staging_of_CKD_modified_2019.pdf).

Kittens have lower TP, albumin, hematocrit, and creatinine levels than adults. Cats over 10 years of age have different creatinine, thyroxine, protein levels, and hematocrit.[6–8]

Individual Reference Intervals/Biologic Variation

Intraindividual variation refers to variation in an individual patient's laboratory values over time and may be of more value in disease interpretation than population

---

Box 1
Reference intervals are not universal

RIs include instrument variation, interindividual variation, and intraindividual variation. Use published RIs sparingly.

- The population definition includes the breed, age, sex, physical characteristics, and region.
- If intervals are established on fasted samples, then all tests for patients should be run on fasted samples.
- The timing of collection and the length of time between collection and processing affect the results.
- Plasma samples may be different from serum samples and can affect the intervals established.
- Machines differ even when the methodology is the same, and the intervals are valid only for the machine used to run the tests.

RIs. This variation is much smaller than the interindividual variation for many analytes; therefore, even correctly established RIs may not identify pathologic changes.[9–12] The indications are that creatinine, blood urea nitrogen (BUN), phosphorus, TP, albumin, cholesterol, ALP, and N-terminal prohormone B-type natriuretic peptide (NT-proBNP) are relatively stable for each individual. Triglycerides, ALP, alanine aminotransferase (ALT), and calcium along with the erythron parameters also are highly conserved within an individual; other analytes are in the intermediate group, where assessment of both population and individual RIs are helpful.

The reference change interval (RCI) describes the variability of the machine and the individual for any given analyte. This can be calculated from the machine bias and a predetermined biological variation for a specific test. Because RCIs are subject to the same caveats (methodology/machine/individual) as RIs, it is a daunting, expensive, and impractical task to establish these for each individual and clinic. But the concept is important for interpreting the results of consecutive samples[13,14] (see example in **Boxes 2** and **3**).

HEMATOLOGY—COMPLETE BLOOD CELL COUNT

All available hematology instruments count particles; computer algorithms correlate the particles to cells (red blood cells, white blood cells, and platelets). Two methods are available for counting; both assume that individual particles are being counted rather than clusters:

1. Impedance (electrical interference across an aperture)
2. Flow cytometry (light scatter across an aperture)

Multidirectional lasers can create a 3-dimensional image and enzymes/dyes/fluorescence can be added to the mix to create patterns and changes in the light passage and to measure reticulocytes. Hemoglobin is measured by spectrophotometry. Techniques are available on some machines that measure the amount of hemoglobin in individual cells using laser-based flow cytometry (cell hemoglobin concentration mean [CHCM]).[15,16]

ERYTHRON

The erythron-measured parameters include red blood cell count, hemoglobin, red blood cell distribution width, and average volume of the red blood cells. These

---

Box 2
Variable methods of interpretation

Machine-determined TAE[a]

    The total allowable error (TEa) for creatinine as published in the American Society for Veterinary Clinical Pathology guidelines is 20% for within RIs and 30% for values greater than the RIs. An ill cat starting with a creatinine value of 6.0 mg/dL (530 μmol/L) and a post–fluid therapy creatinine value of 4.2 mg/dL (371 μmol/L) suggests improvement. The original value at 30% could be anywhere between 4.2 and 7.8 (371–689) (6.0 ± 30% = 6.0 ± 1.8 = 4.2–7.8 [371–689]), whereas the post–therapy value could be 2.94 to 5.46 (260–482). But has the creatinine actually improved? These results would be equivocal but the TEa calculated for in-house machines could be lower than the accepted 30% and, if the value is determined for your machine, the interpretation maybe different.

[a] TEa tables can be found on the on the American Society for Veterinary Clinical Pathology Web site (www.asvcp.org/page/QALS_Guidelines).

Box 3
Impact of reference interval versus reference change interval

Example. If the initial ALP from a patient (from routine wellness screening) falls within the RI but a sample taken when a patient is showing signs of illness has ALP values within RI but greater than the RCI, that result represents a significant change and should be investigated. A compilation of the current veterinary literature regarding RCIs is available at http://vetbiologicalvariation.org/database-table-cat; these data can be used to give approximate percentage changes that aid in interpretations.

---

parameters are used to characterize the red blood cell populations. Calculated parameters used to describe red blood cell characteristics include shape, color, and size but these are not superior to visual examination of the blood smear.[17] Changes in the calculated parameters may help in identifying iron deficiency or identifying a regenerative or nonregenerative anemia. CHCM exhibits a bias that could compromise the interpretation of iron deficiency or result in an inappropriate assessment of normal hemoglobin concentration. CHCM does eliminate the effects of hemolysis and lipemia on hemoglobin, however; the difference between the calculated MCHC and the CHCM provides an accurate assessment of hemolysis within the sample. The use of reticulocyte CHCM to help assess iron status is of some benefit in cats, but the specificity for iron deficiency in at least 1 article is only 76.9%,[18] so the interpretation is incorrect in approximately 25% of the cases.[19,20]

Assessment of whether an anemia is regenerative or nonregenerative requires evaluation of reticulocytes. Automated analyzers can measure reticulocytes but they tend to overestimate the number of reticulocytes in cats. The use of 0.5% for the normal number of circulating reticulocytes in cats is questionable and appears to be subject to breed variation with percentages that range from 0.5% to 3.3%. A cutoff value of 0.5% reticulocytes is sensitive but not specific for anemia (<75%).[21]

Both the maturation time of red blood cells and the effect of anemia on the red blood cell life span are unknown in cats, which affects the utility of the red blood cell production index. At present, it is best to use the reticulocyte percentage and monitor the trends with the reticulocyte counts and hematocrit[20] understanding that recovery from anemia requires the reticulocyte percentage to exceed the normal value.

Nonregenerative Anemia

If a reticulocyte count supports a nonregenerative anemia, then other disease processes must be excluded. Conditions, such as inflammation, renal diseases, and other organ dysfunctions, affect the ability of the marrow to respond to anemia. If other diseases are excluded, a bone marrow cytology must be performed.

Hepcidin is an iron regulatory protein, which, when measured in concert with ferritin, iron, and iron-binding capacity, provides a better understanding of anemia of chronic disease and can provide a rationale for therapeutic responses to nonregenerative anemia[22] (**Box 4**).

Polycythemia

Primary polycythemia (ie, erythrocytosis) is uncommon cats; the most common cause is dehydration, followed by splenic contraction.[23] High erythron values must be verified by repeat sampling and dilution. Plasma should be checked to make sure there

---

Box 4
Hepcidin

Hepcidin is a protein produced by the liver that circulates complexed to albumin or α_1-macro-globulin. It is excreted by the kidney. Its function is to regulate iron uptake by enterocytes, macrophages, and hepatocytes by forming a complex with cellular ferroportin that prevents exportation of iron from the cells. Increased hepcidin levels occur with decreased renal excretion as well as most inflammatory conditions (mediated by interleukin 6). In these scenarios, erythropoiesis is decreased, resulting in functional iron deficiency. Enzyme-linked immunosorbent assays are available in human medicine and, given the similar structure, cross-reacts with feline hepcidin.

---

is no color change (hemolysis/lipemia), which could interfere with the measurement of hemoglobin. The erythron is stable over time in an individual and the RCI is between 15% and 20%.

LEUKON

Hematology machines provide automated differentials that have inherent errors, which differ depending on the machine.[24,25] Techniques have improved and there is better characterization of the cells, so normal is recognized more easily but abnormal remains poorly recognized (**Box 5**).

PLATELETS

Automated platelet numbers are erroneously assumed to be correct. Evaluation of a blood smear is imperative because there are very few samples from cats that do not have platelet clumping (<30%). The blood smear evaluation should include assessment of platelet size, granularity, and whether white blood cell numbers are altered by the clumping. If platelet clumping is present, the cat does not have a clinically significant thrombocytopenia.

Although numerous formulae exist to assess platelet numbers on a blood smear, they all have inherent errors. In a well-spread blood smear, 7 to 9 platelets averaged over 10 high-power fields indicates adequate platelet numbers. Immune-mediated thrombocytopenia is linked to very low platelet counts, less than 1 on average/10 high-power fields.

Increased platelet numbers are not uncommon in cats, but the magnitude often is obscured by the platelet clumping. Levels that exceed 1 million warrant a search for sustained low-grade blood loss or neoplasia, including feline leukemia virus testing (**Box 6**).

Box 5
Common problems associated with machine generated differentials

- There are discrepancies in the assessment of band neutrophils or toxic change.
- The ratio of neutrophils to lymphocytes often is inaccurate if reactive lymphoid cells are present (eg, due to recent vaccination).
- Numerous error messages may develop that negate the value of the automated differential.
- Evaluation of the dot plots for the differentials can be a valuable tool in determining accuracy and can be used to help with the manual differential.

> **Box 6**
> **Hematology summary**
>
> Manual, microscopic assessment of a blood smear remains the gold standard for determination of red blood cell, white blood cell, and platelet morphology. For in-clinic differentials, it is imperative to provide additional technical training, RIs, and a standard protocol for grading morphology along with parameters that instigate a submission to a reference laboratory and review by a pathologist (www.asvcp.org/page/QALS_Guidelines).

SERUM BIOCHEMISTRIES

Critical considerations

1. What type of sample is required for the test? Results are not interchangeable between plasma/serum/whole blood.
2. Lipemia/hemolysis/icterus can cause interference and the degree should be determined and recorded.[26]
3. Although a correlation can exist between machines and methodologies, direct comparisons are inaccurate. Do not compare results between machines and methods; look at where the value lies within the RI.[27,28]
4. RIs must be established for the machine and for the population. Cutoff values and critical decision levels are unique to a practice.
5. Tubes supplied by different manufacturers vary considerably and tube consistency is important; both the tube coating and the rubber stoppers can affect results.[29] See **Box 7**.
6. The order of the blood draw must be maintained. Ethylenediaminetetraacetic acid (EDTA) tubes always are filled last, because EDTA is a calcium chelator and even a small amount removes calcium and interferes with its measurement and those enzyme tests that require calcium in the chemical reaction.
7. The written test procedure (standard operating procedure) must document which test results generate an automatic repeat or when the sample should be diluted and retested.

ELECTROLYTES

In most analyzers, sodium, potassium, and chloride are determined by ion-selective electrodes, which represent the state of the art and are both precise and accurate; chemically based methods show more imprecision. Marked differences are present with different methodologies and between whole blood and serum/plasma. Subtle changes with these electrolytes are important; looking at the RCI helps in determining significant change. A sodium level that is at the high end of, or exceeds, the RI coupled

> **Box 7**
> **Effects of different collection tubes**
>
> Separation gels may decrease phenobarbital, creatine phosphokinase, progesterone, and thyroxine and alter electrolytes measured by ion-selective electrodes; red blood cells may penetrate the gel, which can change enzyme levels and electrolytes. The clot activators and surfactants may affect a multitude of tests; consequently, serum/plasma should be removed from the gel-containing tubes as soon as possible after centrifugation to eliminate effects of the gel and to allow for accurate repeat testing on stored samples.[29]
>
> *Data from* Bowen AR, Remaley AT. Interferences from blood collection tube components on clinical chemistry assays. Biochem Med. 2014; 24(1): 31-44.

with a low potassium should prompt evaluation for hyperaldosteronism, which could be primary or secondary to renal disease.[30]

RENAL DISEASE

A urinalysis is the first step in evaluating renal function (**Box 8**).

SDMA has an advantage over creatinine in that it is not affected by decreased muscle mass; however, both parameters assess glomerular filtration rate and are variably affected by conditions that decrease it (**Box 9**).

Renal disease and its progression involve complex interactions with bone metabolism, the endocrine system, and electrolyte balance (**Fig. 1**). There is no single biochemical test that can be used to determine prognosis. Promising early markers of renal function include serum fibroblast growth factor 23 (FGF-23), indoxyl sulfate, kidney injury molecule 1, and urinary γ-glutamyltransferase (GGT).[37–40]

FGF-23, a fibronectin, is a very early marker of calcium/phosphorus imbalance and renal disease. It is produced by osteoblasts/osteocytes and is up-regulated with the bone turnover that occurs with renal disease. FGF-23 interacts with renal tubular cells to decrease phosphate reabsorption and to down-regulate 1α-hydrolase and increase 24-hydroxylase, resulting in decreased calcitirol.[40] Measurements of P, ionized Ca^{++}, parathyroid hormone (PTH), and FGF-23 allow for both early detection of renal disease and evaluation of treatment interventions.

LIVER DISEASE

Liver enzymes reflect leakage from damaged cells or induction and spillage of excess into the circulation. Bile acids, ammonia, and bilirubin are functional tests because they reflect metabolism by the liver. Bilirubin is a good indicator of cholestasis and hepatic disease. Commonly reported RIs for bilirubin are at the low range of the test methodology, which magnifies the effects of interferences. Serum color changes (hemolysis/lipemia) can cause erroneously increased results, and random high errors also occur due to protein/albumin or paraproteins abnormalities. Bilirubin changes the color of serum/plasma and this is recognized when values exceed the upper limit of RIs

---

Box 8
Urinalysis—the first step in determining renal dysfunction

Refractometer specific gravity is a requirement; dipstick specific gravity is inappropriate for cats. A cutoff of 1.035 for cats is appropriate only if the cat is hydrated and the refractometer is maintained correctly. The use of feline specific refractometers has been questioned but, regardless of the brand, refractometers should be temperature calibrated and tested daily against water and an appropriate urine standard.[31]

Increases in urine protein levels in a sample with an inactive/quiet sediment must be confirmed by biochemical evaluation of protein levels (microprotein) and urine creatinine (urine protein to creatinine ratio).[32]

Sediment evaluation is a critical part in interpretation of a urinalysis. To improve accuracy in evaluating cells and bacteria, a slide should be made of the sediment and stained using Diff-Quik (Wright-Giemsa stain).

Data from Tvedten HW, Norein A. Comparison of a Schmidt and Hasensch refractometer and an Atago Pal-USG cat refractometer for determination of specific gravity in dogs and cats. Vet Clin Pathol 2014; 43(1):63-66 and Giraldi M, Rossie G, Bertazzolo W, et al. Evaluation of the analytical variability of urine protein-to-creatinine ratio in cats. Vet Clin Pathol 2018; 47:448-457.

Box 9
Symmetric dimethylarginine

Asymmetric dimethylarginine (ADMA) is a competitive inhibitor of nitric oxide synthetase, which reduces the generation of nitric oxide (NO), thereby decreasing the effects of NO on vasodilatation and endothelial function. The structural isomer of ADMA, SDMA, appears excreted solely by the kidney and not subject to enzymatic catabolism. Levels of SDMA appear to increase before creatinine levels in cats with renal disease,[33,34] but, similar to creatinine, SDMA elevations occur with anything that decreases the glomerular filtration rate (GFR), including prerenal azotemia.

Glomerular filtration rate, including prerenal azotemia (dehydration). Published RIs exist for this test; they have not been evaluated for breed differences except in Birman cats, where levels were significantly different from the published RIs.[4]

Further data that examine changes with age/diet and altered lipid metabolism are needed. Articles have assessed SDMA in cats with hyperthyroidism, obesity, and diabetes mellitus.[35,36]

Data from Refs.[4,33-36]

(0.7–1.0 mg/dL or 8–17.1 μmol/L). Recording the color of the serum/plasma helps determine if the machine values are accurate. Bilirubinuria is uncommon in cats and has a high specificity to liver disease but color interference from hematuria, high SG, and high pH, may cause false-positive results.

PANCREATIC DISEASE

Feline pancreatitis remains an enigma. Clinical signs are nonspecific; malaise with abdominal pain is present in less than 25% while vomiting is variable (30%–50%).[41] This is not a diagnosis that can be made with the use of 1 test, such as feline pancreatic lipase immunoreactivity (fPLI) or lipase. Diagnosis requires complete blood panels along with clinical observations and perhaps ultrasound.[42] Cholestasis is common in this condition and elevations in ALT, ALP, cholesterol, and/or total bilirubin occur in half of affected cats. Low serum calcium and low sodium and chloride maybe present. Although lipase methodology varies, articles indicate similar sensitivity and specificity to the Spec fPLI.[42] Ultrasound should be used only in those animals with a high index of suspicion for pancreatitis.

Biopsy of the pancreas is the gold standard for diagnosis but biopsies should be taken from multiple sites throughout the pancreas. If an exploratory laparotomy is performed then biopsies should also be taken from the intestine, stomach, liver and lymph nodes as combined organ system involvement is common in cats (**Box 10**).

Exocrine pancreatic insufficiency is not uncommon in the aging cat. Although clinical signs are nonspecific, a poor hair coat and increased appetite along with weight loss occur commonly. Feline trypsin-like immunoreactivity remains the gold standard for diagnosing exocrine pancreatic insufficiency. Cobalamin levels are low with pancreatic insufficiency.[43]

GASTROINTESTINAL DISEASE

Inflammatory bowel disease is common in cats and represents a spectrum of disease and etiologies. Suspicious laboratory findings include low TP, albumin, calcium, and cholesterol. Cobalamin and folate are used to evaluate the degree of gastrointestinal (GI) dysfunction; these are not screening tests. Elevated folate reflects increased bacterial numbers or altered bacterial flora, either primary or secondary to other intestinal

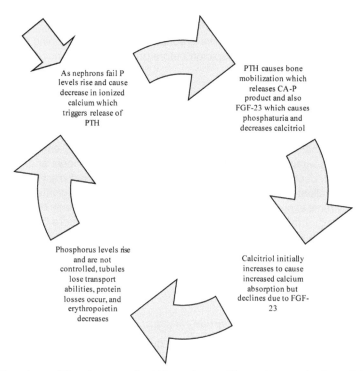

As nephrons fail P levels rise and cause decrease in ionized calcium which triggers release of PTH

PTH causes bone mobilization which releases CA-P product and also FGF-23 which causes phosphaturia and decreases calcitriol

Calcitriol initially increases to cause increased calcium absorption but declines due to FGF-23

Phosphorus levels rise and are not controlled, tubules lose transport abilities, protein losses occur, and erythropoietin decreases

Fig. 1. Phosphorus (P) and progressive kidney disease. The pathogenesis of renal disease is related to the loss of nephrons, which results in decreased P excretion and decreased calcitriol (produced in the renal tubular cells). Calcium (Ca) levels decrease as serum P increases, resulting in increased PTH production which, in turn, causes bone mobilization, releases Ca/P product, and increases FGF-23 to increase Pi lost in the urine. Concurrently, calcidiol production is increased (by the liver) but FGF-23 increases tubular 24-hydroxylase so conversion to calcitriol is diminished. Lower calcitriol levels decrease GI absorption of calcium; more PTH is produced, but the progressive loss of nephrons requires increasing levels of PTH to maintain calcium levels. The end result is renal hyperparathyroidism, which develops to maintain calcium balance at the expense of the skeleton. FGF-23 is a very early marker of Ca/P imbalance and renal disease.

diseases. Cobalamin levels decline with chronic GI disease but RIs may be more dependent on the individual than the population. Sustained low cobalamin levels theoretically could cause other problems, including macrocytosis and neutrophil hyposegmentation.[44,45]

Florescence in situ hybridization may be applied to intestinal biopsies to detect bacteria and provide information as to the mucosal location of these organisms. Bacteria located within enterocytes imply pathogenicity and are detected by this method.

Box 10
Diagnosing pancreatitis

Individual tests for pancreatitis lack specificity and have a poor predictive value. Complete blood panels, imaging, and clinical findings aid in the diagnosis, and, if clinical improvement is lacking, tissue evaluation (ie, by cytology/histopathology) is warranted.

CARDIAC DISEASE

The gold standard with cardiac disease is echocardiography. Screening tests should be used only to confirm clinical suspicion before proceeding to echocardiography.

Cardiac Troponin I

The contractile myofibrils of cardiac muscle include regulatory proteins called troponins. There are 3 protein subunits but troponin I is specific to cardiac muscle and is released in response to myocardial damage and leakage. Although specific time frames for this analyte are not determined in felines, in humans, cardiac troponin I (CTNI) increases within 4 hours of myocardial injury, peaks in 8 hours and, if the injury is not sustained, declines rapidly with low detectable levels for at least 50 hours. This makes it an excellent marker of acute injury and as a prognostic indicator.[46,47] CTNI is eliminated by renal excretion and may be mildly elevated with chronic renal disease.[47] Newer variations of this test (highly sensitive troponin) may be more helpful because the low levels of the test (<0.2 ng/mL) have a high total allowable error (TEa). Modest increases are more likely to be associated with secondary myocardial injury (eg, pulmonary fibrosis, chylothorax, or pyothorax) than a primary myocardial event. This test has the advantage of using serum or plasma and has no special handling procedures (**Fig. 2**).

N-terminal ProB-type Natriuretic Peptide

B-type natriuretic peptide (BNP) is part of a duo of natriuretic peptides produced within atrial myocytes in response to stretching of the fibers (distension/volume overload). It is released into circulation as a nonactive peptide and cleaved to an active form that promotes diuresis and vasodilatation. Unlike cardiac troponin, elevations in NT-proBNP reflect changes in fluid dynamics (such as distension or fluid overload), which result in stretching of the cardiac muscle. Variable reports on sensitivity (67%–100%) and specificity (70%–100%) suggest that this test should be interpreted cautiously.[48] There is median 40% variability and weekly variation of 60%, with increased inaccuracies with age due both to hypertension and to renal disease. BNP is subject to degradation and sample handling is critical. There are 2 methodologies, qualitative and quantitative, with the latter showing the most benefit in monitoring responses to therapy. The SNAP test (qualitative) has reported sensitivity of 89% and specificity of 82% and, when used on pleural fluid, the specificity was 64.7%.[48]

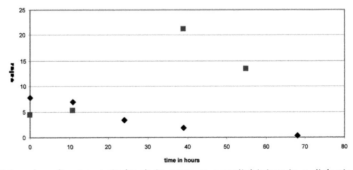

Fig. 2. SAA and cardiac troponin levels in acute myocardial injury in a diabetic cat. Pink blocks: SAA μg/mL, RI 0–5.3 μg/mL; blue blocks: CTNI ng/mL, range 0.02–0.15 ng/mL.

ACUTE INFLAMMATORY MARKERS
Serum Amyloid A

Serum amyloid A (SAA) is an acute-phase protein that is conserved across species. SAA, C-reactive protein, haptoglobin, and α_1-acid glycoprotein all have been studied in cats as markers of inflammation.[49,50] SAA is technically easy to measure and the turbidimetric method has been validated for use in the cat.[51] SAA levels peak rapidly with increases occurring before other acute-phase markers and before changes in white blood cell counts. In humans, levels are elevated within 4 hours to 8 hours, with peak concentrations at 24 hours to 48 hours, and decline within 5 days to 7 days. The relatively rapid decline makes it suitable as prognostic indicator (see **Fig. 2**). Elevated levels are seen with most inflammatory conditions and levels appear proportional to the degree of inflammation.[51–53] Breed-related RIs are needed because levels are higher in Abyssinians and Siamese cats, which may reflect the increased incidence of systemic amyloidosis. C-reactive protein has not proved a reliable marker of inflammation in the cat.[49,50] α_1-Acid glycoprotein is an inflammatory marker, which along with SAA has been elevated with both inflammatory and neoplastic conditions.[50,52] α_1-Acid glycoprotein is more consistently elevated in feline infectious peritonitis effusions than is SAA.[53]

Lactate and D-lactate

Although lactate is not an acute-phase marker, it is useful in critical care situations because elevated levels correspond to a poor prognosis. The test is an indirect measurement of tissue perfusion/hypoxia (ie, shock, sepsis, and systemic inflammatory response syndrome). The serial use of this measurement can guide therapy as well as predicting the likelihood of recovery.[54,55] D-lactate is a different analyte and test procedure that has been used to predict GI necrosis[56] (**Table 1**).

Table 1
Summary of disease, test considerations in a timely sequence after a complete physical examination and history

Disease	Initial	Next	Consider	Perhaps	New
Renal disease	UA	BUN, creatinine	SDMA	PTH, Ca^{++}, P	FGF-23, feline kidney injury molecule 1, hepcidin
Liver disease	ALT/ALP/GGT, bilirubin	UA: bilirubinuria	TP albumin, bile acids	Ammonia SAA	
Pancreatitis	CBC/CHEM	Lipase, fPLI	Ionized Ca, SAA	Ultrasound biopsy or cytology	
Inflammatory bowel disease	TP/albumin/ cholesterol	Vitamin B$_{12}$/ folate	Electrolytes lactate SAA	Biopsy	
Cardiac disease	CTNI	NT-proBNP	CK, SAA	ECHO to confirm	
Diabetes	Serum glucose, UA	Fructosamine	BHB	CGMS	

Abbreviation: CBC, complete blood count; CHEM, chemistry panel; CK, creatine kinase; ECHO, echo cardiography; UA, Urinalysis.

ENDOCRINE DISEASE
Tests for Diabetes Mellitus

Glucose
Monitoring of glucose with glucometers or with continuous glucose monitoring systems (CGMS) is the norm for this condition. CGMSs may detect hypoglycemic periods not identified by the portable glucose monitoring devices.[57]

Fructosamine
Fructosamine reflects average glycemic control over 7 days to 10 days so peaks and valleys are not detected. Values in the middle to low end of the RIs seldom are attained in diabetic cats and, if seen, should prompt evaluation of a glucose curve. Fructosamine levels may be artificially low in hyperthyroid cats, making diagnosis of concurrent diabetes challenging.

β-hydroxybutyrate
The β-hydroxybutyrate (BHB) test remains underutilized in veterinary medicine. Levels are increased, with diabetes, lipidosis, and disease states resulting in cachexia or prolonged anorexia. They are highest with diabetic ketoacidosis but are within RIs in well-controlled diabetic cats.[58,59]

Insulinlike growth factor 1
Insulinlike growth factor (IGF)-1 is a screening test for acromegaly and has been recommended for use in diabetic cats that require high insulin doses or that are difficult to regulate. The RIs described have limitations because cats on insulin therapy have high levels of IGF-1, which are inversely proportional to fructosamine levels and which can exceed the upper limit of reference. Determination of acromegaly requires demonstration of a pituitary mass in concert with high IGF-1 levels and often is not possible until postmortem examination.[60]

Tests for Hyperthyroidism and Hypothyroidism

A majority of cats with clinical signs of hyperthyroidism have elevated thyroxine levels. The methodology used for the measurement of T4 shifted from radioimmunoassay to chemiluminescence and now immunologic/turbidimetric assays are used. Values are not interchangeable between methods.[61] Radioimmunoassay/chemiluminescence remains the gold standard. Results that are discordant with the clinical history or physical examination findings always should be repeated with a different and more-specific assay method. Values normally fluctuate and also are variable with therapy.[62]

Although there is no specific test method available for thyroid-stimulating hormone (TSH) in cats, the use of the canine methodology has been proposed to aid in diagnosis of occult hyperthyroidism and to aid in distinguishing low levels of thyroxine that are due to other disease processes or to iatrogenic causes (medications). In theory, an undetectable level of TSH coupled with a high normal T4 level suggests autonomous production of thyroxine and is consistent with hyperthyroidism. Finding a subnormal T4 level in a cat on methimazole along with a TSH level within RIs may indicate a need to decrease medication, whereas a very high TSH level coupled with subnormal T4 levels supports iatrogenic hypothyroidism. T4 levels near the low end of the RI, however, along with a measurable but low TSH remain difficult to interpret and can reflect euthyroid sick syndrome.[63,64] Difficulties arise because the RI suggested for cats is at the insensitive end of the assay (cutoff values include <0.03 ng/mL and >0.03 ng/mL) with a supposed RI of 0.0 to 0.3 ng/mL in cats without disease. But the assay only measures 40% of the feline TSH moiety, thus errors are not uncommon, and values should be interpreted cautiously (see also Hyperthyroidism and Hypothyroidism in Cats by Peterson in Part 2).

Molecular Diagnostics: Polymerase Chain Reaction

Polymerase chain reaction (PCR) often is suggested for infectious diseases, but clinicians need to be aware of the following[65]:

1. The tests are subject to contamination both in acquiring the specimen and within the laboratory.
2. Licensing is not a requirement for these reagents or for the laboratory doing the tests and there is no standardization. Procedures and primers vary, the use of controls is variable, and results can different significantly between laboratories.
3. Sample quality affects results. Vaccines and/or antibiotics may interfere.
4. The presence of DNA or RNA does not indicate that the organism is alive or the cause of the disease.

PCR can help identify unusual organisms and those that are difficult to culture (eg, *Mycobacterium* and *Bartonella*) or determine whether treatment has eliminated an organism. PCR is helpful in epidemiologic/population studies and in screening blood donors for transmissible infectious organisms (eg, FeLV).

DISCLOSURE

The author has nothing to disclose.

REFERENCES

1. Omar F. Essential laboratory knowledge for the clinician. CME 2012;30(7):244–8.
2. Paltrinieri S, Ibba F, Rossi G. Haematological and biochemical reference intervals of four feline breeds. J Feline Med Surg 2014;16(2):125–36.
3. Paltrinieri S, Giraldi M, Proio A, et al. Serum symmetric dimethylarginine and creatinine in Birman cats compared with cats of other breeds. J Feline Med Surg 2018;20(10):905–12.
4. Reynolds BS, Concordet D, Germain CA, et al. Breed dependency of reference intervals for plasma biochemical values in cats. J Vet Intern Med 2010;24:809–18.
5. Spada E, Antognoni MT, Proverbio D, et al. Hematological and biochemical reference intervals in adult Maine Coon Cats. J Feline Med Surg 2015;17(2):1020–7.
6. Hoskins JD. Clinical evaluation of the kitten from birth to eight weeks of age. Comp Cont Education 1990;12(9):1215–25.
7. Paepe D, Verjans G, Duchateau L, et al. Routine health screening: findings in apparently healthy middle-aged and old cats. J Feline Med Surg 2013; 15(1):8–19.
8. Pineda C, Escolastico A, Guerrero F, et al. Mineral metabolism in growing cats: changes in the values of blood parameters with age. J Feline Med Surg 2013; 15(10):866–71.
9. Trumel C, Monzali C, Geffre A, et al. Hematologic and biologic variation in laboratory cats. J Am Assoc Lab Anim Sci 2016;55(5):503–9.
10. Walton RM. Subject based reference values: biological variation, individuality and reference change values. Vet Clin Pathol 2012;41(2):175–81.
11. Harris AN, Estrada AH, Gallagher AE, et al. Biologic variability of N-terminal pro-brain natriuretic peptide in adult healthy cats. J Feline Med Surg 2017;19(2): 216–23.

12. Baral RM, Dhanol NK, Freeman KP, et al. Biological variation and reference change values of feline plasma biochemistry analytes. J Feline Med Surg 2014; 16(4):317–25.

13. Petersen PH, Sandberg S, Fraser CG, et al. Influence of index of individuality on false positives in repeated sampling from healthy individuals. Clin Chem Lab Med 2001;39(2):160–5.

14. Petersen PH, Fraser CG, Sandberg S, et al. The index of individuality is often a misinterpreted quantity characteristic. Clin Chem Lab Med 1999;37(6):655–61.

15. Moritz A, Fickenscher Y, Meyer K, et al. Canine and feline hematology reference values for the ADVIA 120 hematology system. Vet Clin Pathol 2004;33(1):32–8.

16. Bauer N, Moritz A. Evaluation of three methods for measurement of hemoglobin and calculated hemoglobin parameters with the ADVIA 2120 and ADVIA 120 in dogs, cats and horse. Vet Clin Pathol 2008;37(2):173–9.

17. Bain BJ. Diagnosis from a blood smear. N Engl J Med 2005;353:498–507.

18. Paltrinieri S, Fossati M, Menaballi V. Diagnostic performances of manual and automated reticulocyte parameters in anaemic cats. J Feline Med Surg 2018; 20(2):122–7.

19. Bauer N, Nakagawa J, Dunker C, et al. Evaluation of the automated hematology analyzer Sysmex XT2000iV™compared to the ADVIA 2120 for its use in dogs, cats and horses. Part II: accuracy of leukocyte differential and reticulocyte count, impact of anticoagulant and sample aging. J Vet Diagn Invest 2012;24(1):74–9.

20. Prins M, vanLeeuwen MW, Teske E. Stability and reproducibility of ADVIA 120 measured red blood cell and platelet parameters in dogs, cats and horse and the use of reticulocyte haemoglobin content (CH(R)) in the diagnosis of iron deficiency. Tijdschr Diergeneeskd 2009;134(7):272–8.

21. Perkins PC, Grindem CB, Cullins LD. Flow cytometric analysis of punctuate and aggregate reticulocyte responses in phlebotomized cats. Am J Vet Res 1995; 56(12):1564–9.

22. D'Angelo G. Role of hepcidin in the pathophysiology and diagnosis of anemia. Blood Res 2013;48:10–5.

23. Darcy H, Simpson K, Gajanayake I, et al. Feline primary erythrocytosis: a multi-centre case series of 18 cats. J Feline Med Surg 2018;20(12):1192–8.

24. Papasoullotis K, Cue S, Crawford E, et al. Comparisons of white cell differential percentages determined by the in-house LaserCyte hematology analyzer and a manual method. Vet Clin Path 2006;35(3):295–302.

25. Tvedten HW, Andersson V, Lilliehook IE. Feline differential leukocyte count with ProCyte Dx: frequency and severity of a neutrophil-lymphocyte error and how to avoid it. J Vet Intern Med 2017;31(6):1708–16.

26. Alleman AR. The effects of hemolysis and lipemia on serum biochemical constituents. Vet Med 1990;1272–84.

27. Barel RM, Dhand NK, Morto JM, et al. Bias in feline plasma biochemistry results between three in-house analysers and a commercial laboratory analyser: result should not be directly compared. J Feline Med Surg 2015;17:653–66.

28. Braun JP, Cabe E, Geffre A, et al. Comparison of plasma creatinine values measured by different veterinary practices. Vet Rec 2008;162(7):215–6.

29. Bowen AR, Remaley AT. Interferences from blood collection tube components on clinical chemistry assays. Biochem Med 2014;24(1):31–44.

30. Djajaddiningrat-Laenen S, Galac S, Koolstra H. Primary hyperaldosteronism: expanding the diagnostic net. J Feline Med Surg 2012;13(9):641–50.

31. Tvedten HW, Norein A. Comparison of a Schmidt and Hasensch refractometer and an Atago Pal-USG cat refractometer for determination of specific gravity in dogs and cats. Vet Clin Pathol 2014;43(1):63–6.

32. Giraldi M, Rossie G, Bertazzolo W, et al. Evaluation of the analytical variability of urine protein-to-creatinine ratio in cats. Vet Clin Pathol 2018;47:448–57.

33. Jepson RE, Syme HM, Vallance C, et al. Plasma asymmetric dimethylarginine, symmetric dimethylarginine, L-arginine and Nitrate/Nitrate concentrations in cats with chronic renal disease and hypertension. J Vet Intern Med 2008;22: 317–24.

34. Hall JA, Yerramilli M, Obare E, et al. Comparisons of serum concentrations of symmetric dimethylarginine and creatinine as kidney function biomarkers in cats with chronic kidney disease. J Vet Intern Med 2014;28:1676–83.

35. Buresova E, Stock E, Paepe D, et al. Assessment of symmetric dimethylarginine as a biomarker of renal function in hyperthyroid cats treated with radioiodine. J Vet Intern Med 2019;33(2):516–22.

36. Langhorn R, Kielre IN, Koch J, et al. Symmetric dimethylarginine in cats with hypertrophic cardiomyopathy and diabetes mellitus. J Vet Intern Med 2018;32(1): 57–63.

37. Bland SK, Clark ME, Côté O, et al. A specific immunoassay for detection of feline kidney injury molecule. J Feline Med Surg 2018;21:1069–79.

38. Liao Y, Chou C, Lee Y. The association of indoxyl sulfate with fibroblast growth factor-23 in cats with chronic renal disease. J Vet Intern Med 2019;33:686–93.

39. Geddes RF, Elliott J, Syme HM. Relationship between fibroblast growth factor-23 concentration and survival time in cats with chronic kidney disease. J Vet Intern Med 2015;29(6):1494–501.

40. Galvan JF, Nagode LA, Schneck PA, et al. Calcitriol, calcidiol, parathyroid hormone and fibroblast growth factor-23 interactions in chronic kidney disease. J Vet Emerg Crit Care (San Antonio) 2013;23(2):134–62.

41. Xenoulis PG. Diagnosis of pancreatitis in dogs and cats. J Small Anim Pract 2015; 56:13–26.

42. Opplinger S, Hartnack S, Reusch CE, et al. Agreement of serum feline pancreas-specific lipase and colorimetric lipase assays with pancreatic ultrasonographic findings in cats with suspicion of pancreatitis:161 cases (2008-2012). J Am Vet Med Assoc 2014;244:1060–5.

43. Xenoulis PG, Zoran DL, Fosgate GT, et al. Feline exocrine pancreatic insufficiency; a retrospective study of 150 cases. J Vet Intern Med 2016;30(6):1790–7.

44. Hill SA, Cave NJ, Forsyth S. Effect of age, sex, body weight on the serum concentrations of cobalamin and folate in cats consuming a consistent diet. J Feline Med Surg 2018;20(2):135–41.

45. Jugan MC, August JR. Serum cobalamin concentrations and small intestinal ultrasound changes in 75 cats with clinical signs of gastrointestinal disease: a retrospective study. J Feline Med Surg 2017;19(1):48–56.

46. Borgeat K, Sherwood K, Payne JR, et al. Plasma cardiac troponin I concentration and cardiac death in cats with hypertrophic cardiomyopathy. J Vet Intern Med 2014;28:1731–7.

47. Langhorn R, Jessen LR, Kloster AS, et al. Cardiac troponin I in cats with compromised renal function. J Feline Med Surg 2018;20(1):1–7.

48. Machen MC, Oyama MA, Gordon SG, et al. Multi-centered investigation of a point-of-care NT–proBNP assay to detect moderate to severe occult (per-clinical) feline heart disease in cats referred for cardiac evaluation. J Vet Cardiol 2014; 16(4):245–55.

49. Ceron JJ, Eckersall PD, Martinez-Subiela S. Acute phase proteins in dogs and cats: current knowledge and future perspectives. Vet Clin Pathol 2005;34:85–99.

50. Kajikawa T, Furuta A, Onishi T, et al. Changes in concentrations of serum amyloid A protein, alpha-1-acid glycoprotein, haptoglobin,and C-reactive protein in feline sera due to induced inflammation and surgery. Vet Immunol Immunopathol 1999; 68:91–8.

51. Tamamoto T, Ohno K, Takahashi M, et al. Serum amyloid as a prognostic marker in cats with various diseases. J Vet Diagn Invest 2013;25(3):428–32.

52. Winkel VM, Pavan TLR, Wirthl VABF, et al. Serum α-1 acid glycoprotein and serum amyloid A concentrations in cats receiving anti-neoplastic treatment for lymphoma. Am J Vet Res 2015;76(11):983–8.

53. Hazuchova K, Held S, Neiger R. Usefulness of acute phase proteins in differentiating between feline infectious peritonitis and other diseases in cats with body cavity effusions. J Feline Med Surg 2017;19(8):809–16.

54. Reineke EL, Rees C, Drobatz KJ. Association of blood lactate concentration with physical perfusion variables, blood pressure and outcome for cats treated at an emergency service. J Am Vet Med Assoc 2015;247(1):79–84.

55. Trigg NL, McAlees TJ. Blood lactate concentration as a prognostic indicator in cats admitted to intensive care. Aust Vet Pract 2015;45(1):17-10.

56. Packer RA, Moore GE, Chang CY, et al. Serum D-lactate concentration in cats with gastrointestinal disease. J Vet Intern Med 2012;26(4):905–10.

57. Hoenig M, Pach N, Thomaseth K, et al. Evaluation of long-term glucose homeostasis in lean and obese cats by use of continuous glucose monitoring. Am J Vet Res 2012;73(7):1100–6.

58. Weingart C, Lotz F, Kohn B. Measurement of β-hydroxybutyrate in cats with non-ketotic diabetes mellitus, diabetic ketosis and diabetic ketoacidosis. J Vet Diagn Invest 2012;24(2):295–300.

59. Gorman L, Sharkey LC, Armstrong PJ, et al. Serum beta hydroxybutyrate concentrations in cats with chronic kidney disease, hyperthyroidism or hepatic lipidosis. J Vet Intern Med 2016;30:611–6.

60. Strange EM, Sundberg M, Holst BS, et al. Effect of insulin treatment on circulating insulin-like growth factor 1 and IGF binding proteins in cats with diabetes mellitus. J Vet Intern Med 2018;32:1579–90.

61. Peterson ME, Rishniw M, Bilbrough GE, et al. Comparisons of in-clinic point of care and reference laboratory total thyroxine immunoassays for diagnosis and post-treatment monitoring of hyperthyroid cats. J Feline Med Surg 2018;20(4): 319–24.

62. Peterson ME, Graves TK, Cavanagh I. Serum thyroid hormone concentrations fluctuate in cats with hyperthyroidism. J Vet Intern Med 1987;1:142–6.

63. Peterson ME, Guteri JN, Nichols R, et al. Evaluation of serum thyroid-stimulating hormone concentration as a diagnostic test for hyperthyroidism in cats. J Vet Intern Med 2015;29:1327–34.

64. Aldridge C, Behrend EN, Martin LG, et al. Evaluation of thyroid-stimulating hormone, total thyroxine and free thyroxine concentrations in hyperthyroid cats receiving methimazole treatment. J Vet Intern Med 2015;29:862–8.

65. Tasker S. The polymerase chain reaction in the diagnosis of infectious disease. Vet Clin Pathol 2010;39(3):261–2.

Integrating Science and Well-Being

Bernard E. Rollin, PhD*

KEYWORDS

- Art and science of veterinary medicine • Veterinarians as family members
- Veterinarians as animal advocates • Ethics of specialization • Moral stress • Suicide

KEY POINTS

- Veterinary medicine is a combination of art and science.
- Through routine referral, the advocacy of the individual animal is being lost.
- Just because one can, does not mean one should.
- Moral stress is a consequence of veterinarians losing their position as advocates.

THE ART AND SCIENCE OF PRACTICING FELINE MEDICINE
Introduction

Medicine, human or veterinary, is an admixture of art and science. As Aristotle pointed out, the science part is represented by universal laws that hold in all cases of a given phenomenon. Art, however, represents the understanding of an individual in its individuality.

Historically, human and veterinary medicine were as much art as science. By the second half of the 20th century, however, medicine experienced "scientization," as evidenced by the proliferation of medical specialties. In part for economic reasons, but also for perceived greater status, veterinary graduates ceased to aspire to be general practitioners (GPs), but instead turned to a specialty practice. There have undoubtedly been gains, but there have also been losses not just to the patient and caregiver but also to the profession.

The cost to the patient and client

What was lost was the understanding of animals and clients as individuals. Historically, the GP became part of the family, knowing and treating the animal for its entire life, and relating to the family unit with all of its specific needs and quirks. Like human GPs, veterinarians were friends of the family, often invited to family celebrations and important events. Their advice was sought on all animal matters, and in rural areas, their

Colorado State University, Fort Collins, CO 80525, USA
* Department of Philosophy, Colorado State University, Fort Collins, CO 80523-1781.
E-mail address: Bernard.Rollin@Colostate.Edu

Vet Clin Small Anim 50 (2020) 899–904
https://doi.org/10.1016/j.cvsm.2020.03.009
0195-5616/20/© 2020 Elsevier Inc. All rights reserved.

advice was sought in the absence of physicians. As one cowboy said to me, "If my vet can fix my livestock fractures, he can sure as hell fix mine! Bone is bone."

Perhaps most importantly, veterinarians were familiar with all aspects of the animal's life and behavior. Although important with any patient, this is especially important with cats because of their inherently more solitary nature. They often tolerate handling by strangers with less equanimity than dogs do in a clinic setting. Because many people find cats difficult to read, this can result in problems for cats and clinic staff.[1] To do a proper examination on a cat, a long-term, empathic relationship between practitioner and animal is virtually a *sine qua non*. Knowledge of what constitutes "normal" behavior for that individual in the clinic or at home helps with assessing the severity of any underlying concerns.

Sometimes the opposite is true: what seems to be a behavior problem, may indicate ill health (See Stelow's article, "Behavior as an Illness Indicator," in this issue.) Prolonged experience with an animal under a variety of circumstances helps a veterinarian distinguish between the animal having a psychological/emotional problem and a physical one. As Tony Buffington and others have so elegantly shown, the idea that a sickness is based in one or the other is overly simplified, and in many cases the emotional and physical state are intimately related (See Tony Buffington and Bain's article, "Stress and Feline Health," in this issue.)

Sickness behaviors are nonspecific clinical and behavioral signs that may be a reflection of a change in motivation to one that promotes recovery by inhibiting metabolically expensive activities (eg, hunting) and favoring those that contribute to recovery. They include diarrhea; vomiting; anorexia; decreased food or water intake; fever; lethargy; depression; somnolence; enhanced pain-like behaviors; and decreased activity, grooming, and social interactions.[2,3] Additionally, indoor cats experience a higher prevalence of medical conditions (eg, hyperthyroidism, idiopathic cystitis and other lower urinary tract disorders, diabetes [as a result of boredom and inactivity], and dental resorptive lesions) suggesting a stress component in some cats.[4]

To refer or not to refer

More than 45 years ago I wrote the following on the ethics of referral: "A clear medical example of hearing with one's expectations occurs when a medical professional says, 'cancer.' Patients almost immediately expect a death sentence, preceded by exquisite suffering. While there is no guarantee that the primary practitioner can affect communication, knowing the client certainly provides an advantage the specialist lacks."

Specialists are often prone to perceive with the theoretic biases and predilections of their specialty. For example, the specialty of oncology, especially in human, but possibly also in veterinary medicine, has taken as its goal extending length of life; the oncologist "wins" if the quantity of life is prolonged. Quality of life (QoL) has historically been ignored in human medicine leading many patients to request discontinuation of therapy and an end to their suffering. Patients fear uncontrolled pain and suffering more than death. In the practice of hospice, treatment modalities are initiated by nurses rather than doctors. As one nurse told me: "Physicians worry about cure, we worry about care."

QoL in the present moment is the only thing that matters to an animal, because all indications are the animals do not have the mentational apparatus to understand that current suffering, if treated, can mean extended life later. Insofar as QoL looms large in a client's mind, the GP can and should serve as an animal advocate mediating between specialist and client. Because the primary practitioner knows the client and the animal, and the likely consequences of the treatment modalities for the animal's well-being, he or she can serve as guardian of the animal's QoL, tempering the natural zeal of many specialists to try everything, and the desire of some clients to keep the animal alive at all costs. Additionally, they serve as a voice for the client because of their familiarity with the client's circumstances.

The GP enjoys certain marked advantages over the specialist. By knowing the animal, he or she should be more adept at picking up subtle signs of pain and distress, or other behavioral signs specific to that animal (eg, an idiosyncratic reaction to certain drugs, fear of men but not women, defensive reactions when being touched over their head). The long-term GP also has the advantage of knowing how perceptive is a given client. They know the family unit, the animal's home circumstances, the lifestyle, the owner's personality and degree of medical sophistication, and tensions in the household that may be relevant to the animal's condition.

This is also true in human medicine. Although suffering virtually nightly asthmatic attacks, the level of stress exerted on my psyche was unparalleled. There is little that is as frightening as the perceived inability to breathe. This fear was easily mitigated by the use of tranquilizers. Yet my highly mechanistic and reductionist allergist simply dismissed my request for the alleviation of stress by affirming that tranquilizers were absolutely counterindicated in asthma, because of their effect of creating respiratory depression. Although technically true, this point was phenomenologically and experientially irrelevant, and adherence to this mechanistic dogma caused me many unnecessary days of suffering. It was only when I moved to Colorado and encountered an extremely common sense–based country doctor that I was able to calm down enough not to be gasping for breath.

The same adherence to common sense must be allowed to play out in veterinary medicine, in particular with regard to cats. In addition to possessing a heightened awareness of the patient's unique needs, the GP has a pretty good idea of how and to what extent complex treatment regimens will be adhered to, whereas a specialist new to the case has no idea. The primary practitioner knows, for example, not to expect an owner to give a treatment every 4 hours because the owner works 14-hour days. He or she knows that the household contains six raucous small children, so that there is no hope of the animal resting undisturbed. He or she knows that the doting owner is not going to cut back the quantity of food for an obese cat if their relationship is based on "food is love." He or she knows which owners will never rake through the litter looking for blood in the feces. Perhaps, most important, he or she knows how to translate for the client in question; not only interpreting medical technicalities, but also ensuring that what the specialist says is not only understood, but also heard, not reinterpreted through wishful or pessimistic thinking. What one perceives does not depend on level of medical knowledge alone. We hear not only with our ears, but also with our beliefs, expectations, theories, hopes, biases, and so forth. "Perception is based in theory"[5] and belief.

This sort of intimacy with the cat and the family is core to the practice of veterinary medicine and is virtually gone in a version of veterinary medicine that is dominated by specialty practices often with only brief interactions with the cat and client. Despite this era of fear of litigation, referral should not be a way of passing off difficult cases, or of avoiding responsibility.

The cost to the profession

In 1987, I published what I believe is the first paper on moral stress, defined in ethical terms as the unbridgeable tension between what one aspires to do in a profession, such as veterinary medicine, and what one is called on to actually do.[6,7] In veterinary medicine, the reason for becoming a veterinarian is typically because of the desire to help animals and improve their health and QoL. Too often, veterinarians are asked to euthanize an animal for owner convenience or for other morally unacceptable reasons, such as, "The animal has gotten too old to run with me, so I need to get rid of this one and adopt a younger one." This creates a great deal of moral stress in the practitioner that is not easily resolved. It may well be the case that the animal you are now being called on to euthanize was one you labored tirelessly to save after it had been struck by a car a few years earlier. Not only is intolerable stress created in the current situation, you are led to question your purpose and doubt the reasons you went into veterinary medicine in the first place.

Over the last three decades, it has become increasingly clear that moral stress is a grave and life-threatening occupational hazard. In Britain and in the United States, there are increasing rates of suicide of veterinarians, at least in part as a direct result of moral stress. There are many prominent stories in the press highlighting this tragic state of affairs. For example, according to the Washington Post, on January 1, 2019, the Centers for Disease Control and Prevention released the first account examining veterinarian mortality rates in America. The results were grim: between 1979 and 2015, male and female veterinarians committed suicide between 2 and 3.5 times more often than the national average, respectively.[8]

Moral stress is different than ordinary stress or burnout. Stress management techniques, such as mindfulness or yoga, are ineffective for moral stress. Even talking about the distress with friends or family may not be available to veterinarians asked to perform convenience euthanasia. Animals are archetypally innocent and cannot be seen as deserving what owners are asking for.

One can argue that the "scientization" or medicalization of veterinary practice contributes to psychological damage. Rather than treating an individual animal, one is treating the diseased body system or organ; a broken machine, the way a mechanic approaches a broken transmission. The desire to heal and care for the whole individual, rather than parts of a biologic machine, has gotten lost along the way and this contributes to moral stress. In an email to me, a veterinarian characterized the source of the problem: "Vets are so caught up in the medicine, tests, treatments, and mechanics of being a really good doctor that they have forgotten why they wanted to be vets in the first place. That was their empathic humanity, their awareness of their patient's experience. In addition, every client comes with a certain amount of emotional attachment/empathy, time, and money and this budget has to be spent carefully so that no one part of it depletes the others preventing appropriate care for their cat. That contributes to moral stress and this is killing veterinarians… and the profession" (M. Scherk, Personal Correspondence, 2019).

Which brings us to the crux of this article. Losing the relationship with patients and clients can result in self-harm. Excessive referral is detrimental to the patient and client. Part of burnout may come from practicing in a proscribed manner with no room for the imagination. History taking is often given short shrift when it is extremely important in the quest for a diagnosis. A good diagnostician recognizes that there are many different ways to ask the same question. I recall a period when my wife was experiencing periodic fever of unknown origin. Our GP began to query her on whether she had inhaled anything capable of causing toxic effects. She was angry at him for discounting her intelligence. "Don't you think I would have mentioned something if that were the case?" she asked angrily. He nodded and continued asking diagnostic questions. Some 5 minutes later he asked her if she had smelled anything unusual around the house. She said yes, citing a fungicide I had been using on the wood outside the house. That was a wonderful example of where knowing a patient's thought patterns and asking the same question in different ways revealed highly relevant information.

Obviously, veterinarians cannot verbally question a patient; however, conveying empathy engenders trust and alleviates fear. Communication happens through touch, tone of voice, posture, and numerous subtle cues that are grasped unconsciously. This ability contributes to what a client means when they say "Dr. X is an excellent veterinarian." Empathic rapport with an animal is what leads many people to choose veterinary medicine as a career. There are few satisfactions as profound as establishing a connection across species and earning an animal's trust. It is most unfortunate that this is being lost, or at least, downplayed, as veterinary medicine becomes ever-increasingly mechanistic and devoid of a strong emotional component. As Teddy Roosevelt said: "People don't care how much you know until they know how much you care."

During the years that I have been involved with veterinary medicine, I have watched the veterinary profession increasingly emulate the human medical profession, in its embracing of scientism and in its failure to cherish and preserve "the art of medicine." Some of the impetus for this is pecuniary, with greater financial rewards attendant on specialization. However, what is lost is far more than what is gained. Physicians no longer make house calls except under extraordinary circumstances, and thereby lose the full rapport with patients that characterized medicine until recently. Veterinarians are rapidly losing the deep understanding they used to have of their patients. Health and disease are far more than laboratory diagnostics. To understand the subtle dimensions of health and disease requires more than numbers on a machine, test results, or other data. What is also required is an ability to identify with the individual animal's form of life and the pressures and stresses attendant on them. Not only would this help restore the role of healer, it would move the respective professions away from a mechanistic perception of their patients and back toward empathetic identification that was characteristic of traditional medicine.

If this shift is to take place, there must be a root change in veterinary education. In particular, excessive "scientization" needs to be reversed. We must guard against overzealous diagnostic and treatment plans to avoid losing sight of the well-being of the individual patient in question. "Just because one can, does not mean one should" applies in veterinary medicine and human medicine.[9–11] In addition to graduating with an adequate knowledge of the biochemistry, physiology, and pathology of disease, the veterinary graduate must understand the role of the animal in the relevant family unit.

Illness is not merely physical. In human and veterinary medicine, knowledge of the patient's psychological state is of extreme importance. Through empathic connection with patients and reduced fear of missing a diagnosis come rewarding relationships and, it is hoped, less moral stress.

DISCLOSURE

The author has nothing to disclose.

REFERENCES

1. Dawson L, Niel L, Cheal J, et al. Humans can identify cats' affective states from subtle facial expressions. Anim Welf 2019;28:519–31.
2. Dantzer R. From inflammation to sickness and depression: when the immune system subjugates the brain. Nat Rev Neurosci 2008;9(1):46–56.
3. Hart BL, Hart LA. Sickness behavior in animals: implications for health and wellness. In: Choe JC, editor. Encyclopedia of animal behavior. 2nd edition. Cambridge (MA): Academic Press; 2019. p. 171–5.

4. Buffington CT. External and internal influences on disease risk in cats. J Am Vet Med Assoc 2002;220(7):994–1002.

5. Rollin B. The ethics of referral. Can Vet J 2006;47(7):717–8.

6. Rollin B. Euthanasia and moral stress. Loss, Grief, and Care 1987;1(1):115–26.

7. Reynolds SJ, Owens BP, Rubenstein AL. Moral stress: considering the nature and effects of managerial moral uncertainty. J Bus Ethics 2012;106:491.

8. Leffler D. Suicides among veterinarians become a growing problem. Washington Post 2019. Available at: https://www.washingtonpost.com/national/health-science/suicides-among-veterinarians-has-become-a-growing-problem/2019/01/18/0f58df7a-f35b-11e8-80d0-f7e1948d55f4_story.html?utm_term=14c453dcf285.

9. Scherk M, Rollin B. Palliative medicine, quality of life, and euthanasia decisions. In: Little SE, editor. The cat clinical medicine and management. St. Louis (MO): Elsevier; 2012. p. P1155–63.

10. Ross S, Robert M, Harvey MA, et al. Ethical issues associated with the introduction of new surgical devices, or just because we can, doesn't mean we should. J Obstet Gynaecol 2008;30(6):508–13.

11. Siegal EM. Just because you can, doesn't mean that you should: a call for the rational application of hospitalist comanagement. J Hosp Med 2008;3(5):398–402.

Printed and bound by CPI Group (UK) Ltd, Croydon, CR0 4YY

03/10/2024

01040408-0007